Goodwin and Guze's
Psychiatric Diagnosis

Goodwin and Guze's Psychiatric Diagnosis

Sixth Edition

CAROL S. NORTH, MD, MPE
The Nancy and Ray L. Hunt Chair in Crisis Psychiatry
Director, Program in Trauma and Disaster
VA North Texas Health Care System
Dallas, Texas
Professor, Departments of Psychiatry and
Surgery/Division of Emergency Medicine
University of Texas Southwestern Medical Center
Dallas, Texas

SEAN H. YUTZY, MD
Professor, Department of Psychiatry
University of New Mexico
Albuquerque, New Mexico

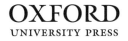

UNIVERSITY PRESS

2010

OXFORD
UNIVERSITY PRESS

Oxford University Press, Inc., publishes works that further
Oxford University's objective of excellence
in research, scholarship, and education.

Oxford   New York
Auckland   Cape Town   Dar es Salaam   Hong Kong   Karachi
Kuala Lumpur   Madrid   Melbourne   Mexico City   Nairobi
New Delhi   Shanghai   Taipei   Toronto

With offices in
Argentina   Austria   Brazil   Chile   Czech Republic   France   Greece
Guatemala   Hungary   Italy   Japan   Poland   Portugal   Singapore
South Korea   Switzerland   Thailand   Turkey   Ukraine   Vietnam

Published by Oxford University Press, Inc.
198 Madison Avenue, New York, New York 10016

www.oup.com

Oxford is a registered trademark of Oxford University Press

Library of Congress Cataloging-in-Publication Data
North, Carol S.
Goodwin and Guze's psychiatric diagnosis. — 6th ed. / by Carol S. North,
Sean H. Yutzy.
p.   ;   cm.
Rev. ed. of: Psychiatric diagnosis / Donald W. Goodwin,
Samuel B. Guze. 5th ed. 1996.
Includes bibliographical references and index.
ISBN 978-0-19-514429-1
1. Mental illness—Classification.   2. Mental illness—Diagnosis.
I. Yutzy, Sean H.   II. Goodwin, Donald W. Psychiatric diagnosis.
III. Title.   IV. Title: Psychiatric diagnosis.
[DNLM: 1. Mental Disorders—diagnosis. WM 141 N864p 2009]
RC455.2.C4N67 2009
616.89—dc22
2009016486

9 8 7 6 5 4 3 2 1

Printed in the United States of America
on acid-free paper

This book is dedicated to those listed on the following pages and to the legions of their assistants and trainees that firmly believed that psychiatry must have a scientific base and who worked diligently to make that belief a reality.

In Memorium

ROBERT A. WOODRUFF, JR.
The inspiration for—and co-author of—the first edition
of this book

ELI ROBINS
Who, as much as any one person, launched a new era in
American psychiatry

SAMUEL B. GUZE
The tough-minded individual who believed that there
was only one model of psychiatry: the medical model—which
must be part of the mainstream of modern medicine

DON GOODWIN
Gifted writer and co-author of editions two through five

Acknowledgment

There is no doubt that Miss Jacquelyn Farrell kept us organized and on track through the early drafts of this manuscript.

Preface to the Sixth Edition

Thirty-five years have elapsed since this text was first published. Over this time period, psychiatry has clearly evolved along two noteworthy lines.

First, most psychiatrists have become diagnosticians. The groundwork was set for this in no small part by the authors and collaborators of the early versions of this text, including Eli Robins, Robert A. Woodruff, Donald W. Goodwin, and Samuel B. Guze at Washington University in St. Louis. In particular, their two-pronged philosophical approach to psychiatric illness/diagnosis was to be "agnostic" about the origin of a mental illness and to draw psychiatric conclusions (including diagnostic criteria) based on reliable, reproducible data. The early studies of this group of psychiatric researchers from the 1960s and 1970s eventually produced formal operational criteria sets for the 12 major mental illnesses. While this overall approach to psychiatric illness was described as "narrow" by some (and less charitably by others) in mainstream psychiatry at the time, the criteria sets formed the early basis for a common language among psychiatrists. The diagnostic approach used an "atheoretical" basis for the origin of psychiatric illness, drawing conclusions and developing criteria based on scientific evidence. This approach gained much wider acceptance (and general acceptance by the field) after publication of the best selling *DSM-III* (*Diagnostic and Statistical Manual of Mental Disorders, 3rd edition*) in 1980. The "similarities" between the *DSM-III* and Washington University approaches were not surprising, as the authors noted above were among the *DSM-III* taskforce contributors, and one-third of the overall taskforce members were trained at Washington University.

Ultimately, the *DSM-III* solidified a widely acceptable common language and explicit criteria for the major mental illness as had long been used in most other areas of medicine. Frustrated by the unknown etiology of most major psychiatric illnesses, young scientifically trained physicians could at least rely upon a published framework as a foundation for communication, research, diagnosis, and treatment. Many well-respected individuals both inside and outside the specialty would attack the approach over the next two decades, but its utility in almost all psychiatric venues remained undeniable.

Of particular interest were that external forces over the ensuing two decades further solidified psychiatry's use of the diagnostic model. Among other developments, diagnoses became a required practice for reimbursement of services (e.g., diagnostic-related groups, or DRGs), with only specific diagnoses (and not others, especially Axis II disorders) generating payment; accreditation requirements compelled diagnostic uniformity in general medicine; and communication among treating professionals increased, particularly across medical specialties.

In sum, both internal and external forces have driven psychiatry to accept the diagnostic or medical model as THE approach to major mental illness.

The second noteworthy line is that the elapse of time with continuing critical review has clarified that this empirically based "approach" to the major psychiatric diagnoses has prevailed. While the *DSM-III* has had several subsequent minor revisions (including the *DSM-III Revised* [*DSM-III-R*] in 1987, *DSM-IV* in 1994, and the latest, *DSM-IV-Text Revision* [*DSM-IV-TR*] in 2000), most would argue that the last (*DSM-IV/DSM-IV-TR*) has become the most widely accepted psychiatric diagnostic text in the world. The stability of this approach first espoused by early authors of the *Psychiatric Diagnosis* text has stood the test of review and time which are a testament to its fundamental inherent strength.

Two years before his untimely death, Sam Guze asked us (C.S.N. and S.H.Y.) to write the sixth edition of *Psychiatric Diagnosis*. We share his vision of the evolution of the field and agree with his view that although neuroscience has evolved over the decades, the fundamentals of psychiatric diagnosis have remained constant. What we tried to achieve in this latest edition was to include the relevant new scientific research which not surprisingly continues to support the fundamental premise of the primacy of psychiatric diagnosis.

For this sixth edition, all the chapters have been updated to include the most recent reliable data and some minor updates to more modern language. Separate chapter subsections have been created to review neurobiological findings relevant to each diagnosis. The reader will clearly be able to see that some diagnoses have not been the subject of intense study over the last 13 years and that a significant collection of biological investigations has not revealed even early convergence of new finding(s) supporting inclusion.

While we remain steadfast in our position that only about a dozen diagnostic entities warrant inclusion (see Preface to the First Edition for this heretical view), the field has been working intensely toward validation of other diagnoses, in particular posttraumatic stress disorder and borderline personality disorder. We include chapters on these two diagnoses because they are of considerable recent interest, and to illustrate the state of the art of the validity and reliability status of these disorders (although not because we consider them to have achieved the same level of validation as the first 12 diagnoses in earlier editions of this text).

The sixth edition comes with some adjustment to the order and arrangement of the chapters. Panic and phobic disorders have been combined into a single chapter, because the former is now defined in terms of a form of the latter, and vice versa. Because posttraumatic stress disorder and obsessive-compulsive disorder, like panic and phobic disorders, are classified as anxiety disorders, it is natural to present these diagnoses consecutively. Antisocial personality disorder now follows somatization disorder, because of the historical evidence that these two classes of disorders may constitute a spectrum of psychopathology partly determined by gender. The new chapter on borderline personality disorder was placed after the chapter on the only personality disorder included in previous editions of this text. An introductory chapter was added to review the history and evolution of development of evidence-based criteria for diagnosis. Its intent is to orient readers to the origins of the diagnostic material that is fundamental to the rest of this text.

We have updated references extensively, replacing many of the citations for original research articles with recent review articles to direct readers to currently accessible sources of the material for further study. Readers pursuing historical study of the original work may find the citations in the earlier editions of this text.

The current authors remain staunchly aligned with the original goal of *Psychiatric Diagnosis*: to provide a concise compendium of current knowledge in psychiatry, with abundant citations, not much theory, and as little personal opinion as possible.

C. S. N.
Dallas, Texas
S. H. Y.
Albuquerque, New Mexico

Preface to the First Edition

> A rose is a rose is a rose.
> GERTRUDE STEIN

Because it remains a rose.

Classification has two functions: communication and prediction. A rose can be defined precisely. It has pinnate leaves, belongs to the rose family, and so forth. When you say "rose" to a person who knows something about the definition, communication results.

A rose also has a predictable life history: It stays a rose. If it changes into a chrysanthemum, if may not have been a rose in the first place. If roses routinely change into chrysanthemums, like caterpillars into butterflies, well and good. Natural history may include metamorphoses but they must be routine to be "natural."

Classification in medicine is called "diagnosis," and this book is about diagnosis of psychiatric conditions. Diagnostic categories—diseases, illnesses, syndromes—are included if they have been sufficiently studied to be useful. Like roses, they can be defined explicitly and have a more or less predictable course.

In choosing these categories, the guiding rule was: *Diagnosis is prognosis.* There are many diagnostic categories in psychiatry, but few are based on a clinical literature where the conditions are defined by explicit criteria and follow-up studies provide a guide to prognosis. Lacking these features, such categories resemble what sociologists call "labeling." Two examples are "passive-aggressive personality" and "emotionally unstable personality," which, like most personality diagnoses, have been inadequately studied for us to know whether they are useful or not.

Not every patient can be diagnosed by using the categories in this book. For them, "undiagnosed" is, we feel, more appropriate than a label incorrectly implying more knowledge than exists. Terms like "functional" and "psychogenic" and "situational reaction" are sometimes invoked by physicians to explain the unexplained. They usually mean "I don't know," and we try to avoid them.

Because classification in psychiatry is still at a primitive stage, there are reasonable grounds for questioning our choice of categories. It general, we lump rather than split. Hence we have two affective disorders—primary and secondary—rather than the half-dozen affective disorders cited in the official nomenclature. Schizophrenia is divided into "good prognosis" and "bad prognosis" schizophrenia rather than sliced more finely, as some prefer. Our justification for this is "the literature," meaning primarily follow-up studies.

"The follow-up is the great exposer of truth, the rock on which many fine theories are wrecked and upon which better ones can be built," wrote P. D. Scott. "It is to the psychiatrist what the postmortem is to the physician." Not all such studies are perfect, but we feel they are better than no studies. And inevitably there are instances where our "clinical judgment" has prevailed in evaluating the merit of individual studies. No text in psychiatry could be written today without a certain amount of this, but we have tried to limit personal opinion to a minimum. Many if not most assertions have a citation, and the reader can check the references to form his own judgment.

When the term "disease" is used, this is what is meant: A disease is a cluster of symptoms and/or signs with a more or less predictable course. Symptoms are what patients tell you; signs are what you see. The cluster may be associated with physical abnormality or may not. The essential point is that it results in consultation with a physician who specializes in recognizing, preventing, and sometimes, curing diseases.

It is hard for many people to think of psychiatric problems as diseases. For one thing, psychiatric problems usually consist of symptoms—complaints about thoughts and feelings—or behavior disturbing to others. Rarely are there signs—a fever, a rash. Almost never are there laboratory tests to confirm the diagnosis. What people say changes from time to time, as does behavior. It is usually harder to agree about symptoms than about signs. But whatever the psychiatric problems are, they have this in common with "real" diseases—they result in consultation with a physician and are associated with pain, suffering, disability, and death.

Another objection to the disease or medical "model" arises from a misconception about disease. Disease often is equated with physical abnormality. In fact, a disease is a category used by physicians, as "apples" is a category used by grocers. It is a useful category if precise and if the encompassed phenomena are stable over time. Diseases are conventions and may not "fit" anything in nature at all. Through the centuries, diseases have come and gone, some more useful than others, and there is no guarantee that our present "disease"—medical or psychiatric—will represent the same clusters of symptoms and signs a hundred years from now that they do today. On the contrary, as more is learned, more useful clusters surely will emerge.

There are few explanations in this book. This is because for most psychiatric conditions there *are* no explanations. "Etiology unknown" is the hallmark of psychiatry as well as its bane. Historically, once etiology is known, a disease stops being "psychiatric." Vitamins were discovered, whereupon vitamin-deficiency psychiatric disorders no longer were treated by psychiatrists. The spirochete was found, then penicillin, and neurosyphilis, once a major psychiatric disorder, became one more infection treated by nonpsychiatrists.

Little, however, is really known about most medical illnesses. Even infectious diseases remain puzzles in that some infected individuals have symptoms and others do not.

People continue to speculate about etiology, of course, and this is good if it produces testable hypotheses and bad if speculation is mistaken for truth. In this book, speculation largely is avoided, since it is available so plentifully elsewhere.

A final word about this approach to psychiatry. It is sometimes called "organic." This is misleading. A better term, perhaps, is "agnostic." Without evidence, we do not believe pills are better than words. Without evidence, we do not believe chemistry is more important than upbringing. Without evidence, we withhold judgment.

Advocacy is not the purpose of this book. Rather, we hope it will be useful in applying current knowledge to those vexatious problems—crudely defined and poorly undertood—that come within the jurisdiction of psychiatry.

D. W. G.

Saint Louis

December 1973

Contents

Looking Back

It is a distinct pleasure to write a foreword for the 6th edition of *Psychiatric Diagnosis* that reflects the uniform philosophy of the Department of Psychiatry at Washington University School of Medicine in St. Louis that laid the groundwork for all editions of this text.

I began medical school at Washington University in 1956. In my second year in our introduction to psychiatry, we were taught, with determination, by Eli Robins, Sam Guze, George Winokur, and others about 11 very specific psychiatric disorders. Since the mid 1950s, these three men had developed sets of criteria, based on published data and their own research, for the diagnosis and treatment of these mental disorders. In particular the focus was on data supporting diagnostic criteria, signs and symptoms, course, family history, outcomes, and response to treatment that validated these disorders. They termed their endeavor "the medical model for psychiatric disorders." Their approach produced a vast amount of information supporting what ultimately became the "gold standard" for psychiatric validity (1) and formed the basis for the first edition of *Psychiatric Diagnosis* in 1974 by Robert Woodruff, Donald Goodwin, and Samuel Guze.

Their thinking was logical and progressive, but certainly out of sync with the rest of psychiatry at the time, which was dominated by psychoanalytic thinking. I recall as a resident going with Drs. Hudgens and Winokur to my first regional meeting in Chicago on the establishment of Community Mental Health

Centers (there were none at the time). A psychoanalyst was promoting the centers on the premise that they would prevent mental illnesses. Dr. Hudgens pointed out that in psychiatry we did not have a vaccine, as they did, to prevent polio or even a method, as they did, to prevent pregnancy, so it was irresponsible to believe that anything they proposed to establish would prevent mental illnesses. They established the Community Mental Health Centers anyway, and as this book emphasizes, almost 50 years later we still have no methods to prevent mental illnesses much less a validated test to diagnose any mental disorder. In my day, at least we could confirm cerebral syphilis, which is now thankfully almost extinct.

While the battle for the mainstream of psychiatry raged, those who accepted the premise of the medical model for psychiatry continued their research mainly using structured interviews for assessment, follow-up, and genetic studies to support the validity and reliability of the 12 diagnoses identified in the original edition of *Psychiatric Diagnosis*. This necessitated revision for the 2nd and 3rd editions. Eventually, this body of scientific work formed the basis for the development of diagnostic criteria for the selected major mental disorders identified in the *Diagnostic and Statistical Manual of Mental Disorders, Third Version (DSM-III)*, published by the American Psychiatric Association in 1980 (2). The work also lead to a host of validated structured interviews, a method for testing new drugs, a method for validating psychiatric diagnoses, an emphasis on the importance of genetics to psychiatry, and many important clinical findings (3).

Research and clinical support for the major mental disorders grew after the introduction of *DSM-III* and the next editions of *Psychiatric Diagnosis* took into account these changes as well as additional pharmacologic and behavioral treatments for them.

Clearly, this 6th edition by two "newer" Washington University psychiatrists follows the original principles laid down by the authors and their colleagues more than 40 years ago. Until such time as the basic research arm of psychiatry identifies a "marker" for an illness or a precise mechanism of the dysfunction or an absolutely unique, specific treatment (other than lithium for mood disorders), the establishment of a psychiatric diagnosis remains the best method for evaluation, assessment, and treatment that science can provide.

Paula J. Clayton, MD
American Foundation for Suicide Prevention
New York

REFERENCES

1. American Psychiatric Association. *Diagnostic and Statistical Manual of Mental Disorders*, 3rd edition. Washington, DC: Author, 1980.
2. Clayton, P. Training at Washington University School of Medicine in Psychiatry in the late 1950's, from the perspective of an affective disorder researcher. J. Affect. Disord., 92:13–17, 2006.
3. Robins, E., and Guze, S. B. Establishment of diagnostic validity in psychiatric illness: Its application to schizophrenia. Am. J. Psychiat., 6:983–987, 1970.

Looking Forward

Diagnosis is the cornerstone of medicine. It allows physicians to communicate effectively with their patients and other health-care professionals and serves as a predictor of the future. It is the means by which physicians make treatment decisions and are able to assess whether an intervention has an effect. In the absence of accurate diagnosis, medicine largely becomes a "Tower of Babel" where no one understands what is going on. This lesson has been learned more slowly in psychiatry than in other fields of medicine, but thanks to a group of psychiatrists at Washington University in St. Louis, the field has moved to a reliable, criteria-based system of classification over the past 30–40 years. Early pioneers included Eli Robins, Sam Guze, George Winokur, and a host of others at Renard Hospital in the 1960s and 1970s. Their efforts were highlighted with the publication of a set of criteria for psychiatric diagnoses by John Feighner et al. in 1972 (1). Subsequently, Bob Woodruff, Don Goodwin, and Sam Guze published the first edition of this text, *Psychiatric Diagnosis*, in 1974 (2). The book has undergone several revisions over the years and the three original authors are now deceased. Based on efforts dating almost a decade and surviving their move from Washington University to institutions in Texas and New Mexico, Carol North and Sean Yutzy have taken up the mantle and have done the field a major service by providing us with an outstanding and thoroughly updated version of this classic text.

It is interesting to note that with the publication of this 6th edition of *Psychiatric Diagnosis*, psychiatry once again finds itself at a crossroad. As described in greater detail by Paula Clayton in her Preface, psychiatry in the 1960s and 1970s was digging itself out of the morass that was *Diagnostic and Statistical Manual of Mental Disorders, First Version (DSM-I)* and *DSM-II*. At the time of the first edition, *Psychiatric Diagnosis* featured the 11 major disorders that Woodruff et al. believed had sufficient reliability and validity to be included in a diagnostic system (2). Sexual problems were included as a separate chapter. The authors did not believe that these were the only diagnoses possible, rather these were the most reliable and valid at that time. Furthermore, the first edition included the criteria of Feighner et al. (1) for making these diagnoses—criteria that were meant to guide research, not to be treated as gospel. This was a necessary first step allowing reliability, that is, agreement among examiners, to move to the forefront. Validity of psychiatric diagnoses was more problematic and was determined on the basis of criteria described by Robins and Guze in a paper on schizophrenia in 1970 (3). To this day, the Robins–Guze criteria remain the "gold standard" for establishing the validity of psychiatric diagnoses. With the publication of *DSM-III* in 1980 (4), psychiatry moved to a criteria-based diagnostic system, a system that has evolved to be as reliable as any in medicine. Unfortunately, the validity issue (i.e., whether a disorder/syndrome reflects specific pathology or pathophysiology) remains highly problematic. I point this out not to rehash the past, but to indicate where we stand today as we contemplate the future of the field. We have reliability . . . but we sorely lack validity for many common diagnoses. North and Yutzy deal very effectively with these issues in this revised text.

How is psychiatry at another crossroad? Since the arrival of *DSM-I* (4), diagnosis has become a "growth industry" for the field. We have gone from about 100 disorders in *DSM-I* in the 1950s to about 270 disorders in *DSM-III* in 1980 to nearly 300 disorders and about 500 diagnoses in the current version of *DSM-IV* (5). From this one might conclude that either the field has advanced greatly or we now have generated a system that codifies many poorly studied and poorly validated "descriptors." Both factors likely contribute, although the latter seems to play the lead. Again, reliability is not the issue—we can effectively codify all kinds of categories with high interrater reliability; we suffer from a lack of the hard work and insight required to validate these categories.

There are a number of other disturbing trends in the field that threaten to weaken the diagnostic system further. Critics of the current system rightfully complain that many categories are indistinct. That is, patients meet criteria for multiple diagnoses. This is clearly the case with regard to personality disorders, but also involves axis I disorders, including well-validated disorders like schizophrenia and psychotic mood disorders in some cases. Thus, we have seen an explosion in the diagnosis of "comorbid conditions," meaning that the same patient may now carry multiple diagnoses . . . in some cases five or more. At times this seems legitimate (e.g., a person with major depression who also has alcoholism), but in others, comorbidity reflects a lack of syndromic thinking and a failure to use parsimonious logic and a longitudinal perspective for describing the illness course. We are also seeing a movement in the field to consider more "sub-syndromal" disorders and weakened versions of major diagnoses (e.g., some subtypes of posttraumatic stress disorder and watered-down versions of bipolar disorder). Along this line, others in the field advocate a more drastic move to consider psychiatric disorders from a "continuum" perspective, that is, viewing symptoms as continuously distributed in the population and disorder as the extreme of the population distribution. This would result in psychiatric disorders being diagnosed more like hypertension and diabetes. This is an interesting idea that requires systematic study, including careful longitudinal follow-up studies. A major concern about the continuum idea is that, unlike the medical disorders diagnosed this way, psychiatric syndromes are still diagnosed based on patient (and/or informant) history. This adds uncertainty in determining how symptoms are distributed in the population, given that human memory is not a truth-generating device and is subject to numerous biases, not the least of which are simple forgetfulness and retrospective change. Compounding these issues is now the reified importance of the diagnostic system for clinical billing purposes. Here third-party payers are reluctant to accept uncertainty, requiring clinicians to force patients into "neat" but not necessarily appropriate categories. This is easiest to observe in the frequent inclusion of "not otherwise specified" (NOS) categories for purposes of reimbursement. These trends significantly weaken and challenge the field. Again, North and Yutzy are on the right path in bringing us back to tough-minded logic and science.

Today we are on the verge of *DSM-V*, a tome that will likely be published in 2012. This has been met by mixed responses. Some view it as a significant advance, giving the field a chance to clean up prior mistakes and to start the process of reconceptualizing psychiatric symptoms and syndromes. This includes better incorporation of disabilities into clinical thinking. The latter is much needed, given the contribution of psychiatric disorders to disability and death. Others are less enthused about *DSM-V* and do not believe the field has advanced far enough based on systematic and longitudinal studies to warrant significant changes. What is clear is that validation of many current disorders has not advanced to the level that we can be more confident in the quality of information conveyed by certain diagnostic labels (e.g., some personality disorders and dissociative identity disorder, among others).

North and Yutzy have done an impressive job bringing us up to date on where we are with regard to the major and best-validated diagnoses; the field has made significant advances and we can have great confidence in the information provided in this text. This is a big help for clinicians and researchers. It would be interesting to hear North and Yutzy's thoughts about other disorders in *DSM-IV* and how they view those disorders from a validation perspective. Given their thoughtful selections in the current text, it seems clear where they stand and silence speaks volumes. It is in these areas that the field must focus its attention if our diagnostic system is to advance.

Where do we go from here? Again, psychiatry seems to be at a crossroad. Most importantly, the field must decide whether or not it is really a branch of neuroscience. For this discussion, it is critical to remember that psychiatry deals with "mental" (mind) disorders. In turn, "mind," from any meaningful scientific perspective, is a product of the brain. Thus, a major challenge is how to get brains back into clinical psychiatry and into our diagnostic system. As practiced today, much of psychiatry is "brainless"; that is, diagnosis and treatment are done much like they have been done for at least the past 30 years (actually the past 100 years or longer). Understanding what is wrong in the brain is not a major factor in diagnosis or treatment. As a result, psychiatry relies on psychometrics and tries to build better "mousetraps" based on clinical histories (e.g., *DSM-IV*), but we are only scratching the surface of the big questions that could radically change our thinking about these illnesses. Eventually, the scientific hope is that we will revise our diagnostic system based on neuroscience and genetics. Under such a scenario, we may start to understand how syndromes are distinct, how symptoms overlap, how molecular pathologies play a role, whether we need to redefine certain disorders, and why comorbid symptoms are so common.

How do we get there? First and foremost, we need to understand how "brain" generates "mind." This is not a philosophical discussion—mind is what results from the operation of specific brain networks that underlie thinking (cognition), emotion, and motivation—the so-called mental trilogy in the words of Joseph LeDoux (6). As we move forward in the twenty-first century, understanding the operations of neural networks involved in generating "mind" is a tractable problem and understanding how these systems go awry in illnesses has the potential to contribute a real pathophysiology to psychiatry. Psychiatry must embrace these changes and this will alter how we train future clinicians and researchers. Subsequent versions of *Psychiatric Diagnosis* (and maybe the DSM) will result in different approaches to how we diagnose, validate, and treat psychiatric disorders, based on neuroscience and perhaps molecular mechanisms. This will not be the case in *DSM-V*.

In 2009, psychiatry is actively investigating several areas of particular interest that may result in major advances. The ability to visualize the functioning human brain, including imaging activity in socially relevant and emotionally provocative situations, offers a lot of hope for unraveling the neural defects that underlie psychiatric disorders. Early examples include the work of Read Montague examining how individuals with borderline personality disorder (a syndrome that North and Yutzy point out is not as well validated as many think) (7) or high-functioning autism spectrum disorders (8) interact with others while playing social/economic games. This work has begun to highlight differences in processing that may contribute to symptoms and disabilities. Similarly, advances in cellular, synaptic, and network biology, coupled with the ability to develop more meaningful animal models of certain behaviors, offer a great deal of hope. Here, work on animal models of chronic mild stress by Karl Deisseroth and colleagues (9) are starting to unravel how information flow in the hippocampus, a region involved in several major psychiatric disorders, may be altered and how psychiatric treatments affect those changes. Network dynamics are now being considered in patient groups, as evidenced by hippocampal gene expression studies done by Francine Benes and colleagues (10) in patients with bipolar disorder and schizophrenia. One can argue that we are probably furthest along in studying how the brain becomes addicted to various drugs. Many scientists, including Eric Nestler, Rob Malenka, and others, have contributed significantly to this effort, and there is hope that insights from this cellular and molecular work will translate into diagnostic and treatment strategies. Similarly, we are learning a lot about how emotions are generated in brain networks (fear being the best example at present) and such work has the hope of defining "emotional endophenotypes" in the words of Jaak Panksepp (11).

One of the things we are learning that seems most relevant to human illnesses is how the brain is organized into specific processing networks. Based on temporally coordinated fluctuations in functional imaging signals, it appears there are intrinsic connectivity networks (ICNs) in our brains that are designed to process certain types of information (12). These include ICNs for language, attention, executive decision making, and various emotions, among others. This is not terribly surprising at first glance, but what is perhaps surprising is how pathology can be localized to and percolate within a specific network, possibly via synaptic pathways. What is also critical for psychiatry is that these ICNs can be imaged in real time and their actions can be determined doing real tasks. A network that may be critical to psychiatry goes under the name of the "default processing network" (13). This system involves several structures, including the medial prefrontal cortex, retrosplenial/precuneal regions, lateral temporal cortex, and hippocampus. The system is so named because it is the "default" state that our brains relax to when not doing other tasks. This system is highly active at rest and appears to process internal information, letting us know how we are doing and updating and reflecting upon our memories and thoughts. When we focus attention on a task, we must exit this default state and use the ICNs required for the selected task. Several studies indicate that patients with psychiatric disorders, including major depression, have problems shifting out of the default state (14). In effect, these persons appear to be stuck in processing their current internal mood state and thoughts ... not a far cry from what is observed clinically. Why this occurs is not clear, but recent observations by Myrna Weissman and colleagues (15) showing that thinning of neocortex in patients with highly familial major depression is correlated with illness risk and severity are an interesting lead. Importantly, cortical thinning was associated with problems in focusing attention—a finding that may be related to the defects in shifting out of the default state observed by Yvette Sheline and colleagues (14) in depressed subjects. I point out these recent results not because they are the "answer" or explain major depression, but rather because they are innovative concepts that crystallize a direction for understanding neural network defects in psychiatric disorders. Against this background, I would also inject a note of strong caution as the field moves down the path of more sophisticated imaging studies. The work by the Sheline and Weissman groups used highly selected and carefully diagnosed subjects with major depression. This is to be applauded. As North and Yutzy note, depression is a heterogeneous group of disorders and extremely careful classification is mandatory if we are to make any sense of neuroimaging (or genetic) results. The field sometimes loses sight of this and poorly characterized and poorly selected subject groups can result in uninterpretable results, as evidenced by the oddities and uncertainties that pepper many of the field's clinical trials.

Work on the pathophysiology of neural networks is in its infancy and is only one example of how things might progress. My comments about this work are emboldened by recent findings linking subtypes of dementia to pathology in specific ICNs (16). Importantly, clinical dementia syndromes, including syndromes with marked behavioral changes, aren't tied to their molecular pathology but rather result from the specific ICNs that are involved. The latter observation may help us understand why there is seemingly so much overlap in the genetics of major psychiatric disorders. That is, molecular/synaptic mechanisms may be more generic and point to potential therapeutic targets, but it is the specific networks and how they are affected that lead to specific clinical symptoms, syndromes, and disabilities. Why certain ICNs are vulnerable to dysfunction in certain individuals is a major unanswered question.

North and Yutzy are to be congratulated for their efforts in this updated edition of *Psychiatric Diagnosis*. Their work has profound implications for our field and how we think about psychiatric illnesses. As they clearly state, we have a very reliable diagnostic system, but we validate our diagnoses using criteria developed nearly 40 years ago (3). Nonetheless, those validating criteria are as important today as they were when first published. What is missing and must be added is meaningful biomarkers and pathophysiological understanding. When that is accomplished we will be in a position to develop a more refined diagnostic system ... not just a better mousetrap.

In closing, I would note that this book originated in St. Louis but now carries Dallas and Albuquerque as points of origin. Life circumstances and opportunities change all of us, but those of us in St. Louis still view this as a "Washington University" contribution to the field. North and Yutzy spent their formative years in our department and are dyed-in-the-wool "Renardians," as good of diagnosticians as exist in the field. Their crisp and critical thinking is a source of pride to us. From a St. Louis perspective, it is great to see what they have accomplished and how they have enhanced the Robins–Guze legacy. Diagnostic systems may come and go, but tough mindedness is never out of style.

Charles F. Zorumski, MD
Washington University in St. Louis

REFERENCES

1. Airan, R. D., Meltzer, L. A., Roy, M., Gong, Y., Chen, H., and Deisseroth, K. High-speed imaging reveals neurophysiological links to behavior in an animal model of depression. Science, *317*:819–823, 2007.
2. American Psychiatric Association. *Diagnostic and Statistical Manual of Mental Disorders*, 3rd edition. Washington, DC: Author, 1980.
3. American Psychiatric Association. *Diagnostic and Statistical Manual of Mental Disorders*, 4th edition. Washington, DC: Author, 1994.
4. Benes, F. M., Lim, B., Matzilevich, D., Subburaju, S., and Walsh, J. P. Circuitry-based gene expression profiles in GABA cells of the trisynaptic pathway in schizophrenics versus bipolar. Proc. Natl. Acad. Sci. USA, *105*:20935–20940, 2008.

5. Buckner, R. L., Andrews-Hanna, J. R., and Schacter, D. L. The brain's default network. Anatomy, function and relevance to disease. Ann. NY Acad. Sci., 1124:1–38, 2008.

6. Chiu, P. H., Kayali, M. A., Kishida, K. T., Tomlin, D., Klinger, L. G., Klinger, M. R., and Montague, P. R. Self responses along cingulate cortex reveal quantitative phenotype for high-functioning autism. Neuron, 57:463–473, 2008.

7. Feighner, J. P., Robins, E., Guze, S. B., Woodruff, R. A., Winokur, G., and Munoz, R. Diagnostic criteria for use in psychiatric research. Arch. Gen. Psychiat., 26:57–63, 1972.

8. King-Casas, B., Sharp, C., Lomax-Bream, L., Lohrenz, T., Fonagy, P., and Montague, P. R. The rupture and repair of cooperation in borderline personality disorder. Science, 321:806–810, 2008.

9. LeDoux, J. Synaptic Self: How Our Brains Become Who We Are. New York: Viking Press, 2002.

10. Mesulam, M. Defining neurocognitive networks in the BOLD new world of computed connectivity. Neuron, 62:1–3, 2009.

11. Panksepp, J. Emotional endophenotypes in evolutionary psychiatry. Prog. Neuropsychopharmacol. Biol. Psychiat., 30:774–784, 2006.

12. Peterson, B. S., Warner, V., Bansal, R., Zhu, H., Hao, X., Liu, J., Durkin, K., Adams, P. B., Wickramaratne, P., and Weissman, M. M. Cortical thinning in persons at increased familial risk for major depression. Proc. Natl. Acad. Sci. USA, 106:6273–6278, 2009.

13. Robins, E., and Guze, S. B. Establishment of diagnostic validity in psychiatric illness: Its application to schizophrenia. Am. J. Psychiat., 126:983–987, 1970.

14. Seeley, W. W., Crawford, R. K., Zhou, J., Miller, B. L., and Greicius, M. D. Neurodegenerative diseases target large-scale human brain networks. Neuron, 62:42–52, 2009.

15. Sheline, Y. I., Barch, D. M., Price, J. L., Rundle, M. M., Vaishnavi, S. N., Snyder, A. Z., Mintun, M. A., Wang, S., Coalson, R. S., and Raichle, M. E. The default mode network and self-referential processes in depression. Proc. Natl. Acad. Sci. USA, 106:1942–1947, 2009.

16. Woodruff, R. A., Goodwin, D. W., and Guze, S. B. Psychiatric Diagnosis. New York: Oxford University Press, 1974.

I

Evolution of Psychiatric Diagnosis

The diagnostic approach in psychiatry does not have a long and illustrious tradition in the United States. Historically, Freud and his influential psychoanalytic school in Europe during the late 1800s focused on symptoms that were felt to be of "psychogenic" origin. Subsequently, the fundamental principles of psychoanalysis were imported into the United States, where they predominated for almost three-quarters of the twentieth century.

The American Psychiatric Association (APA) published the first *Diagnostic and Statistical Manual of Mental Disorders* (*DSM*) in 1952 (1), moving American psychiatry incrementally toward a descriptive approach. Although that text included various psychiatric conditions with diagnostic labels, it did not provide explicit criteria, and most symptoms were conceptualized in a framework of a reaction to a situation or stressor. Consistent with the predominating Freudian approach at that time in America, symptoms were considered to originate from underlying dynamic conflicts, representing symbolic meaning. Understanding a patient's symptoms required exploration of that individual's own developmental history and life experiences (14). Problematic to scientific advancement of the field within this approach was the flaw that such prevailing assumptions about the etiology of psychiatric problems were scientifically untestable (18). Further, problems of unreliability plagued symptom interpretation, a process unique to the individual patient and inconsistent from one clinician to the next. Definition of psychiatric problems using these approaches poorly differentiated healthy from ill individuals and hampered communication among clinicians about their cases. In 1968, the APA published the second edition of the text (*DSM-II*) (2), which embraced the disease concept for mental illness—but again without explicit criteria. Diagnostic reliability was not yet a feature of the proffered labels. To find its place among the medical sciences, psychiatry needed to develop an epidemiological system for classifying disease, known as "nosology" (14).

Several European physicians specializing in problems of psychiatry (Kraepelin, Kahlbaum, Bleuler, and others) who predated or were contemporaries of Freud found it more useful to describe the phenomenology of mental illness as clustering in "syndromes" according to their unique symptoms, course, and outcome over time. These physicians followed an earlier and evolving approach to disease initiated by Sydenham in the late 1600s and further developed over the centuries by Koch, Pasteur, Virchow, and others. The relevant assumption by most of these investigators was that identification of a syndrome would lead to a better understanding of the illness and possibly etiology. Kraepelin considered mental disorders to be commensurate with physical diseases. He followed medical traditions of careful observation of many cases to describe overt characteristics of illness, rather than relying on unproven etiological theories. Kraepelin predicted that empirical research would eventually provide evidence of biological origins of mental illness (18, 20).

The classification/diagnostic approach and attendant scientific methods were not systematically applied in American psychiatry until the advent of the "descriptive school" in the latter half of the twentieth century, whose traditions were founded on the earlier work of Sydenham, Kraepelin, and others. During the 1960s and early 1970s, the Washington University group in St. Louis, described as "an outpost of diagnostically oriented thinking" (p. 259) (18), refined the descriptive approach to psychiatry and distinguished themselves as radically different from the prevailing psychoanalytic school. In American psychiatry at that time, the belief that mental disorders were a subset of medical disorders was controversial (18) if not heretical. Members of this group, often referred to as "neo-Kraepelinians," were described by some as "organic" or "biological" in orientation, but their position regarding the origin of symptoms was simply "what the evidence or reproducible data demonstrated."

In 1970, Robins and Guze (17) at Washington University in St. Louis published their proposal for the phases necessary to establish the validity and reliability of a psychiatric diagnosis. The five phases included the following:

1. *Clinical description.* The first step is to describe the clinical picture. Race, sex, age at onset, precipitating factor(s), and other items may be used to define the disorder. The clinical picture described in the United States should be the same as in the United Kingdom, Russia, and elsewhere.
2. *Laboratory studies.* These include any laboratory test of a chemical, physiological, radiological, or anatomical (biopsy or autopsy) nature that could reproducibly demonstrate a finding.
3. *Delimitation from other disorders.* Symptoms of the disorder of interest must be distinguishable from other potentially overlapping disorders.
4. *Follow-up studies.* The first diagnosis is reconfirmed at follow-up (usually years later), supporting the original diagnosis.
5. *Family studies.* Most psychiatric illnesses have been shown to run in families, whether of genetic or environmental origin. Identification of the illness in the family supports the validity of the diagnosis.

Feighner et al. in 1972 (10) outlined the diagnoses and criteria that met these phases. Included were the following: primary affective disorder (mania/ depression), secondary affective disorder, schizophrenia, anxiety neurosis, obsessive-compulsive neurosis, phobic neurosis, hysteria, antisocial personality disorder, alcoholism, drug dependence, mental retardation, organic brain syndrome, anorexia nervosa, and several others. It should be noted that with the possible exception of brain syndrome(s), laboratory studies still have not been developed that reproducibly demonstrate pathological lesions. However, thoughtful and careful completion, with replication, of most of the phases (1, 3, 4, and 5) firmly established the bases for the validity of the major mental illnesses.

To gain a foothold in the published literature, this group published their early work in diagnostic psychiatry in British and other European literature, outside the reach of American hostility to their ideas (Samuel B. Guze, personal communication). In 1974, the first edition of *Psychiatric Diagnosis*, co-authored by Robert A. Woodruff, Jr., Donald W. Goodwin, and Samuel B. Guze, was published by Oxford University Press (19). Although written for the education of medical students, it became an icon for the field. At the time, this text was the most authoritative source of diagnostic psychiatry, as the current diagnostic manual of the APA had not yet incorporated empirically based criteria.

In the late 1970s, Robert Spitzer, with remarkable political finesse, convened meetings (Samuel B. Guze, personal communication) of members of the two formal psychiatric schools, psychoanalytic and evidence-based/biological (18) to generate the third edition of the *Diagnostic and Statistical Manual* (*DSM-III*) (3). The text was generally intended to be atheoretical in orientation regarding the origin of most psychopathology. (Of note, to appease an opposition that threatened to block the document's approval, the word *neurosis*, a concept fundamental to Freudian psychoanalysis, was retained parenthetically after the word *disorder* (18). *Neurosis* did not survive the next revision of the diagnostic text.) *DSM-III* was the first of the APA's diagnostic manuals to embrace the Washington University (St. Louis) group's emphasis that medical diagnosis is the keystone of medical practice and research (18). The *DSM-III* text included practically en bloc the Feighner criteria for the diagnoses of the major mental illnesses. Unfortunately for validity and reliability considerations, the text also included approximately 213 other "mental disorder" labels with essentially untested criteria. Nonetheless, the creation of a common language utilizing valid and reliable psychiatric diagnoses, as well as defining explicit criteria, was an important advance.

While some considered the advances of *DSM-III* a revolution, many data-oriented psychiatrists saw it as simply a move to align with the substantially evolved general medical model of the time. With *DSM-III*, psychiatric diagnosis became practical and useful to clinicians as well as researchers. Psychiatrists now had psychiatric diagnoses that provided clear boundaries for major psychiatric illnesses within dichotomies rather than dimensions that blurred boundaries between normal and abnormal. These diagnoses were based on documented observations of psychopathology rather than on unsupported theoretical etiologic mechanisms (18). Of particular note was the fact that diagnostic reliability (measured by the *kappa* statistic designed to measure diagnostic concordance or agreement about diagnosis among examinations) of the major diagnoses moved into the good to excellent range, equaling the established reliability of medical diagnoses made on clinical grounds. The data/evidence-based school continued describing its approach to psychiatric nosology simply as "medical model" (dating back to 1973). This term is broader than "biological" (implying limitation within purely physical processes such as genes and brain chemistry). The medical model is more descriptive of the categorical/diagnostic approach, which encompasses all aspects of illness, including environmental and social aspects, within medical definitions and descriptions.

At first, the academicians involved with the development of *DSM-III* and those embracing the new medical model of psychiatry were alleged to constitute an "invisible college" of professionals trained at Washington University dispersed to leadership positions at the University of Iowa, the University of Minnesota, the University of Kansas, and Columbia University in New York

City, among other sites. As their numbers and their publications grew and these clinician/scientists blended into the landscape of American psychiatry under the aegis of *DSM-III* and its predecessors, the invisible college grew into the mainstream institution.

Prevailing forces in medicine and psychiatry at the time facilitated and embraced the changes brought about with *DSM-III* (18). Prior to *DSM-III*, psychiatry had largely fallen outside the mainstream of the science and practice of medicine. Psychologists, social workers, and other mental health professionals threatened to replace psychiatrists. Critics of psychiatry claimed that definitions of mental illnesses did not have objective criteria, asserting that psychiatric illness did not even exist. *DSM-III* provided objective diagnostic criteria and positioned psychiatric diagnosis within the medical purview. Psychiatry re-asserted its place in medicine as a medical specialty. Evolving computer technology contributed substantially to the investigation of empirical aspects of disease. Advances in diagnosis provided powerful incentives for the pharmaceutical industry and independent researchers to develop new drugs and other treatments targeted for treatment of specific disorders. Insurance companies sought diagnostic structure to guide reimbursement for treatment of validated disorders with demonstrable evidence of specified treatments for them. The achievement of diagnostic reliability led to new research opportunities and directions (18).

Subsequent versions of the APA textbook (*DSM-III-R* (4), *DSM-IV* (5), and *DSM-IV-TR* (6)) further solidified and reaffirmed the transformation of American psychiatry to an empirically based system of classification of diagnosis that *DSM-III* initiated (18). They also, however, further increased and expanded the number of labeled mental disorders (5, 6). Unfortunately, the new labels promulgated have not met the phases noted above, which over time have become the "gold standard" for establishing validity and reliability of a psychiatric diagnosis. In sum, the vast majority of diagnostic labels in the latest version (*DSM-IV-TR*) have not met the diagnostic gold standard. Not surprisingly, research on many of the coded non-major "mental disorders" or labels during the 1990s and later have led to significant questions about comorbidity (problems with delimitation). (For specific examples of these problems, see also Chapters 5 and 10 on posttraumatic stress disorder and borderline personality disorder.)

The effects of the medical model movement in psychiatry have been substantial. The National Institute of Mental Health embraced the *DSM-III* and subsequent versions of this text as the authoritative text for psychiatric disorder classification. Shortly after the publication of *DSM-III*, students and physicians from American medical schools and residency programs were expected to pass qualifying examinations based on APA diagnostic criteria. Scholarly journals and federal research granting agencies similarly assumed conformation to current diagnostic conventions as delineated in APA criteria. Colleagues in different locales, even different countries, could finally collaborate using a common diagnostic language (18).

Through this history, the *Psychiatric Diagnosis* textbook stayed alive—and grew—not in numbers of diagnoses, but in size. Accumulated data in support of the valid major mental illnesses over half a century were slowly and painstakingly gathered into the second, third, fourth, fifth, and now sixth editions. The original authors have all passed away: first Bob Woodruff (1976), later Don Goodwin (1999), and finally Sam Guze (2000). The text's new authors were trained by the original members of the Washington University group, Eli Robins and Sam Guze, and, as students, read *Psychiatric Diagnosis* along with the hundreds and thousands of other students educated with this text over the years.

The subsequent chapters in this text review the accumulated wealth of data over the years relevant to the diagnoses included in it. The information is not meant to comprise a cutting-edge review of the latest findings in research. Rather, it is meant to provide fundamental and time-tested evidence for psychiatric disorders to teach and support the principles of psychiatric diagnosis so eloquently constructed through established empirical research.

This chapter would not be complete without addressing and placing in proper perspective newer trends that are buffeting the field of psychiatry. Evolving developments in biological technology are increasingly providing new directions for scientific exploration. Many such leads, holding promise of fundamental advances in the understanding of psychopathology, have disappointingly not delivered as anticipated. A classic example is the dexamethasone suppression test, introduced in the early 1980s, which was hoped to be psychiatry's first laboratory test (8). This putative marker generated great interest and hundreds of articles; however, low sensitivity of the test limited its clinical utility (7), although it has remained a useful research tool.

Psychiatric genetics is another area that was hoped to translate into nosologic insights that could further revolutionize conceptualization and utility of psychiatric diagnosis. It has been predicted that increasing elucidation of genotype–phenotype relationships may eventually force the abandonment of traditional Kraepelinian dichotomy in the classification of psychiatric illness (9). Continuing research, however, has yielded growing frustration and no indications that genetic research findings will fundamentally alter empirically based classification of psychiatric illness any time soon. First, no "Mendelian-like" genes have been found for the major psychiatric disorders, and it is generally recognized that none will be found. Second, efforts to carve nature at its joints are not destined to cleave psychiatric disorders using purely genetic tools, because the psychiatric phenotype is more than a product of its genes. Kendler (12) recently concluded that even genes known to be involved in the generation of psychopathology cannot provide the basis for construction of psychiatric diagnoses. He predicted that molecular genetics, like traditional genetics, will offer disappointingly little in terms of advancing conceptualization of psychiatric diagnosis.

Advances in biological science continually challenge the field of psychiatry to evolve. Although an empirical approach to classification in psychiatry was revolutionary in the 1970s when a small group of academicians and their text *Psychiatric Diagnosis* were instrumental in changing the field, the current classification system has now been generally accepted for many years. Pressures to change have persisted, however, during the period of exponential growth in research since the first edition of this text was published. Not surprisingly, critics of the current classification system have replayed and amplified suggestions of past eras for a "dimensional construction" of diagnostic concepts.

Although past and some new voices continue to advocate for the inclusion of dimensional methodology in definition of psychopathology, no clearly compelling reason has been advanced to eliminate the categorical process of diagnostic assessment. Academic proponents of dimensional components of psychiatric classification continue to champion the categorical system of diagnosis while emphasizing advantages of adding dimensional measurements to diagnostic taxonomies (11, 13). In many contexts, categorical and dimensional measurements are interrelated and are sometimes equivalent. Further, while a dimensional approach may, to a degree, enhance data, statistical power, and measurement of psychiatric change, it does not contemplate in many forms the actual validity of the diagnostic assessment. Categorical considerations remain unarguably vital in establishing inclusion criteria for research studies and for making clinical decisions about treatment (13).

Critics of the categorical diagnostic approach rightfully point to the inflation of number of recognized psychiatric diagnoses as problematic (15). Others who are troubled by the inability to classify symptomatic individuals not meeting diagnostic criteria promote concepts of "partial" or "spectrum" diagnoses. Continuing concerns about lack of clear demarcation between diagnostic cases and others (16) have not recognized the original authors' specification that approximately one out of five cases assessed in the Washington University tradition is not cross-sectionally classifiable in a diagnostic structure. Thus, uncertainties in estimation of boundaries were built into the diagnostic classification process, circumventing otherwise unsolvable problems of diagnostic decision making.

In addition to movements to dimensionalize psychiatric classification systems, the field has encountered significant external pressures to assess psychopathology in short time frames and develop outcome measures to justify pharmaceutical/psychotherapeutic interventions. These trends have encouraged the use of brief screening instruments for identification of psychiatric disorders and self-report questionnaires in both clinical and research settings. These shortcuts, however, cannot substitute for careful establishing of a psychiatric diagnosis. Although some screening tools may have utility in overall patient assessment, they do not rely upon or yield adequate information for a formal diagnosis. Screening instruments may be appropriate and useful for identifying a high-risk subgroup when the population of interest is too large to permit full diagnostic assessment of all its members and to identify a subset of individuals at high risk for illness who can then be further assessed using the full diagnostic criteria. Screening instruments without formal interview, however, should not be relied upon for assigning a psychiatric diagnosis that can be the basis for treatment decisions. Further, screening instruments are inadequate for assessing general population prevalence rates of psychopathology. Unfortunately, the research literature is fraught with examples of studies inappropriately using screening instruments to diagnose cases and estimate population prevalence.

Overall, psychiatric diagnosis is of paramount importance, and there is no shortcut to diagnosis using screening tools to estimate likelihood within individual patients or entire populations. Further, while dimensional aspects of illness may add to our understanding of psychiatric disorders, they cannot replace psychiatric diagnosis. For the foreseeable future, psychiatrists and other medical doctors must continue to rely on established psychiatric diagnoses and gathering information the old-fashioned way—through clinical interviews with patients—to guide assessment and treatment decisions.

Finally, the current edition of this text flows from the original and seminal work by its predecessors to establish and validate psychiatric diagnoses that support the mainstream activities of medical practice and research. We do not entertain the recently popular screening tools, notions of "partial" diagnosis, dimensional classifications, or disorders outside those considered sufficiently validated and useful within empirical traditions of psychiatric diagnosis. Clearly the diagnostic traditions based on empirical findings over approximately five decades—sufficiently revised in this text to accommodate new knowledge and the changing field—will instruct future generations of students in the fundamental concepts of psychiatric diagnosis.

REFERENCES

1. American Psychiatric Association. *Diagnostic and Statistical Manual of Mental Disorders*, 1st edition. Washington, DC: Author, 1952.

2. American Psychiatric Association. *Diagnostic and Statistical Manual of Mental Disorders*, 2nd edition. Washington, DC: Author, 1968.

3. American Psychiatric Association. *Diagnostic and Statistical Manual of Mental Disorders*, 3rd edition. Washington, DC: Author, 1980.

4. American Psychiatric Association. *Diagnostic and Statistical Manual of Mental Disorders*, 3rd edition, revised. Washington, DC: Author, 1987.

5. American Psychiatric Association. *Diagnostic and Statistical Manual of Mental Disorders*, 4th edition. Washington, DC: Author, 1994.

6. American Psychiatric Association. *Diagnostic and Statistical Manual of Mental Disorders*, 4th edition, text revision. Washington, DC: Author, 2000.

7. American Psychiatric Association Task Force on Laboratory Tests in Psychiatry. The dexamethasone suppression test: an overview of its current status in psychiatry. Am. J. Psychiat., *144*:1253–1262, 1987.

8. Carroll, B. J. The dexamethasone test for melancholia. Br. J. Psychiat., *140*:292–304, 1982.

9. Craddock, N., O'Donovan, M. C., and Owen, M. J. Genes for schizophrenia and bipolar disorder? Implications for psychiatric nosology. Schizophr. Bull., *32*:9–16, 2006.

10. Feighner, J. P., Robins, E., Guze, S. B., Woodruff, R. A., Winokur, G., and Muñoz, R. Diagnostic criteria for use in psychiatric research. Arch. Gen. Psychiat., *26*:57–62, 1972.

11. Helzer, J. E., Kraemer, H. C., and Krueger, R. F. The feasibility and need for dimensional psychiatric diagnoses. Psychol. Med., *36*:1671–1680, 2006.

12. Kendler, K. S. Reflections on the relationship between psychiatric genetics and psychiatric nosology. Am. J. Psychiat., *163*:1138–1146, 2006.

13. Kraemer, H. C., Noda, A., and O'Hara, R. Categorical versus dimensional approaches to diagnosis: methodological challenges. J. Psychiat. Res., *38*:17–25, 2004.

14. Mayes, R., and Horwitz, A. V. DSM-III and the revolution in the classification of mental illness. J. Hist. Behav. Sci., *41*:249–267, 2005.

15. Mullen, P. E. A modest proposal for another phenomenological approach to psychopathology. Schizophr. Bull., *33*:113–121, 2007.

16. Neese, R. M., and Jackson, E. D. Evolution: psychiatric nosology's missing biological foundation. Clin. Neuropsychiat., *3*:121–131, 2006.

17. Robins, E., and Guze, S. B. Establishment of diagnostic validity in psychiatric illness: its application to schizophrenia. Am. J. Psychiat., *126*:983–987, 1970.

18. Rogler, L. H. Making sense of historical changes in the Diagnostic and Statistical Manual of Mental Disorders: five propositions. J. Health Soc. Behav., *38*:9–20, 1997.

19. Woodruff, R. A., Jr., Goodwin, D. W., and Guze, S. B. *Psychiatric Diagnosis*. New York: Oxford University Press, 1974.

20. Young, A. *The Harmony of Illusions: Inventing Post-traumatic Stress Disorder*. Princeton, NJ: Princeton University Press, 1996.

2

Mood (Affective) Disorders

There is a pitch of unhappiness so great that the goods of
nature may be entirely forgotten, and all sentiment of their
existence vanish from the mental field. For this extremity of
pessimism to be reached, something more is needed than
observation of life and reflection upon death. The individual
must in his own person become the prey of pathological
melancholy.... Such sensitiveness and susceptibility to
mental pain is a rare occurrence where the nervous constitu-
tion is entirely normal; one seldom finds it in a healthy subject
even where he is the victim of the most atrocious cruelties of
outward fortune ... it is positive and active anguish, a sort of
psychical neuralgia wholly unknown to healthy life.

William James
The varieties of religious experience.
In *The Epidemiology of Depression*

Depression and euphoria are the primary symptoms of mood disorders, but not the only ones. Associated with low moods are such
symptoms as insomnia, anorexia, suicidal thoughts, and feelings of
worthlessness or of being a burden to others; associated with euphoria
are such symptoms as hyperactivity, decreased need for sleep, and
flight of ideas. The extent of depression or euphoria is often inappropriate to the patient's life situation, a fact sometimes as obvious to
patients as to their relatives and friends. Formerly known as "affective
disorders," these conditions were renamed "mood disorders" in the
1987 edition of the American Psychiatric Association's diagnostic
manual, *DSM-III-R.*

Whatever the name, the definition remains unchanged. It refers to a group of disorders characterized by prolonged disturbances of mood accompanied by several symptoms as described above. Mood disorders have been divided and subdivided endlessly as investigators endeavor to distinguish "normal" from "abnormal" mood and to create clinical clusters with distinct natural histories, familial prevalence, course and prognoses, and response to treatment. After more than a century there is still disagreement about the most satisfactory classification.

Amid all this diversity, there is a common theme: Mood disorders are primarily characterized by depressed mood, elevated mood (mania), or alterna-tions of depressed and elevated moods. Severe depression is termed "major depression." The building blocks for defining mood disorders are mood epi-sodes, which represent a distinct and persistent change from a person's typical mood with accompanying symptoms, lasting 2 weeks for a major depressive episode and 1 week for a manic episode.

The most recent classification of mood disorders is provided by *DSM-IV-TR*, published by the American Psychiatric Association in 2000. Criteria for major depressive and manic episodes are presented in Tables 2.1 and 2.2, respectively.

Manic and major depressive episodes by themselves do not constitute diagnoses, because a patient with a mood disorder may experience different types of mood episodes over the course of a single illness, and the different episodes would not be diagnosed as separate disorders. This is illustrated by the classical term for manic mood disorder, "manic depressive illness," reflecting the presence of both manic and major depressive episodes as part of the disorder. A newer term, "bipolar disorder," also expresses this same central feature of the disorder. The two terms are interchangeable.

Mood disorders are defined as bipolar when mania occurs, regardless of whether depressions occur. When the disorder involves solely depression, the term "unipolar" or major depression is often used. (A natural initial impression of the terms "bipolar" and "unipolar" is that bipolar disorder implies a history of both mania and depression, whereas unipolar implies a history of one or the other alone. "Bipolar" actually refers to a history of mania regardless of whether depression has also been present. "Unipolar" refers to episodes of depression without mania.)

As many as 40% of patients meeting criteria for bipolar disorder have episodes with both depressive and manic features, called mixed episodes. Bipolar illness with four or more episodes of mania within 12 months is specified as rapid cycling.

Milder depressive syndromes are called "dysthymia"; milder forms of mania are called "hypomania." Milder expressions of bipolar disorder with

TABLE 2.1 Diagnostic Criteria for Major Depressive Episode

A. Five (or more) of the following symptoms have been present during the same 2-week period and
    represent a change from previous functioning; at least one of the symptoms is either (1)
    depressed mood or (2) loss of interest or pleasure.

Note: Do not include symptoms that are clearly due to a general medical condition, or mood-
incongruent delusions or hallucinations.

  (1) Depressed mood most of the day, nearly every day, as indicated by either subjective report
       (e.g., feels sad or empty) or observation made by others (e.g., appears tearful).
       Note: In children and adolescents, can be irritable mood
  (2) Markedly diminished interest or pleasure in all, or almost all, activities most of the day,
       nearly every day (as indicated by either subjective account or observation made by others)
  (3) Significant weight loss when not dieting or weight gain (e.g., a change of more than 5% of
       body weight in a month), or decrease or increase in appetite nearly every day
       Note: In children, consider failure to make expected weight gains
  (4) Insomnia or hypersomnia nearly every day
  (5) Psychomotor agitation or retardation nearly every day (observable by others, not merely
       subjective feelings of restlessness or being slowed down)
  (6) Fatigue or loss of energy nearly every day
  (7) Feelings of worthlessness or excessive or inappropriate guilt (which may be delusional)
       nearly every day (not merely self-reproach or guilt about being sick)
  (8) Diminished ability to think or concentrate, or indecisiveness, nearly every day (either by
       subjective account or as observed by others)
  (9) Recurrent thoughts of death (not just fear of dying), recurrent suicidal ideation without a
       specific plan, or a suicide attempt or a specific plan for committing suicide

B. The symptoms cause clinically significant distress or impairment in social, occupational, or
    other important areas of functioning.
C. The symptoms are not due to the direct physiological effects of a substance (e.g., a drug of abuse,
    a medication) or a general medical condition (e.g., hypothyroidism).
D. The symptoms are not better accounted for by bereavement (i.e., after the loss of a loved one).

Adapted from diagnostic criteria in the *DSM-IV-TR* (234).

both hypomanic and depressive episodes in the absence of manic or psychotic
episodes are referred to as "cyclothymia" or bipolar II disorder.

For all these terms, more than disturbed mood is required. There must be a
syndrome, a group of characteristic clinical features that distinguish one disorder from another.

Historical Background

Descriptions of mood disorders began with Hippocrates. The term "melancholia" is usually attributed to him, as is the notion that it results from the
influence of black bile and phlegm on the brain "darkening the spirit and
making it melancholy" (133).

TABLE 2.2 Diagnostic Criteria for Manic Episode

A. A distinct period of abnormally and persistently elevated, expansive, or irritable mood, lasting at least 1 week (or any duration if hospitalization is necessary)

B. During the period of mood disturbance, three (or more) of the following symptoms have persisted (four if the mood is only irritable) and have been present to a significant degree:

    (1) Inflated self-esteem or grandiosity

    (2) Decreased need for sleep (e.g., feels rested after only 3 hours of sleep)

    (3) More talkative than usual or pressure to keep talking

    (4) Flight of ideas or subjective experience that thoughts are racing

    (5) Distractibility (i.e., attention too easily drawn to unimportant or irrelevant external stimuli)

    (6) Increase in goal-directed activity (either socially, at work or school, or sexually) or psychomotor agitation

    (7) Excessive involvement in pleasurable activities that have a high potential for painful consequences (e.g., engaging in unrestrained buying sprees, sexual indiscretions, or foolish business investments)

C. The mood disturbance is sufficiently severe so as to cause marked impairment in occupational functioning or in usual social activities or relationships with others, or to necessitate hospitalization to prevent harm to self or others, or there are psychotic features.

D. The symptoms are not due to the direct physiological effects of a substance (e.g., a drug of abuse, a medication, or other treatment) or a general medical condition (e.g., hyperthyroidism).

Adapted from diagnostic criteria in the *DSM-IV-TR* (234).

About 500 years later, early in the second century A.D., Aretaeus of Cappadocia recognized and recorded an association between melancholia and mania:

> Those affected with melancholia are not everyone of them affected according to one particular form; they are either suspicious of poisoning or flee to the desert from misanthropy, or turn superstitious, or contract a hatred of life. If at any time a relaxation takes place, in most cases hilarity supervenes ... the patients are dull or stern, dejected or unreasonably torpid, without any manifest cause ... they also become peevish, dispirited, sleepless, and start up from a disturbed sleep. Unreasonable fear also seizes them, if the disease tends to increase ... they complain of life, and desire to die (114). Aretaeus observed that affective disorder was often episodic but also occurred in a chronic, unremitting form. Like Hippocrates, he attributed the cause to a humoral imbalance: If it [black bile] be determined upwards to the stomach and diaphragm, it forms melancholy, for it produces flatulence and eructations of the fetid and fishy nature, and it sends rumbling wind downwards and disturbs the understanding (133).

The nineteenth-century French physician Falret described an episodic variety of depression with remissions and attacks of increasing duration, an illness occurring more frequently among women than men, sometimes associated with precipitating events, sometimes alternating with mania (*la folie circulaire*). Falret and his contemporary Baillarger (who also described recurring attacks of mania and melancholia) probably influenced Kraepelin's later concept of manic depressive psychosis.

In 1896 Kraepelin made his major contribution to psychiatry by separating the functional psychoses into two groups, dementia praecox and manic depressive psychosis. Dementia praecox was chronic and unremitting with a generally bad prognosis. Manic depressive psychosis, on the other hand, did not usually end in chronic invalidism. After publishing the sixth edition of his textbook in 1896, Kraepelin continued to define the limits of dementia praecox narrowly, but he expanded those of manic depressive psychosis to include almost all abnormalities of mood. Chronic depression was included as well as episodic illness; mania was included as well as depression (126, 221).

Kraepelin had insisted that manic depressive psychosis was generally independent of social and psychological forces, that the cause of the illness was "innate." Freud and the psychoanalysts assumed the opposite. Freud in *Mourning and Melancholia*, published in 1917, outlined his theories of the psychodynamic genesis of depression (70). He hypothesized that depression had in common with the process of mourning a response to the loss of a "love-object," that is, the loss of something greatly valued. Grief, a healthy response, differed from melancholia in that the latter involved direction of unresolved, negative feelings inward, resulting in despair, a sense of worthlessness, thoughts of self-harm, and other depressive symptoms.

Since early in the twentieth century there has been considerable controversy over the distinction between "endogenous" depression and "reactive" depression. This controversy had its origin partially in the differing viewpoints of the Kraepelinians and Freudians toward mental phenomena in general. Kraepelin and his followers searched for the limits of pathological behavior by describing the symptoms of syndromes in keeping with the traditions of nineteenth-century German medicine. Freud and his pupils searched for mental mechanisms that might be most obvious in pathological states but were not limited to those states. Such differences in attitude were augmented by the fact that Kraepelinian psychiatrists dealt chiefly with severely ill, hospitalized patients, whereas Freudian psychiatrists tended to treat mildly ill, nonhospitalized patients. The differences have never been fully resolved. Over the years, the field has seen classification after classification of the mood disorders, most frequently in terms of dichotomies: endogenous opposed to reactive, psychotic opposed to neurotic, agitated opposed to retarded.

For centuries, it was assumed tacitly that two major forms of depression exist, "reactive" and "endogenous" depression (53). Reactive depression was considered a direct result of precipitating events or unique individual responses of social and psychological stress, and equated with neurotic features. Endogenous depression, in contrast, was equated with psychotic features. Reactive depression was considered to be less responsive to somatic therapies yet milder than endogenous forms of depression, although empirical research has not confirmed these assumptions (168). The current diagnostic classification of depressive disorders in *DSM-IV-TR* does not mention reactive/endogenous subtypes. However, controversy persists about the validity of this distinction. Recent discovery of a genetic variant of serotonin regulation in individuals prone to major depression in the context of stressful situations has stimulated further interest in the role of stressful environment in the etiology of depression in biologically vulnerable individuals (41).

An alternative subclassification of major depressive disorder that avoids inference about cause is the concept of *primary or secondary* disorders. "Primary affective disorder" applies to major depression in individuals who have had no previous psychiatric disorder aside from episodes of depression or mania. "Secondary affective disorder" refers to major depressive disorder in patients with a preexisting psychiatric illness other than depression or mania. In other words, if the first onset of a mood disorder precedes other psychiatric disorders within an individual it is considered primary, and if it follows onset of any other disorder it is considered secondary. Patients with mild or severe depression, with or without psychotic symptoms such as hallucinations or delusions, with many episodes or with few, and regardless of age of onset, may be diagnosed as having either primary or secondary affective disorder.

Although *DSM-IV-TR* does not distinguish between "primary" and "secondary" affective disorder, we make the distinction for the following reason: The symptoms of primary and secondary affective disorder are similar, but the two conditions have different prognostic and therapeutic implications (60, 180, 182, 224). Primary affective disorder, which occurs in the absence of a preexisting psychiatric disorder or a chronic debilitating medical illness, consists of discrete episodes interspersed with periods of normality. In the case of secondary affective disorders, when the preexisting illness is chronic, which is usually the case, the patient is *not* well between episodes.

Depressive syndromes that are indistinguishable symptomatically from primary affective disorder occur commonly in association with obsessive-compulsive disorder, phobic disorders, panic disorder, somatization disorder, alcohol and drug dependence, and antisocial personality. In fact, almost all psychiatric disorders, including schizophrenia and brain syndromes, are associated with an increased risk of secondary depression. (Secondary mania is much less common.)

A further advantage of the primary-secondary distinction is that some studies indicate that primary affective disorder involves a higher risk of suicide than does secondary affective disorder (except for cases with comorbid alcoholism, which adds considerable suicide risk) (203, 211). Finally, decisions about treatment will be influenced by distinguishing primary from secondary affective disorder; the preexisting illness as well as the depressive syndrome must be treated in the latter (87).

The separation of mood disorders into unipolar and bipolar subtypes was first proposed by Leonhard et al. (131). Support for the separation has emerged from several decades of supporting research evidence from studies in Europe and the United States (18, 19, 23, 155, 176, 222, 223). Patients with bipolar illness have a somewhat earlier age of onset than unipolar patients. Their histories are characterized by more frequent and shorter episodes, which is true for depressive as well as manic episodes. There is a greater prevalence of mood disorder among relatives of bipolar patients than among relatives of unipolar patients.

Many of the questions about the classification of mood disorders that have plagued investigators are still unresolved. At present there is no way to evaluate the importance of precipitating events in either bipolar or unipolar illness. An abiding problem is an old question of how to separate the experience of bereavement from that of depression.

Epidemiology

Estimates of the prevalence of primary affective disorder depend on the sample or population studied and on the definition of the illness. Older studies have estimated the lifetime prevalence of major depression at 5%–9% in the general population (69, 91, 162). The Epidemiologic Catchment Area study, a national household study of psychiatric disorders conducted a quarter of a century ago using structured diagnostic interviews, provided a 5% lifetime prevalence of major depression in the U.S. general population (220). A much higher rate of 17% was reported by a more recent national household study of psychiatric disorders, the National Comorbidity Survey, which used a different diagnostic instrument, provided memory cues, and studied a younger sample (119, 219). Such methodological differences in these studies make it difficult to know which data are most accurate (218, 219). A recent systematic review of 18 population prevalence studies determined pooled lifetime prevalence rates to be 6.7% for major depression and 0.8% for bipolar disorder (218). The authors were unable to account for all of the variability across studies on the basis of common methodological differences.

Another potential explanation for the variability is that cultural and genetic differences may be important in determining the actual prevalence of affective disorders. For example, a 1983 study of 12,500 Amish individuals in Pennsylvania yielded a prevalence rate of 1% for primary affective disorder (59). The Amish are a culturally and genetically homogeneous population consisting of large extended families living in a socially cohesive environment in which alcoholism, drug abuse, and sociopathy are virtually absent. It is conceivable that reports of higher rates of affective disorder were based on samples "contaminated" by individuals with other psychiatric disorders or possibly that the Amish have a smaller genetic propensity for affective disorders than other populations. Finally, as the Amish study was one of the first to use *DSM-III* criteria, a third potential explanation is that previous studies used looser criteria that produced inflated rates because of false-positives.

In any case, private psychiatric hospitals report that major depression is the problem for which patients are most frequently admitted, and the same is true of many psychiatric clinics. Furthermore, whatever the chief diagnosis, depression is a common reason for psychiatric consultation. Among patients with panic disorder in one study, for example, one-third presented with a secondary depression (11). Secondary depression is also frequently the reason for psychiatric consultation in alcoholism, somatization disorder, and other disorders seen in psychiatric practice (130, 151, 232). Depression—primary and secondary—is clearly the most common diagnosis in psychiatry (120, 124, 218, 233).

Most studies show that mood disorders are more common in women than men. However, this may only apply to unipolar disorder where women, in some studies, outnumber men by two to one (68, 127, 218). Apparently, men and women share about equally the risk of suffering bipolar disorder (68, 92, 218). Among patients with bipolar disorder, however, women have more depressive episodes and men have more manic episodes (127).

There is growing evidence of increasing prevalence of major depression in successively younger birth cohorts in the last century (68, 119, 218). The age of onset has been dropping, and the likelihood of recurrent episodes has increased (68).

A number of studies in both humans and animals have concluded that early adverse life events result in lifelong brain changes mediated by the HPA axis that may relate to vulnerability to depression later in life (84, 164). Early adverse environmental factors have been implicated in adult development of mood disorders (75, 90). Much of the evidence supporting theories of the role of adverse early childhood experiences in the development of mood disorders either comes from animal studies without adequate human equivalents, or it is confounded by associations of risk factors for early adverse experience with other risk factors for development of adult psychopathology.

Although a link between bipolar affective disorder and above-average occupational or educational achievement has been suggested (225), studies have demonstrated lower socioeconomic levels in bipolar patients compared to the rest of the population (81, 190). Their relatives may also have a socio-economic advantage (217).

Depressive disorders are more prevalent in industrialized countries and in urban settings (68). Reviews of population studies internationally have reported that lifetime rates of both unipolar and bipolar disorder are highest in European studies and lowest in Asian studies (218).

Clinical Picture

The chief complaints of patients with a depressive episode are usually psycho-logical: feelings of worthlessness, despair, or ideas of self-harm. But it is also common for depressed patients to complain chiefly of pains, tachycardia, breathing difficulty, gastrointestinal dysfunction, headache, or other somatic disturbances (17, 110, 112, 202).

The dysphoric mood experienced by patients with depressive illness is usually characterized as sadness or despondency, but some patients describe themselves as feeling hopeless, irritable, fearful, worried, or simply discour-aged. Occasionally, patients will present with what seems to be major depres-sion, though they report minimal feelings of dysphoria. Such patients may complain of insomnia and anorexia. They may even cry profusely while telling the examining physician that they do not feel sad. These patients are unusual, but not unknown to psychiatrists. Regardless, a patient with depressive illness can have no symptoms of sadness or low mood if anhedonia is predominant during the episode (3). It may seem counterintuitive that major depression can present without depressed mood, but recognition of this possibility can help the clinician identify cases like these, which may occur more often in medical settings.

Other characteristic symptoms of depression are anorexia with weight loss; insomnia; early morning awakening; loss of energy, described as general tired-ness or fatigability; agitation or (its opposite) psychomotor retardation; loss of interest in usual activities, including loss of interest in sex; feelings of self-reproach or guilt, which may be delusional in intensity; inability to focus one's thoughts, often with a simultaneous awareness of slowed thinking; and recurrent thoughts of death or suicide.

It is common for patients with major depression to say, "Something is wrong with my mind." Patients will often tell their physician that they fear they are losing their mind or have a sense of emotions out of control. It is also common for depressed patients to have a low expectancy of recovery. Such a pessimistic outlook should serve as a warning that the patient may be depressed. Medically ill patients seldom give up all hope of improvement, even if seriously ill.

In some depressed patients agitation is so overwhelming that other symptoms go almost unnoticed. These patients are brought to physicians when they are found by relatives or friends pacing, wringing their hands, bemoaning their fate, clinging to anyone who will listen. They ask for reassurance, they beg for help, yet nothing satisfies them.

In other patients retardation is prominent. Marked slowing of both thought and motor behavior occurs. Tasks that once took minutes may require hours. These patients may be so slowed that it is painful to listen to their conversation. Psychomotor retardation can be so severe that a patient becomes mute or even stuporous (63, 207).

Paranoid symptoms can occur among patients with major depression. There are usually exaggerated ideas of reference associated with notions of worthlessness. Characteristic delusions of patients with depression are those of a hypochondriacal or nihilistic type. Some severely ill depressed patients seem to feel they are so guilty and evil that they have become the focus of universal abhorrence or even that the world is disintegrating because of their terrible inadequacies and failures.

Hallucinations may also occur in major depression. These commonly involve accusatory voices or visions of deceased relatives associated with feelings of guilt. Delusions and hallucinations occurring in major depression are usually "mood congruent," their content consistent with the person's dominant mood. If delusions and hallucinations occur during major depression, the themes are commonly guilt, disease, poverty, death, or deserved punishment. Delusions and hallucinations occurring as part of mania are often of inflated worth, power, or special relationship to a deity or famous person.

DSM-IV-TR includes mood-congruence as a diagnostic feature of mood disorders. Mood-*in*congruent psychotic features are more often seen in schizophrenia, where, for example, the patient may seem cheerful and relaxed while describing terrifying, delusional experiences. The importance of mood-congruence is based mainly on a widespread clinical impression rather than systematic studies.

Depressed patients may or may not mention events that they consider important in producing their illness. When a precipitating event is described, it is sometimes surprisingly trivial and difficult for the examining physician to take seriously. Furthermore, some symptoms actually began before the so-called precipitating event. This suggests that some patients who begin to feel depressed search for reasons to explain their depression, unable or unwilling to believe they could feel as they do for no apparent reason.

Stressful events frequently mentioned by women as precipitants of depression are pregnancy and childbirth. In a series of women with mood disorders, the first episode of depression occurred during pregnancy or postpartum in 37% of bipolar and 17% of unipolar cases (101).

A change in drinking habits often accompanies depressive illness (93, 194). Middle-aged individuals with no previous history of alcoholism who begin to drink heavily may be suffering from depression. On the other hand, some individuals drink less than usual when depressed.

A physician (178) has written movingly about how it feels to have the illness:

> Firstly, it is very unpleasant: depressive illness is probably more unpleasant than any disease except rabies. There is constant mental pain and often psychogenic physical pain too. If one tries to get such a patient to titrate other pains against the pain of his depression one tends to end up with a description that would raise eyebrows even in a medieval torture chamber.
>
> Naturally, many of these patients commit suicide. They may not hope to get to heaven but they know they are leaving hell. Secondly, the patient is isolated from family and friends, because the depression itself reduces his affection for others and he may well have ideas that he is unworthy of their love or even that his friendship may harm them. Thirdly, he is rejected by others because they cannot stand the sight of his suffering.
>
> There is a limit to sympathy. Even psychiatrists have protective mechanisms for dealing with such cases: the consultant may refer the patient to an outpatient clinic; he may allow too brief a consultation to elicit the extent of the patient's suffering; he may, on the grounds that the depression has not responded to treatment, alter his diagnosis to one of personality disorder—comforting, because of the strange but widespread belief that patients with personality disorders do not suffer.
>
> Fourthly, and finally, the patient tends to do a great cover-up. Because of his outward depression he is socially unacceptable, and

because of his inward depression he feels even more socially unacceptable than he really is. He does not, therefore, tell others how bad he feels.

Most depressives, even severe ones, can cope with routine work—initiative and leadership are what they lack. Nevertheless, many of them can continue working, functioning at a fairly low level, and their deficiencies are often covered up by colleagues. Provided some minimal degree of social and vocational functioning is present, the world leaves the depressive alone and he battles on for the sake of his god or his children, or for some reason which makes his personal torment preferable to death.

Psychologist Kay Jamison (100) described the emotional suffering of her own experience with bipolar depression:

Profound melancholia is a day-in, day-out, night-in, night-out, almost arterial level of agony. It is a pitiless unrelenting pain that affords no window of hope, no alternative to a grim and brackish existence, and no respite from the cold undercurrents of thought and feeling that dominate the horribly restless nights of despair. (p. 114)

Jamison also described her experience of mania:

...the seductiveness of these unbridled and intense moods is powerful; and the ancient dialogue between reason and the senses is almost always more interestingly and passionately resolved in favor of the senses. The milder manias have a way of promising—and, for a very brief while, delivering—springs in the winter and epochal vitalities. In the cold light of day, however, the reality and destructiveness of rekindled illness tend to dampen the evocativeness of such selective remembered, wistful, intense, and gentle moments. Any temptation that I now may have to recapture such moods by altering my medication is quickly hosed down by the cold knowledge that a gentle intensity soon becomes first a frenetic one and then, finally, an uncontrolled insanity. (p. 212)

The cardinal features of mania are euphoria, hyperactivity, and flight of ideas. Not all manic moods are euphoric; some are irritable instead. Flight of ideas is a rapid digression from one idea to another. One's response to a patient with mania is often that of sympathetic amusement. In fact, experienced clinicians who find themselves amused by a patient immediately consider the possibility that the patient's condition is either mania or hypomania (mild mania). Flight of ideas, unlike the incoherence and tangentiality of schizophrenia, is usually understandable, even though some connections between ideas may be tenuous. (Comedians often use a well-controlled flight of ideas to amuse audiences.) Attention is often called to this symptom by a push of speech, that is, speech in which a great deal is said in a short period of time. Such speech may exhibit rhyming, punning, and jocular associations.

Psychotic symptoms also occur: persecutory and grandiose delusions, hallucinations, and ideas of reference. They are usually mood-congruent. Some patients exhibit depression and mania simultaneously. They may cry while speaking euphorically or show other unusual combinations of symptoms.

The currently accepted dichotomy of mood disorders into bipolar and unipolar forms is based on fundamental differences in the characteristics of these two forms. Compared to unipolar disorders, bipolar disorders tend to have an earlier age of onset, cyclical depressions, a higher frequency of postpartum onsets, and a greater tendency for suicide attempts. Unipolar cases have a somewhat older age of onset and are more likely to have single episodes and confounding with anxiety (64, 181, 188, 217, 224). Bipolar disorder cases are more likely to be psychotic and to manifest psychomotor retardation and anhedonia. Unipolar cases more often have agitated depressions and accompanying anxiety and somatization (50, 155, 157).

Some children have episodes of depression that resemble major depression in adulthood: crying, social withdrawal, hypersensitivity, and behavioral problems (200). It is not clear whether such episodes are an early manifestation of primary affective disorder. Two observations suggest that they may not be: (1) unlike adult depression, childhood depression is not more common in females (200); (2) the sleep of depressed children does not differ from that of age-matched normal children, whereas depressed adults differ from normal subjects in taking longer to fall asleep, awakening more often throughout the night, and experiencing greater early morning wakefulness (27, 216).

Depression in adults is also associated with a reduction in slow-wave sleep (stages 3 and 4), shortened rapid eye movement (REM) latency, and increased REM density (12, 216). Sleep studies of depressed children demonstrate none of these differences (27).

This suggests either that a sleep disorder makes a rather abrupt appearance within the depressive syndrome or that the depressive disorders of children and adults differ in important ways. Because human growth hormone (HGH) is excreted mostly during sleep, sleep has an additional function in children not present in adults. As a physiological state, sleep may be more protected in children than in adults. In any event, it appears that sleep measures are less useful as markers for childhood depression than for depressive illness in later years.

Biological Findings

Over the last two decades, a monoamine model of depression has evolved, primarily implicating serotonin and noradrenaline. Various other brain neurotransmitter systems have also been implicated in both mania and depression: dopamine, glutamate, and GABA (107). It has been pointed out, however, that abnormalities in these systems are not proven fundamental to the etiology of mood disorders, and they may instead reflect sequelae of the disorder or risk factors for it (54).

Neuroimaging studies have demonstrated abnormalities in blood flow and glucose metabolism in limbic, prefrontal, and anterior cingulate cortex as well as in the hippocampus and amygdala (107). Cryoarchitectural changes have been identified in prefrontal cortex, especially involving glial loss and reduced neuronal size and density, and in hippocampal and subcortical structures involving synaptic terminals and dendrites, in neuropathological studies of mood disorder (89). Reduced hippocampal volume has been found to be proportional to depressive illness duration (137). Increased neurogenesis has been demonstrated in rodent hippocampus in response to antidepressant treatment (189). These findings have stimulated theories of impaired neuroplasticity and hippocampal neurogenesis in mood disorders, but further research is needed to determine how such processes might be involved.

For decades, researchers have sought to identify biological correlates of bipolar and unipolar mood disorders. Scores of studies have investigated neurochemical measures such as platelet imipramine binding, monoamine oxidase activity, catechol-O-methyltransferase activity, brain dopamine activity, cerebrospinal serotonin and metabolites, plasma GABA and cortisol levels, urinary norepinephrine and metabolites, insulin tolerance, mitochondrial energy transduction, and platelet intracellular calcium levels. Despite scattered reports of significant findings, no consistent replicable evidence of biological differences between unipolar and bipolar depression has emerged (50, 158, 228). Brain imaging studies have also demonstrated strong parallels rather than consistent distinctions between bipolar and unipolar depression (50). Few studies, however, have compared unipolar and bipolar depression directly, most comparisons being drawn between separate studies.

The dexamethasone suppression test (DST), introduced by Carroll (39), was heralded as psychiatry's first laboratory test. For more than two decades, DST generated both enthusiasm and criticism while establishing itself as the most used biomarker for mood disorders (64, 97). The DST is only fairly sensitive for mood disorders: About 50% of patients with depression test positive, that is, resist suppression of blood cortisol levels following a dose of dexamethasone. The *specificity* of the test is higher. Only about 10% of *normal* control subjects are nonsuppressors. However, the specificity drops to less than 70% in some psychiatric conditions—including dementia and alcohol abuse—and in medical conditions involving weight loss. Initial DST status in depression does not predict antidepressant response sufficiently to guide treatment decisions (6).

More recently, a combined dexamethasone/corticotrophin-releasing hormone (dex/CRH) test was developed as a tool for assessing hypothalamic-pituitary-adrenal (HPA) axis changes associated with depressive disorders (97). With effective antidepressant treatment, the dex/CRH normalizes, suggesting potential utility of this test for predicting drug efficacy and treatment response. Another laboratory diagnostic test proposed for depression involves administering thyroid-releasing hormone (TRH) to patients suspected to have depression. Results vary, but in some studies half or more of unipolar patients have a "blunted" response of thyroid-stimulating hormone (TSH) secretion following a challenge with TRH. To date, neither the dex/CRH nor the TRH tests have provided consistent biological markers for depression (98).

Natural History

The natural history of mood disorders is variable. The age of risk extends throughout life. Together with the usual episodic nature of the illness, this distinguishes mood disorders from most other psychiatric illnesses.

The average age of onset of major depression is in the fourth decade (57). For bipolar disorder, the average age of onset is in the third decade (181). Studies have found a significant correlation between family members in age of onset (135).

A longstanding view that mania in children is extremely rare or nonexistent has been increasingly replaced with a view that the disorder is much more common than previously recognized. Part of the reason for its lack of recognition is thought to relate to difficulty in diagnosis of the disorder. Pediatric mania is atypical by adult standards in its characteristic presentation and longitudinal course, comorbidity patterns, and response to treatment (29).

How often do patients experience a single episode of mood disorder without recurrence? Most patients who have a manic episode have multiple recurrences of depression and mania (77). About 50%–75% of patients who have a major depressive episode will have one or more subsequent episodes of depression in their lifetime (9, 95). Thus, mood disorders are increasingly being recognized as lifetime disorders, as opposed to the historical cross-sectional focus on isolated episodes of illness (82, 111, 119, 177). In about 10% of patients presenting with a depressive episode, the illness will eventually declare itself as bipolar, with the appearance of subsequent episodes of full mania in about 5% and hypomania in about 5% (2, 46). About 20% of patients with mood disorders develop a chronic illness difficult for physicians to manage (47, 68, 78, 129).

Between episodes of major depression, residual symptoms are not uncommon (116, 117). Analysis of data from the NIMH National Collaborative Depression Study demonstrated that patients may experience some symptoms more than half of the time when not experiencing full depressive episodes (104). Bipolar disorder exhibited a similar pattern: Patients continued to have residual symptoms about half the time between episodes, with depressive symptoms predominating over manic symptoms (105). With treatment, episodes are much diminished in frequency and intensity, and bipolar patients often return to completely healthy functioning between episodes of illness (78, 213).

The length of individual episodes of major depression is extremely variable, ranging from a few days to many years. About half of patients recover within 6 months and 80% recover by 2 years (9). By 6 years, 90% have recovered, but recovery is unlikely thereafter (111).

The period for highest risk of relapse is shortly after recovery. The longer the patient remains well, the lower is his or her current risk of relapse. A long-term follow-up study reviewed by Angst (9) showed that within 6 months, 13% of patients with major depression relapsed. The risk of relapse doubled by 1 year and tripled by 2 years following which the rate declined; by 5 years, three-quarters of patients had relapsed. With each subsequent episode of depression, the next episode is likely to occur sooner and be more severe than previous episodes (82, 118). Increased risk of relapse is associated with (1) length of the index episode of depression, (2) residual symptoms, (3) number of episodes, and (4) psychiatric comorbidity (9, 118). Treatment differences may account for different rates of relapse.

Complications

Primary depression and suicide are clearly connected: 50%–70% of those who commit suicide can be found retrospectively to have had symptoms characteristic of depression. A review of 17 studies of suicide in major depression found that 15% will eventually die by suicide (85). However, the patients studied were severe cases in inpatient settings, and not necessarily representative of all depressed patients, who may have substantially lower rates (184). Suicide rates have not been studied in more representative populations. Regardless, the specific suicide rate in relation to mood disorders is elevated 10 to 30 times the rate in the general population (10, 169).

Although a large proportion of people who commit suicide have made previous suicide attempts, only a fraction of attempters eventually kill themselves. About 1 out of 10 or 20 attempters will be found dead by suicide within 5 to 10 years after an attempt (73, 171, 208). The period of highest risk appears to be during the first 2 follow-up years (73, 208). The medical seriousness of the attempt is a weak predictor at best; medically trivial attempts are also sometimes followed by completed suicide. In the end, prior suicide attempts are not a robust predictor of suicide completion.

The risk of suicide is not necessarily correlated with symptom severity. Suicide risk is associated with psychiatric illness, age greater than 65 years, being male, living alone, recent stressors (especially major losses), access to firearms, hopelessness, prior attempts, and communication of suicidal intent (76). The two disorders most frequently associated with suicide are primary affective disorder and substance use disorders, but schizophrenia and personality disorders are also prominently represented among completed suicides (28, 99, 214).

Folklore that patients who talk of suicide do not commit suicide is untrue. Suicidal communication may impart increased risk. However, those who are serious about completing the act often do not convey intent to others in their final days (99).

Most of the increased mortality that is found among patients from primary affective disorder is from unnatural causes, especially suicide, accounting for 55% of excess deaths and conveying a mortality risk 8 times more than expected. Patients with primary affective disorder may also have an increased mortality from causes other than suicide compared with matched members of the general population (99). Deaths from natural causes account for 45% of excess deaths with a risk 1.3 times more than expected, with infections, mental, nervous, circulatory, and respiratory system disorders accounting for most of the excess risk (88).

Alcoholism may be a complication of primary affective disorder. This is particularly true when a person begins to drink heavily in mid or late life, because "primary" alcoholism usually begins earlier. Drug abuse may also be a complication of primary affective disorder.

Poor judgment is another complication of primary affective disorder. Poor judgment, spending sprees, and impulsive, unrealistic decisions are characteristic of manic episodes. Bad decisions also commonly accompany depressive episodes. Decisions to leave a job, to move to a different city, or to separate from a spouse may result from the restless dissatisfaction associated with depression. Clinicians often advise depressed patients not to make major life decisions until they are clearly in remission.

Studies of psychiatric illness in the postpartum period indicate that bipolar women are more likely to have episodes of depression or mania during the puerperium than at other times in their lives. Having had a postpartum episode of depression, the likelihood that a woman with bipolar illness will have another episode after subsequent pregnancy is high. Studies have demonstrated episodes of puerperal mania or psychosis in 20%–30% of bipolar women after delivery; a family history of puerperal psychosis increases the rate to more than 50% of bipolar women after delivery (42, 103).

Three recent studies have demonstrated that major depression is significantly related to poor academic performance, including college dropout (8, 96, 150). In one study at a large university, diagnosed depression was associated with a drop of half a letter grade point average, but those who received treatment for depression evidenced a nearly equivalent gain in grade point average (96). In another study at a major university, students who withdrew from school because of depression did not fare as well on return to classes as other returning students who did not have depression (150).

On cognitive testing, patients with major depression may show impaired attention, deficits in explicit verbal and visual memory (but implicit memory appears to be preserved), impairment in executive functioning, and slowing in motor and cognitive domains. Severity of depression is associated with degree of cognitive impairment (146). These abnormalities are more pronounced in the elderly (13, 80, 154).

Sometimes the memory impairment with depression is so profound that a mistaken diagnosis of dementia is made. The true identity of the problem is revealed when memory returns to normal after recovery from the depression. Memory impairment owing to depression is called "pseudodementia," a century-old term that has garnered recent controversy because it implies that the syndrome is reversible or at least distinct from other forms of dementia. Particularly in the elderly, findings from brain imaging studies have implied some blurring of these distinctions (167, 230).

Cognitive difficulties have been observed in manic as well as depressive phases of bipolar illness (146, 179). Several studies have suggested that reversal of cognitive impairments in mood disorders may not always accompany recovery from the mood episode (13, 45, 143–145). The cognitive impairments in bipolar disorder are thought to represent trait markers that may also be somewhat state modulated. During bipolar episodes, cognitive impairment may be as severe as that observed in schizophrenia; however, between episodes, cognitive functioning in patients with bipolar disorder is far superior than in patients with schizophrenia (45, 179).

Family and Genetic Studies

Several studies in the 1960s reached similar conclusions about familial patterns of affective disorders: Affective disorders tend to be familial and can be subdivided into bipolar and unipolar types. Before 1960, family studies did not differentiate between unipolar depression and bipolar disorder, but demonstrated that mood disorders in general tend to be inherited in families (196). In general, bipolar patients have bipolar relatives and unipolar patients have unipolar relatives (102, 193, 206).

These relationships may be more complex than previously realized. Family studies consistently find bipolar illness more often in relatives of patients with bipolar illness than in relatives of unipolar depression, but unipolar depression is observed with equal frequency in relatives of patients with unipolar depression and relatives of patients with bipolar illness (7, 148, 153, 193). Overall, these findings support conceptual distinctions between unipolar and bipolar mood disorders (7).

Meanwhile, data from adoption and twin studies have provided strong evidence for the role of genetic factors in mood disorders (153, 193, 196). There have been numerous twin studies of mood disorders (4), the first conducted in 1928 (196). Twin studies of both bipolar disorder and unipolar depression have consistently shown far higher rates of concordance among monozygotic than among dizygotic twin pairs (148, 153, 193, 196). The heritability of unipolar depression has been estimated at 30%–45%, while the heritability estimates for bipolar disorder are considerably higher, 60%–80% (115, 148, 153, 193). Thus, bipolar illness appears to be more strongly influenced by genetic factors than unipolar illness.

Adoption studies are the most powerful design for testing the relative contributions of genetic and environmental factors to heredity by comparing rates of disorders in biologic and adoptive family members (153, 196). The few adoption studies that have been conducted on mood disorders have demonstrated significant associations between unipolar depression in adoptees and their biological but not their adoptive relatives; the same pattern was found for bipolar disorder (153, 193).

An association between unipolar depression and alcoholism was proposed by Winokur and his coworkers more than a quarter of a century ago (109). In a series of publications they contrasted "pure depressive illness" with "depressive spectrum disease." The latter refers to families with a high prevalence of alcoholism and sociopathy among the men and a high prevalence of early-onset unipolar depression among the women. Four adoption studies reviewed by Cadoret (36) demonstrated that daughters of alcoholics who were not adopted away showed significantly greater depression than control subjects and their female siblings who had been adopted away, and, conversely, more alcoholism among biological relatives of depressed than among nondepressed adoptees. These findings suggest that the association of depression with alcoholism in family members may be influenced by environmental factors.

A family history of severe psychiatric illness in a first-degree relative of a patient with major depression may predict poor long-term outcome (56). Research indicates that when a patient with primary affective disorder or alcoholism has a family history of suicide attempt, the risk of suicide is increased (187). A family history of attempted suicide does not seem to predict successful suicide, however, in patients with sociopathy, hysteria, or opiate addiction. The mode of genetic transmission in mood disorders is non-Mendelian and almost certainly polygenic.

The first genome-wide linkage analysis for bipolar disorder was conducted in 1993, and since that time another 20 such studies have been performed to search for cosegregation of the disorder with genetic markers or mutations. Neither susceptibility gene linkage nor association studies have yielded consistently replicable results (170, 175). Two meta-analyses suggested two regions of potential significance, 13q32 and 22q12-13, and three other regions of possible interest, 9p21-22, 10q11-22, and 14q24-32 (15, 192). Leading authors have concluded that there is not a single locus for bipolar disorder (i.e., accounting for at least half of the vulnerability in at least half of people with bipolar disorder) (139). Bipolar disorder must result from the effects of several genes interacting with one another and with environmental factors. Heterogeneity, phenotypes, and incomplete penetrance likely provide further pieces in the genetic puzzle of bipolar disorder (138, 175).

Genetic studies in major depression have not fared any better over two decades of study (38, 226). Fourteen different gene region candidates have emerged from replication in at least two studies (1p, 1q, 2q, 3centr, 4q, 5q, 6q, 7p, 8p, 11q [2], 12q, 15q and 18q), but no region has been universally identified (38, 226). Chromosome q33-34 is of particular interest because it has been identified in women in both linkage and association studies (226). Studies of sex specificity and genetically distinct subtypes may help to unravel the genetic basis of major depression (38).

Differential Diagnosis

Making the distinction between grief and major depression can be difficult. Bereaved people may present with symptoms of both grief and depression to some degree (134, 212). During the first 2 months after the loss of a loved one, depressive symptoms are common, and even if the individual would otherwise meet full criteria for a diagnosis of major depression, diagnosis of depression is deferred and the syndrome is considered bereavement. After 2 months, major depression is diagnosed. A diagnosis of major depression is appropriate at any time, however, if the symptom picture involves markedly impaired functioning, preoccupations of worthlessness, suicidality, psychosis, or psychomotor retardation, or if the symptoms persist longer than 2 months (3, 134). Symptoms of grief are not generally responsive to antidepressant treatment, but depressive symptoms in the context of bereavement are (134).

Differential diagnosis between panic disorder and primary affective disorder can be difficult because anxiety symptoms occur frequently in primary affective disorder and depressive symptoms occur frequently in panic disorder. The distinction depends chiefly on chronology. If anxiety symptoms antedate the depressive symptoms, the diagnosis is panic disorder. If depressive symptoms appeared first, the diagnosis is primary affective disorder. Panic disorder almost always begins relatively early in life. Current evidence suggests that in primary affective disorder, secondary panic appears to represent a severity marker more than a separate comorbid condition (121). Conversely, when depression is secondary to panic disorder, the depression appears not to represent a separate condition but an epiphenomenon of the panic disorder (52).

Patients with primary affective disorder often report somatic symptoms. Conversely, affective symptoms are often reported as part of somatization disorder. If depressive and anxiety symptoms predominate, the diagnosis of somatization disorder should be made with caution, particularly if the illness did not occur until the patient was 30 years or older. Though patients with primary affective disorder may report many somatic symptoms, these symptoms are seldom spread throughout the system review. Furthermore, the hallmark combination of conversion symptoms (unexplained neurological symptoms) and menstrual symptoms of somatization disorder occurs only infrequently in primary affective disorder.

Obsessions are common in primary affective disorder. The distinction between obsessional illness and primary affective disorder is also made on the basis of chronology. If obsessions and compulsions antedate depressive symptoms, a diagnosis of primary affective disorder should not be made.

Distinguishing between schizophrenia and primary affective disorder is usually not a problem. Schizophrenia, a chronic illness of insidious onset, is not characterized by the remitting course found in primary affective disorder. Patients with primary affective disorder do not develop the formal thought disorder characteristically seen in schizophrenia. Occasionally, the distinction between mania and schizophrenia may be difficult. Bizarre and dramatic hallucinations, delusions, and other abnormalities of mental content like those seen in schizophrenia may occur in mania. A previous history of episodic illness with remission or the presence of euphoria, hyperactivity, or flight of ideas indicates that the diagnosis may be mania rather than schizophrenia. Although schizophrenia and bipolar disorder are well documented to segregate separately in families, overlap of these two disorders in some families is also known to occur, especially in psychotic forms of bipolar illness (26, 48, 49, 139). Thus, a family history of bipolar disorder in a patient presenting with psychosis should encourage the clinician to consider the possibility of an affective disorder in the differential diagnosis of schizophrenia, although it does not necessarily rule against schizophrenia.

For many years, clinicians assumed that both schizoaffective psychosis and schizophreniform illness were more closely related to schizophrenia than to primary affective disorder (22, 113). Longitudinal studies have demonstrated that schizophreniform disorder, which is defined as a brief and milder version of the psychotic symptoms of schizophrenia (3), sometimes evolves into a schizophrenic disorder and sometimes into a mood disorder (22). Patients with good prognosis features (sudden onset, good premorbid functioning, and lack of flat affect) appear to have family histories and course more consistent with mood disorders; those without good prognosis features appear to have family histories and course more consistent with schizophrenia. Schizoaffective disorders, defined by the presence of both prominent psychotic and mood features, were previously divided into predominantly schizophrenic and predominantly affective illnesses (113). A recent review affirmed that the illness of patients with schizoaffective disorders more closely resembles schizophrenia (e.g., positive symptoms of psychosis) in some ways, and bipolar disorder (e.g., mood symptoms and distress) in other ways (14). Increasing evidence now suggests that the characteristics of this psychiatric illness occupying a diagnostic space somewhere between schizophrenia and bipolar illness are unstable over time and tend to evolve to either predominantly schizophrenic or bipolar illness (14, 22, 43). Today, both schizophreniform illness and schizoaffective psychosis are classified as part of the schizophrenia-related psychotic disorders rather than with the mood disorders (3, 113).

Depressive symptoms may accompany chronic and acute brain syndromes. Patients with vascular disease have elevated rates of associated depression. Vascular depression is especially pernicious, being more disabling and resulting in poorer outcomes compared to other kinds of depression (106). Patients with depression of clearly vascular origins do not have the associated family history of major depression observed in patients with major depressive disorder (106). Gross memory impairment in severely depressed and elderly patients may create diagnostic dilemmas in determining the primary source of the problem—the depression or the dementia (230). Although guidelines have been proposed to help make this distinction (230), it may ultimately prove more useful to pursue understanding of the neuroanatomical substrates that underlie both depression and cognitive impairment than to try to differentiate them clinically (167).

Psychiatric symptoms are side effects of certain drugs. It has long been known that steroids can precipitate psychotic, manic, and depressive states (174). Other medications implicated in the emergence of depressive syndromes are antihypertensive agents, lipid-lowering drugs (statins), and estrogen-receptor modulators (125, 174). Available evidence implicates interferon-alpha, interleukin-2, gonadotropin-releasing hormone agonists, mefloquine, progestin-releasing contraceptives, and propranolol in the occurrence of depressive-like symptoms. Studies utilizing diagnostic instruments, however, do not support a role for these agents in generating major depression (125, 174).

Bipolar disorder should always be considered in the differential diagnosis of patients with unipolar depression, because approximately 1 out of 10 depressions will eventually declare themselves as part of a bipolar illness (2, 79, 218). Switching from apparent unipolar to bipolar illness is most common early in the course of the illness in individuals with onset before the age of 25 years (68). Bipolar disorder must be differentiated from substance use disorders and personality disorders, and, in children, from conduct disorder and attention-deficit/hyperactivity disorder.

Clinical Management

The management of major depressive disorder always involves supportive psychotherapy (4). Many clinicians believe that *insight-directed* psychotherapy, involving examination of motives and deep feelings, is probably not wise because it tends to increase the patient's feelings of guilt. Available evidence, however, indicates that certain types of psychotherapy may be useful for mild or moderate depression. The studies are of three types: *(1)* psychotherapy alone compared with control group, *(2)* psychotherapy compared with antidepressant drugs, and *(3)* combined psychotherapy and drugs compared with psychotherapy alone and drugs alone. Five main types of psychotherapy have been employed in the studies: *(1)* cognitive therapy, *(2)* behavioral therapy, *(3)* interpersonal therapy, *(4)* group therapy, and *(5)* marital therapy.

The goal of *cognitive therapy* is to identify existing negative cognitions and replace them with more positive functionally adaptive ones (21, 128, 231). In *behavior therapy*, the patient learns new behavioral and interpersonal skills to achieve desired responses from others (195). "Social skills training" is a type of behavior therapy that emphasizes assertiveness training and verbal and nonverbal competencies, utilizing role play for developing proficiency (21, 105, 195). *Interpersonal psychotherapy* facilitates return to healthy functioning by focusing on the present rather than the past and interpersonal rather than intrapsychic processes; goals are development of coping, problem solving, and social and interpersonal skills (58, 142). In *group therapy*, a psychotherapist and a group of patients attempt to effect changes in the emotional states and behavior of the patients. *Marital therapy* may be conducted with an individual, a couple or family, or a group of couples.

Several comprehensive reviews of studies comparing psychotherapy, pharmacotherapy, and/or combinations of these therapies for the treatment of less severe forms of major depression have concluded that psychotherapy alone and pharmacotherapy alone are both efficacious and superior to nontreatment (40, 71, 94, 172). Studies concluding that psychotherapy and antidepressant medication have similar efficacy have been criticized for selective inclusion of patients who are especially good psychotherapy candidates and not representative of most patients with major depression (54). Thus, both psychotherapy and pharmacotherapy may be considered first-line treatments in mild to moderate depression in general medical practice and outpatient mental health practice (40). Medication provides benefits of rapid and robust response (94). Psychotherapy appears to help keep patients engaged in therapy and reduce relapse, especially after medication discontinuation (71, 94). Further, psychotherapy appears to be associated with gains in interpersonal skills, social adjustment, well-being, and treatment satisfaction not provided by pharmacotherapy alone (94, 172). Reviews of studies comparing combinations of treatment with pharmacotherapy and psychotherapy have concluded that combined treatment appears to have small but consistent advantages over either treatment alone (71, 94, 172).

Some patients may not be good candidates for one therapy or another. Pregnancy and intolerable side effects may deter the use of medications (40). Some patients may resist psychotherapy; others may not accept medications (40). Fortunately, the research findings indicate that patients with less severe depression can generally be offered the treatment alternative they find most suitable, because outcomes of pharmacotherapy and psychotherapy are generally similar. Among patients with severe depression, however, combined pharmacotherapy and psychotherapy are recommended (71). The two major somatic approaches to the management of depressive episodes are pharmacotherapy and electrotherapy.

The first antidepressant medications were of the monoamine oxidase inhibitor-A (MAO-A) inhibitor class (229). Initially developed for the treatment of tuberculosis, these medications were found to have energizing effects. Monoamine oxidase inhibitors (MAOIs) have potentially serious side effects. Foods and beverages containing tyramine (a pressor substance)—particularly cheese, some wines, and beer—should be avoided because of the danger of a hypertensive crisis. To avoid hypertensive crises, patients taking MAOIs should also not take drugs containing amphetamines or sympathomimetic substances. Over the years, safety concerns have limited the broad use of MAOI antidepressants (185).

Selegiline is a recently FDA-approved treatment for depression, packaged in a transdermal system. Selegiline is a selective MAO-B inhibitor at low doses, but at higher doses it also inhibits MAO-A (66, 185). The tyramine dietary modifications are not needed at lower doses (up to 6 mg per 24 hours), but more experience is needed before recommending higher doses without tyramine avoidance. The main side effects of the transdermal preparation are dermal reactions and insomnia; classic MAOI side effects such as sexual dysfunction and excessive weight gain are fortunately uncommon with selegiline (185).

For many years, tricyclic antidepressants (e.g., imipramine and amitriptyline) supplanted MAOIs as the mainstay of pharmacotherapy for depression. Tricyclic antidepressants have several unpleasant side effects: dry mouth, orthostatic hypotension, tremor, oversedation, and weight gain. These effects often diminish as the drug is continued. Less common, but potentially serious side effects, are cardiac arrhythmias.

Individuals vary widely in their ability to metabolize tricyclic antidepressants; as much as a 40-fold difference has been reported between fast and slow metabolizers. What a physician assumes to be a therapeutic dose may actually produce toxic plasma levels or, alternatively, subtherapeutic levels of the drug. For this reason, monitoring plasma levels of tricyclics is advised when a seemingly therapeutic dose produces either no improvement or significant side effects.

In the late 1980s a new class of antidepressants became available. The selective serotonin-uptake inhibitors (SSRIs) were developed because of evidence that serotonin is involved in depression (191). This class includes fluoxetine (Prozac), sertraline (Zoloft), paroxetine (Paxil), and citalopram (Celexa), among many others. These medications are as effective as tricyclic antidepressants but have fewer serious side effects (e.g., cardiotoxicity is nearly nonexistent) (20). Subsequently, classes of antidepressants were developed with dual actions to block not only norepinephrine but also serotonin (venla-faxine [Effexor]) or dopamine (bupropion [Wellbutrin]) (191). All these antide-pressant medications, regardless of class, must be administered for at least 3 or 4 weeks before significant antidepressant effects can be anticipated.

Following symptom remission in depression, there is believed to be a period of increased risk of symptom recurrence. Because there is no way to determine the length of this period, it is common practice to continue anti-depressant medication for at least 6 months after the remission of acute symptoms.

Unlike their well-appreciated utility for treatment of major depression, antidepressants do not seem to be particularly beneficial for bipolar depression (165, 166). Antidepressants can precipitate mania in approximately one-third of depressed bipolar patients and may induce mixed episodes (with simultaneous features of mania and depression) and "rapid cycling" between states of mania and depression (65, 79, 132, 160). Hence, antidepressants, the treatment of choice for unipolar depression, may be deleterious in bipolar depression, especially for continuing treatment of bipolar depressive episodes. Caution is recommended for use of antidepressants for either acute or prophylactic treat-ment of bipolar depression (65). Tricyclic antidepressants and venlafaxine may be more likely to precipitate switches to mania and bupropion, and SSRIs may be less likely to do so (67, 74, 79, 132). When possible, therefore, it is recom-mended that antidepressants should be discontinued during the maintenance phase of bipolar disorder (67), or at least be used in conjunction with a mood stabilizer, which may help prevent switching to mania (79).

Although lithium is a strong choice for the treatment of mania, its utility as a primary treatment for unipolar depression is limited, with response rates of only 30%–40% (61, 141, 165, 166, 197, 197). Addition of lithium has been well documented, however, as effective in augmenting the therapeutic effects of antidepressant medication in unipolar illness (61, 197). If the unipolar patient has a positive family history of bipolar disorder or hypomanic symptoms, lithium may exert a more antidepressant effect than if neither of these features exists (55).

Some patients experience depression during certain times of the year, especially in the fall and early winter. *DSM-IV-TR* includes seasonal affective disorder (SAD) as a subcategory of major depressive disorder (30). Criteria for SAD include a temporal relationship between the onset of bipolar disorder, or recurrent major depression, and a specific period of the year (e.g., regular appearance of depression in the fall). A growing body of literature indicates that an effective treatment may exist for the condition. This involves prolonged exposure in the fall and winter months to fluorescent lighting with wavelengths similar to sunlight (209). Devices currently on the market provide such lighting. There is disagreement about the length of exposure or the time of day when exposure is most efficacious (209). The effectiveness of the treatment—if definitely shown to exist—may depend on suppressing nighttime melatonin production or some other manipulation of biological rhythms (186). Investigators recommend that patients sit for as long as 4 hours within a few feet of the light. The possibility of resultant cataracts or retinal damage has not been fully assessed.

The drug literature is replete with warnings against combining alcohol with psychotropic drugs used in treatment of depression. In the case of alcohol and barbiturates, the combination may be lethal. There is less additive effect between alcohol and benzodiazepine tranquilizers. Combining alcohol with tricyclic antidepressants increases sedative effects of both. Acute alcohol ingestion increases plasma concentrations of tricyclic antidepressants, increasing the likelihood of fatal poisoning (205). Alcoholics, however, metabolize antidepressant medications at an accelerated rate, resulting in generally reduced blood levels (205).

Choosing the most suitable antidepressant agent for a particular patient is informed by science (210), but it is also an art. Effectiveness of various antidepressant agents is essentially comparable; therefore, the decision is essentially based on the drug's side effect profile (4). Antidepressant medications vary in side effect profiles, allowing the clinician to tailor the side effects to the patient's specific situation. For example, bupropion (Wellbutrin) has an energizing effect and may interfere with sleep. Mirtazepine (Remeron) causes sedation, a property that may be useful in the treatment of depression associated with sleeplessness or agitation. Mirtazepine may significantly increase body weight; if anything, bupropion may be associated with weight loss. When weight gain is undesirable and alertness is desirable, bupropion may be a reasonable choice. For treatment of depression in emaciated or apprehensive cancer patients, the weight gain and sedation associated with mirtazepine favor this drug as a treatment option.

Antidepressant drugs—demonstrated in controlled studies to shorten depressive episodes, reduce the intensity of symptoms, and possibly prevent recurrence—have not demonstrably reduced suicide among patients with mood disorders (16, 159, 215). Suicide-prevention centers, established in many cities during the 1960s, had no apparent effect on the suicide rate. In contrast, lithium maintenance treatment has been demonstrated to yield a distinct suicide reduction advantage (16, 86, 159).

A placebo-controlled study found significant improvement in depressive symptoms with the *N*-methyl-D-aspartate (NMDA) receptor antagonist drug ketamine within 72 hours of intravenous administration, suggesting a potential role for drugs of this type in the treatment of depression (25). Replication is needed with larger controlled studies to verify this finding, which was a serendipitous result and not the primary aim of this study (147). The clinical applicability of NMDA antagonist medications may be limited by their psychotomimetic effects and the potential for abuse with many of these agents.

Electroconvulsive therapy (ECT) is still considered the most effective form of treatment available for depression and one of the most efficacious of all medical treatments, with documented efficacy rates as high as 80%–90% (58, 83). However, the use of ECT declined after effective medications for the treatment of depression became accessible. Despite the fact that ECT has been making a comeback in recent years (44), it still tends to be reserved for patients who do not respond to antidepressants or who are so ill that they cannot be treated outside a hospital (140). In part, this is because of unfavorable public perception and continuing negative media depiction of the practice (44). When ECT was first introduced into clinical practice in the early 1940s, it frequently caused vertebral and other fractures. As advances in the medical modification of electrotherapy have been made, the treatment has evolved into a technologically sophisticated procedure with a proven track record of safety (83). Now the procedure is less frightening to patients and is less commonly associated with complications. Patients are anesthetized briefly with a very rapid-acting barbiturate and then are given a muscle relaxant, usually succinylcholine. Electrodes are placed in the frontotemporal regions and a small, measured amount of electricity is passed between them (1, 5).

The most troublesome side effect of ECT is memory loss (83). This undesirable aspect of the treatment typically applies to the treatment interval, a brief period before initiating treatment, and several weeks after the course. Most patients do not find this to be a problem (5, 83). Delivering unilateral ECT to the nondominant side of the brain minimizes this side effect (58, 83).

Electroconvulsive therapy is generally considered the safest procedure performed under general anesthesia (83). Risk of death following ECT is increased with recent myocardial infarction or states of elevated intracranial pressure. These concerns should be weighed against the risk of not treating severe depression. Electroconvulsive therapy may be the safest and most effective treatment of mood disorders for women in their first trimester of pregnancy or postoperatively (92) and for severely depressed patients with various medical illnesses (44). It is safely used in children under age 18 and the elderly (83, 108, 183, 204). First-line treatment with ECT should be considered when risks of the psychiatric illness are greater than the risks of the procedure, especially in the context of life-threatening psychiatric situations such as those involving suicidality or severe nutritional compromise (140). Additionally, because response to ECT is generally more rapid and robust than to antidepressant medication, it should be considered when fast response is important (83, 122, 140). It should also be considered first for patients with a history of poor medication response and good ECT response, and for patients expressing a preference for ECT.

Repetitive transcranial magnetic stimulation (rTMS), a procedure that applies alternating electromagnetic fields to stimulate brain cortex without producing seizures, has been investigated for the treatment of major depression. Recent research has demonstrated statistically significant, though not clinically large, therapeutic effects of rTMS in the treatment of depression (35, 136, 173). Studies to date have generally been small and inconsistent in key methodological features, limiting comparisons of findings. rTMS has recently received U.S. Food and drug Administration (FDA) approval for use with major depression. Vagal nerve stimulation has also been shown effective in the treatment of refractory depression and also in preventing relapse (163). This method has been approved by the FDA for treatment-resistant depression.

Lithium carbonate has historically been the drug of choice in the treatment of mania (152, 197). Some clinicians began to treat mania with both a neuroleptic and lithium, stopping the neuroleptic after 4 or 5 days when lithium has begun to take effect. Economic pressures to achieve improvement quickly so that the patient can be discharged from hospital reduced enthusiasm for lithium, which is not effective until at least 1 week and often 2 or 3 weeks of treatment (31). Mixed, rapid-cycling, secondary, and comorbid mania are not as responsive as pure mania is to lithium.

Optimal serum levels of lithium for effective maintenance therapy of bipolar disorder are in the range of 0.8–1.0 mEq/l (149). Lower doses may allow subthreshold symptoms to persist (149) but may be effective in preventing depressive episodes; higher doses appear to be more effective against mania (123). Generally, total doses of 1,200–2,400 mg of lithium per day in divided form (300 to 600 mg per dose) are required to achieve such serum levels. Many patients find the once-daily dosing of Lithobid and Eskalith CR preferable and have better compliance with taking it. Because lithium is a potentially toxic drug, its use must be monitored by repeatedly checking serum levels, particularly early in treatment. Most patients experience a fine tremor of the hands at therapeutic levels of lithium (0.8 to 1.5 mEq/l). At higher levels, ataxia, disorientation, somnolence, seizures, and finally circulatory collapse may occur.

The usefulness of lithium is not limited to the treatment of acute mania. It also has a robust response rate of about 70%–80% in bipolar depression (197). Lithium is effective at preventing bipolar depressive as well as manic episodes (67). There is considerable evidence that lithium reduces morbidity and may have specific anti-suicide properties in bipolar illness (32, 159, 213, 215).

Anticonvulsant drugs are used in mania for their mood-stabilizing properties. The divalproex form of valproate is approved by the FDA for treatment of acute mania. Valproate appears to be effective in mixed, secondary, comorbid, rapid-cycling, and psychotic forms of acute mania as well as in pure mania (25). Most patients respond to doses of 15 mg/kg in divided doses two to three times a day. Serum levels must be followed and maintained in the 45–60 µg/mL range, up to 125 µg/mL for patients not achieving full symptom resolution at lower serum levels. Above 125 µg/mL, adverse effects of nausea, vomiting, and asthenia become more likely (33). Risk for thrombocytopenia increases with these higher valproate levels. The sustained release preparation of valproate, divalproex (Depakote) is prefer-able for most patients due to better tolerance and a once-daily dosing schedule. The sprinkle form of divalproex may be associated with fewer gastrointestinal side effects (72).

Use of the anticonvulsant drug carbamazepine in treatment of mania requires slow dosage escalation and has a slow onset of action of 5 to 28 days. Treatment is begun at 200 mg once or twice daily and increased every 5 days until levels of 12–14 µg/mL are reached. Neuromuscular and cognitive side effects are common, especially with rapid dosage escalation. Other adverse effects occur relatively early in treatment, including rashes often with a vascular component, hypothyroidism, thrombocytopenia, low white blood count, and elevated hepatic enzymes, necessitating close clinical and labora-tory monitoring (25).

Both depressive and manic symptoms improved in a trial of lamotrigine and an antipsychotic for patients with refractory bipolar disorder (201). FDA-approved for the adjunct treatment of partial seizures, lamotrigine decreases glutamate release. Other promising anticonvulsant medications used in the treatment of bipolar disorder as adjunctive agents and for treatment-resistant cases include gabapentin, topiramate, and zonisamide, but not tiagabine as adjunctive treatment, but further study is needed to confirm their efficacy (34, 37, 51, 227).

Neuroleptics provide rapid benefit for psychosis and agitation in mania, especially for the one-third of patients with mania who have psychotic symp-toms. However, in randomized comparisons, neuroleptics have been consis-tently less effective than lithium. Although lower dosages of neuroleptics may

be required in the treatment of mania than for schizophrenia, tardive dyskinesia more commonly occurs in patients with bipolar disorder (25). Olanzapine
has more evidence of efficacy in mania than other atypical antipsychotic agents,
although evidence is emerging for the use of risperidone and ziprasidone as
well in the treatment of mania (24).

When treatment with a single agent fails, two or more medications may be
used in combination. Although such polypharmacy is common practice, supporting data from controlled trials are lacking (199).

High-potency benzodiazepines, especially clonazepam and lorazepam, are
commonly used to augment pharmacotherapy of acute mania by providing
sedation and reducing anxiety (156, 199). Because sleep disturbance may
predispose to manic episodes, judicious short-term use of benzodiazepines
may help prevent episodes.

As with unipolar depression, ECT is considered a very effective treatment
for bipolar depression (92, 122, 197). It is also useful in the treatment for
mania, and it may be more effective than medications (62, 161, 197, 198).

REFERENCES

1. Abrams, R. *Electroconvulsive Therapy*, 4th edition. New York: Oxford University
   Press, 2002.
2. Akiskal, H. S., Maser, J. D., Zeller, P. J., Endicott, J., Coryell, W., Keller, M.,
   Warshaw, M., Clayton, P., and Goodwin, F. Switching from "unipolar" to bipolar
   II. An 11-year prospective study of clinical and temperamental predictors in 559
   patients. Arch. Gen. Psychiat., 52:114–123, 1995.
3. American Psychiatric Association. *Diagnostic and Statistical Manual of Mental
   Disorders*, 4th edition, text revision. Washington, DC: Author, 2000.
4. American Psychiatric Association. Practice guideline for the treatment of patients
   with major depressive disorder (revision). Am. J. Psychiat., 157:1–45, 2000.
5. American Psychiatric Association Committee on Electroconvulsive Therapy. *The
   Practice of Electroconvulsive Therapy: Recommendations for Treatment, Training, and
   Privileging: A Task Force Report of the American Psychiatric Association*.
   Washington, DC: Author, 2001.
6. American Psychiatric Association Task Force on Laboratory Tests in Psychiatry.
   The dexamethasone suppression test: an overview of its current status in psychiatry. Am. J. Psychiat., 144:1253–1262, 1987.
7. Andreasen, N. C., Rice, J., Endicott, J., Coryell, W., Grove, W. M., and Reich, T.
   Familial rates of affective disorder. A report from the National Institute of Mental
   Health Collaborative Study. Arch. Gen. Psychiat., 44:461–469, 1987.
8. Andrews, B., and Wilding, J. M. The relation of depression and anxiety to life-
   stress and achievement in students. Br. J. Psychol., 95:509–521, 2004.
9. Angst, J. Major depression in 1998: are we providing optimal therapy? J. Clin.
   Psychiat., 60 Suppl 6:5–9, 1999.

10. Angst, J., Angst, F., and Stassen, H. H. Suicide risk in patients with major depressive disorder. J. Clin. Psychiat., 60 Suppl 2:57–62, 1999.

11. Apfeldorf, W. J., Spielman, L. A., Cloitre, M., Heckelman, L., and Shear, M. K. Morbidity of comorbid psychiatric diagnoses in the clinical presentation of panic disorder. Depress. Anxiety, 12:78–84, 2000.

12. Argyropoulos, S. V., and Wilson, S. J. Sleep disturbances in depression and the effects of antidepressants. Int. Rev. Psychiat., 17:237–245, 2005.

13. Austin, M. P., Mitchell, P., and Goodwin, G. M. Cognitive deficits in depression: possible implications for functional neuropathology. Br. J. Psychiat., 178:200–206, 2001.

14. Averill, P. M., Reas, D. L., Shack, A., Shah, N. N., Cowan, K., Krajewski, K., Kopecky, C., and Guynn, R. W. Is schizoaffective disorder a stable diagnostic category: a retrospective examination. Psychiat. Q., 75:215–227, 2004.

15. Badner, J. A., and Gershon, E. S. Meta-analysis of whole-genome linkage scans of bipolar disorder and schizophrenia. Mol. Psychiat., 7:405–411, 2002.

16. Baldessarini, R. J., Tondo, L., and Hennen, J. Lithium treatment and suicide risk in major affective disorders: update and new findings. J. Clin. Psychiat., 64 Suppl 5:44–52, 2003.

17. Ballas, C. A., and Staab, J. P. Medically unexplained physical symptoms: toward an alternative paradigm for diagnosis and treatment. CNS Spectr., 8:20–26, 2003.

18. Barbini, B., Colombo, C., Benedetti, F., Campori, E., Bellodi, L., and Smeraldi, E. The unipolar-bipolar dichotomy and the response to sleep deprivation. Psychiat. Res., 79:43–50, 1998.

19. Baumann, B., Danos, P., Krell, D., Diekmann, S., Wurthmann, C., Bielau, H., Bernstein, H. G., and Bogerts, B. Unipolar-bipolar dichotomy of mood disorders is supported by noradrenergic brainstem system morphology. J. Affect. Disord., 54:217–224, 1999.

20. Beasley Jr, C. M., Nilsson, M. E., Koke, S. C., and Gonzeles, J. S. Efficacy, adverse events, and treatment discontinuations in fluoxetine clinical studies of major depression: a meta-analysis of the 20-mg/day dose. J. Clin. Psychiat., 61:722–728, 2000.

21. Beck, A. Cognitive Therapy and the Emotional Disorders. New York: International Universities Press, 1976.

22. Benazzi, F. Outcome of schizophreniform disorder. Curr. Psychiat. Rep., 5:192–196, 2003.

23. Berk, M., Malhi, G. S., Mitchell, P. B., Cahill, C. M., Carman, A. C., Hadzi-Pavlovic, D., Hawkins, M. T., and Tohen, M. Scale matters: the need for a Bipolar Depression Rating Scale (BDRS). Acta Psychiat. Scand. Suppl., 422:39–45, 2004.

24. Berk, M., Segal, J., Janet, L., and Vorster, M. Emerging options in the treatment of bipolar disorders. Drugs, 61:1407–1414, 2001.

25. Berman, R. M., Cappiello, A., Anand, A., Oren, D. A., Heninger, G. R., Charney, D. S., and Krystal, J. H. Antidepressant effects of ketamine in depressed patients. Biol. Psychiat., 47:351–354, 2000.

26. Berrettini, W. Evidence for shared susceptibility in bipolar disorder and schizo-phrenia. Am. J. Med. Genet. C Semin. Med. Genet., 123:59–64, 2003.

27. Bertocci, M. A., Dahl, R. E., Williamson, D. E., Iosif, A. M., Birmaher, B., Axelson, D., and Ryan, N. D. Subjective sleep complaints in pediatric depression: a con-trolled study and comparison with EEG measures of sleep and waking. J. Am. Acad. Child Adolesc. Psychiat., 44:1158–1166, 2005.

28. Bertolote, J. M., Fleischmann, A., De Leo, D., and Wasserman, D. Psychiatric diagnoses and suicide: revisiting the evidence. Crisis, 25:147–155, 2004.

29. Biederman, J., Mick, E., Faraone, S. V., Spencer, T., Wilens, T. E., and Wozniak, J. Pediatric mania: a developmental subtype of bipolar disorder? Biol. Psychiat., 48:458–466, 2000.

30. Blazer, D. G., Kessler, R. C., and Swartz, M. S. Epidemiology of recurrent major and minor depression with a seasonal pattern: the National Comorbidity Survey. Br. J. Psychiat., 172:164–167, 1998.

31. Bowden, C. L. Dosing strategies and time course of response to antimanic drugs. J. Clin. Psychiat., 57:4–9, 1996.

32. Bowden, C. L. The ability of lithium and other mood stabilizers to decrease suicide risk and prevent relapse. Curr. Psychiat. Rep., 2:490–494, 2000.

33. Bowden, C. L. Valproate. Bipolar Disord., 5:189–202, 2003.

34. Brambilla, P., Barale, F., and Soares, J. C. Perspectives on the use of anticonvul-sants in the treatment of bipolar disorder. Int. J. Neuropsychopharmacol., 4:421–436, 2001.

35. Burt, L., Lisanby, S. H., and Sackeim, H. A. Neuropsychiatric applications of transcranial magnetic stimulation: a meta analysis. Int. J. Neuropsychopharmacol., 5:73–103, 2002.

36. Cadoret, R. J., Winokur, G., Langbehn, D., Troughton, E., Yates, W. R., and Stewart, M. A. Depression spectrum disease, I: The role of gene-environment interaction. Am. J. Psychiat., 153:892–899, 1996.

37. Calabrese, J. R., Shelton, M. D., Rapport, D. J., and Kimmel, S. E. Bipolar disorders and the effectiveness of novel anticonvulsants. Am. J. Psychiat., 63:5–9, 2002.

38. Camp, N. J., and Cannon-Albright, L. A. Dissecting the genetic etiology of major depressive disorder using linkage analysis. Trends Mol. Med., 11:138–144, 2005.

39. Carroll, B. J. The dexamethasone test for melancholia. Br. J. Psychiat., 140:292–304, 1982.

40. Casacalenda, N., Perry, J. C., and Looper, K. Remission in major depressive disorder: a comparison of pharmacotherapy, psychotherapy, and control condi-tions. Am. J. Psychiat., 159:1354–1360, 2002.

41. Caspi, A., Sugden, K., Moffitt, T. E., Taylor, A., Craig, I. W., Harrington, H., McClay, J., Mill, J., Martin, J., Braithwaite, A., and Poulton, R. Influence of life stress on depression: moderation by a polymorphism in the 5-HTT gene. Science, 301:386–389, 2003.

42. Chaudron, L. H., and Pies, R. W. The relationship between postpartum psychosis and bipolar disorder: a review. J. Clin. Psychiat., 64:1284–1292, 2003.

43. Chen, Y. R., Swann, A. C., and Johnson, B. A. Stability of diagnosis in bipolar disorder. J. Nerv. Ment. Dis., 186:17–23, 1998.

44. Christopher, E. J. Electroconvulsive therapy in the medically ill. Curr. Psychiat. Rep., 5:225–230, 2003.

45. Clark, L., and Goodwin, G. M. State- and trait-related deficits in sustained attention in bipolar disorder. Eur. Arch. Psychiat. Clin. Neurosci., 254:61–68, 2004.

46. Coryell, W., Endicott, J., Maser, J. D., Keller, M. B., Leon, A. C., and Akiskal, H. S. Long-term stability of polarity distinctions in the affective disorders. Am. J. Psychiat., 152:385–390, 1995.

47. Coryell, W., Turvey, C., Endicott, J., Leon, A. C., Mueller, T., Solomon, D., and Keller, M. Bipolar I affective disorder: predictors of outcome after 15 years. J. Affect. Disord., 50:109–116, 1998.

48. Craddock, N., O'Donovan, M. C., and Owen, M. J. The genetics of schizophrenia and bipolar disorder: dissecting psychosis. J. Med. Genet., 42:193–204, 2005.

49. Craddock, N., O'Donovan, M. C., and Owen, M. J. Genes for schizophrenia and bipolar disorder? Implications for psychiatric nosology. Schizophr. Bull., 32:9–16, 2006.

50. Cuellar, A. K., Johnson, S. L., and Winters, R. Distinctions between bipolar and unipolar depression. Clin. Psychol. Rev., 25:307–339, 2005.

51. DeLeon, O. A. Antiepileptic drugs for the acute and maintenance treatment of bipolar disorder. Harv. Rev. Psychiat., 9:209–222, 2001.

52. Dindo, L., and Coryell, W. Comorbid major depression and panic disorder: significance of temporal sequencing to familial transmission. J. Affect. Disord., 82:119–123, 2004.

53. Drake, R. E., McHugo, G. J., and Biesanz, J. C. The test-retest reliability of standardized instruments among homeless persons with substance use disorders. J. Stud. Alcohol., 56:161–167, 1995.

54. Drevets, W. C., and Todd, R. D. Depression, mania, and related disorders. In *Adult Psychiatry*, 2nd edition, Rubin, E. H., Zorumski, C. F. (eds.). Malden, MA: Blackwell, pp. 91–129, 2005.

55. Duffy, A., Grof, P., Robertson, C., and Alda, M. The implications of genetics studies of major mood disorders for clinical practice. J. Clin. Psychiat., 61:630–637, 2000.

56. Duggan, C., Sham, P., Minne, C., Lee, A., and Murray, R. Family history as a predictor of poor long-term outcome in depression. Br. J. Psychiat., 173:527–530, 1998.

57. Eaton, W. W., Anthony, J. C., Gallo, J., Cai, G., Tien, A., Romanoski, A., Lyketsos, C., and Chen, L. S. Natural history of Diagnostic Interview Schedule/DSM-IV major depression. The Baltimore Epidemiologic Catchment Area follow-up. Arch. Gen. Psychiat., 54:993–999, 1997.

58. Ebmeier, K. P., Donaghey, C., and Steele, J. D. Recent developments and current controversies in depression. Lancet, 367:153–167, 2006.

59. Egeland, J. A., and Hostetter, A. M. Amish study, I: affective disorders among the Amish, 1976-1980. Am. J. Psychiat., 140:56–61, 1983.

60. Enns, M. W., Swenson, J. R., McIntyre, R. S., Swinson, R. P., and Kennedy, S. H. Clinical guidelines for the treatment of depressive disorders. VII. Comorbidity. Can. J. Psychiat., *46 Suppl 1*:77S–90S, 2001.

61. Fawcett, J. A. Lithium combinations in acute and maintenance treatment of unipolar and bipolar depression. J. Clin. Psychiat., *64 Suppl 5*:32–37, 2003.

62. Fink, M. Convulsive therapy in delusional disorders. Psychiat. Clin. N. Am., *18*:393–406, 1995.

63. Fink, M., and Taylor, M. A. The many varieties of catatonia. Eur. Arch. Psychiat. Clin. Neurosci., *251 Suppl 1*:8–13, 2001.

64. Fountoulakis, K., Iacovides, A., Fotiou, F., Karamouzis, M., Demetriadou, A., and Kaprinis, G. Relationship among Dexamethasone Suppression Test, personality disorders and stressful life events in clinical subtypes of major depression: an exploratory study. Ann. Gen. Hosp. Psychiat., *3*:15, 2004.

65. Fountoulakis, K. N., Grunze, H., Panagiotidis, P., and Kaprinis, G. Treatment of bipolar depression: an update. J. Affect. Disord., *109*:21–34, 2008.

66. Frampton, J. E., and Plosker, G. L. Selegiline transdermal system: in the treatment of major depressive disorder. Drugs, *67*:257–265, 2007.

67. Frances, A. J., Kahn, D. A., Carpenter, D., Docherty, J. P., and Donovan, S. L. The expert consensus guidelines for treating depression in bipolar disorder. J. Clin. Psychiat., *59*:73–79, 1998.

68. Frank, E., and Thase, M. E. Natural history and preventative treatment of recurrent mood disorders. Annu. Rev. Med., *50*:453–468, 1999.

69. Fremming, K. The expectation of mental infirmity in the sample of the Danish population. In *Occasional Papers of Eugenics, no. 7*. London: Cassell, 1951.

70. Freud, S. Mourning and Melancholia. In *The Complete Psychological Works of Sigmund Freud*. London: Hogarth Press, 1957, vol. 14, pp. 237–259.

71. Friedman, M. A., Detweiller-Bedelle, J. B., Leventhal, H. E., Horne, R., Keitner, G. I., and Miller, I. W. Combined psychotherapy and pharmacotherapy for the treatment of major depressive disorder. Clin. Psychiat. Sci. Pract., *11*:47–68, 2004.

72. Genton, P. Progress in pharmaceutical development presentation with improved pharmacokinetics: a new formulation for valproate. Acta. Neurol. Scand. Suppl., *182*:26–32, 2005.

73. Gibb, S. J., Beautrais, A. L., and Fergusson, D. M. Mortality and further suicidal behaviour after an index suicide attempt: a 10-year study. Aust. N. Z. J. Psychiat., *39*:95–100, 2005.

74. Gijsman, H. J., Geddes, J. R., Rendell, J. M., Nolen, W. A., and Goodwin, G. M. Antidepressants for bipolar depression: a systematic review of randomized, controlled trials. Am. J. Psychiat., *161*:1537–1547, 2004.

75. Gilmer, W. S., and McKinney, W. T. Early experience and depressive disorders: human and non-human primate studies. J. Affect. Disord., *75*:97–113, 2003.

76. Gliatto, M. F., and Rai, A. K. Evaluation and treatment of patients with suicidal ideation. Am. Fam. Physician, *59*:1500–1506, 1999.

77. Goldberg, J. F., Garno, J. L., and Harrow, M. Long-term remission and recovery in bipolar disorder: a review. Curr. Psychiat. Rep., 7:456–461, 2005.

78. Goldberg, J. F., and Harrow, M. Consistency of remission and outcome in bipolar and unipolar mood disorders: a 10-year prospective follow-up. J. Affect. Disord., 81:123–131, 2004.

79. Goldberg, J. F., and Truman, C. J. Antidepressant-induced mania: an overview of current controversies. Bipolar Disord., 5:407–420, 2003.

80. Goodwin, G. M. Neuropsychological and neuroimaging evidence for the involvement of the frontal lobes in depression. J. Psychopharmacol., 11:115–122, 1997.

81. Grant, B. F., Stinson, F. S., Hasin, D. S., Dawson, D. A., Chou, S. P., Ruan, W. J., and Huang, B. Prevalence, correlates, and comorbidity of bipolar I disorder and axis I and II disorders: results from the National Epidemiologic Survey on Alcohol and Related Conditions. J. Clin. Psychiat., 66:1205–1215, 2005.

82. Greden, J. F. The burden of recurrent depression: causes, consequences, and future prospects. J. Clin. Psychiat., 62 Suppl 22:5–9, 2001.

83. Greenberg, R. M., and Kellner, C. H. Electroconvulsive therapy: a selected review. Am. J. Geriat. Psychiat., 13:268–281, 2005.

84. Gutman, D. A., and Nemeroff, C. B. Persistent central nervous system effects of an adverse early environment: clinical and preclinical studies. Physiol. Behav., 79:471–478, 2003.

85. Guze, S. B., and Robins, E. Suicide and primary affective disorders. Br. J. Psychiat., 117:437–438, 1970.

86. Guzzetta, F., Tondo, L., Centorrino, F., and Baldessarini, R. J. Lithium treatment reduces suicide risk in recurrent major depressive disorder. J. Clin. Psychiat, 68:380–383, 2007.

87. Hanna, E. Z., and Grant, B. F. Gender differences in DSM-IV alcohol use disorders and major depression as distributed in the general population: clinical implications. Compr. Psychiat., 38:202–212, 1997.

88. Harris, E. C., and Barraclough, B. Excess mortality of mental disorder. Br. J. Psychiat., 173:11–53, 1998.

89. Harrison, P. J. The neuropathology of primary mood disorder. Brain, 125:1428–1449, 2002.

90. Heim, C., and Nemeroff, C. B. The role of childhood trauma in the neurobiology of mood and anxiety disorders: preclinical and clinical studies. Biol. Psychiat., 49:1023–1039, 2001.

91. Helgason, T. Epidemiology of mental disorders in Iceland. A psychiatric and demographic investigation of 5395 Icelanders. Acta Psychiat. Scand., 40:173, 1964.

92. Hiltry, D. M., Brady, K. T., and Hales, R. E. A review of bipolar disorder among adults. Psychiat. Serv., 50:201–213, 1999.

93. Holahan, C. J., Moos, R. H., Holahan, C. K., Cronkite, R. C., and Randall, P. K. Unipolar depression, life context vulnerabilities, and drinking to cope. J. Consult. Clin. Psychol., 72:269–275, 2004.

94. Hollon, S. D., Jarrett, R. B., Nierenberg, A. A., Thase, M. E., Trivedi, M., and Rush, A. J. Psychotherapy and medication in the treatment of adult and geriatric

depression: which monotherapy or combined treatment? J. Clin. Psychiat., 66:455–468, 2005.

95. Hollon, S. D., Shelton, R. C., Wisniewski, S., Warden, D., Biggs, M. M., Friedman, E. S., Husain, M., Kupfer, D. J., Nierenberg, A. A., Petersen, T. J., Shores-Wilson, K., and Rush, A. J. Presenting characteristics of depressed out-patients as a function of recurrence: preliminary findings from the STAR*D clinical trial. J. Psychiat. Res., 40:59–69, 2006.

96. Hysenbegasi, A., Hass, S. L., and Rowland, C. R. The impact of depression on the academic productivity of university students. J. Ment. Health Policy Econ., 8:145–151, 2005.

97. Ising, M., Kunzel, H. E., Binder, E. B., Nickel, T., Modell, S., and Holsboer, F. The combined dexamethasone/CRH test as a potential surrogate marker in depression. Prog. Neuropsychopharmacol. Biol. Psychiat., 29:1085–1093, 2005.

98. Isogawa, K., Nagayama, H., Tsutsumi, T., Kiyota, A., Akiyoshi, J., and Hieda, K. Simultaneous use of thyrotropin-releasing hormone test and combined dexa-methasone/corticotropine-releasing hormone test for severity evaluation and outcome prediction in patients with major depressive disorder. J. Psychiat. Res., 39:467–473, 2005.

99. Isometsä, E. T. Psychological autopsy studiesa review. Eur. Psychiat., 16:379–385, 2001.

100. Jamison, K. An Unquiet Mind. New York: Knopf, 1995.

101. Johnson, G. F. S., and Leeman, M. M. Onset of illness in bipolar manic-depres-sives and their affectively ill first-degree relatives. Biol. Psychiat., 12:733–741, 1977.

102. Johnson, L., Andersson-Lundman, G., Aberg-Wistedt, A., and Mathe, A. A. Age of onset in affective disorder: its correlation with hereditary and psychosocial factors. J. Affect. Disord., 59:139–148, 2000.

103. Jones, I., and Craddock, N. Familiality of the puerperal trigger in bipolar disorder: results of a family study. Am. J. Psychiat., 158:913–917, 2001.

104. Judd, L. L., and Akiskal, H. S. Delineating the longitudinal structure of depressive illness: beyond clinical subtypes and duration thresholds. Pharmacopsychiat., 33:3–7, 2000.

105. Judd, L. L., Akiskal, H. S., Schettler, P. J., Endicott, J., Maser, J., Solomon, D. A., Leon, A. C., Rice, J. A., and Keller, M. B. The long-term natural history of the weekly symptomatic status of bipolar I disorder. Arch. Gen. Psychiat., 59:530–537, 2002.

106. Kales, H. C., Maixner, D. F., and Mellow, A. M. Cerebrovascular disease and late-life depression. Am. J. Geriat. Psychiat., 13:88–98, 2005.

107. Kalia, M. Neurobiological basis of depression: an update. Metabolism, 54:24–27, 2005.

108. Kamat, S. M., Lefevre, P. J., and Grossberg, G. T. Electroconvulsive therapy in the elderly. Clin. Geriatr. Med., 19:825–839, 2003.

109. Kasperowicz-Dabrowiecka, A., and Rybakowski, J. K. Beyond the Winokur con-cept of depression spectrum disease: which types of alcoholism are related to primary affective illness? J. Affect. Disord., 63:133–138, 2001.

110. Katon, W. J., and Walker, E. A. Medically unexplained symptoms in primary care. J. Clin. Psychiat., *59 Suppl 20*:15–21, 1998.

111. Keller, M. B. Rationale and options for the long-term treatment of depression. Hum. Psychopharmacol., *17 Suppl 1*:S43–S46, 2002.

112. Kelly, R. H., Russo, J., and Katon, W. Somatic complaints among pregnant women cared for in obstetrics: normal pregnancy or depressive and anxiety symptom amplification revisited? Gen. Hosp. Psychiat., *23*:107–113, 2001.

113. Kempf, L., Hussain, N., and Potash, J. B. Mood disorder with psychotic features, schizoaffective disorder, and schizophrenia with mood features: trouble at the borders. Int. Rev. Psychiat., *17*:9–19, 2005.

114. Kendell, R. E. *The Classification of Depressive Illnesses*, Maudsley Monogr. no. 18 edition. London: Oxford University Press, 1968.

115. Kendler, K. S., Gatz, M., Gardner, C. O., and Pedersen, N. L. A Swedish national twin study of lifetime major depression. Am. J. Psychiat., *163*:109–114, 2006.

116. Kennedy, N., and Foy, K. The impact of residual symptoms on outcome of major depression. Curr. Psychiat. Rep., *7*:441–446, 2005.

117. Kennedy, N., and Paykel, E. S. Residual symptoms at remission from depression: impact on long-term outcome. J. Affect. Disord., *80*:135–144, 2004.

118. Kessing, L. V., Hansen, M. G., and Andersen, P. K. Course of illness in depressive and bipolar disorders. Naturalistic study, 1994–1999. Br. J. Psychiat., *185*:372–377, 2004.

119. Kessler, R. C., Berglund, P., Demler, O., Jin, R., Koretz, D., Merikangas, K. R., Rush, A. J., Walters, E. E., and Wang, P. S. The epidemiology of major depressive disorder: results from the National Comorbidity Survey Replication (NCS-R). JAMA, *289*:3095–3105, 2003.

120. Kessler, R. C., Chiu, W. T., Demler, O., Merikangas, K. R., and Walters, E. E. Prevalence, severity, and comorbidity of 12-month DSM-IV disorders in the National Comorbidity Survey Replication. Arch. Gen. Psychiat., *62*:617–627, 2005.

121. Kessler, R. C., Stang, P. E., Wittchen, H. U., Ustun, T. B., Roy-Burne, P. P., and Walters, E. E. Lifetime panic-depression comorbidity in the National Comorbidity Survey. Arch. Gen. Psychiat., *55*:801–808, 1998.

122. Kho, K. H., Zwinderman, A. H., and Blansjaar, B. A. Predictors for the efficacy of electroconvulsive therapy: chart review of a naturalistic study. J. Clin. Psychiat., *66*:894–899, 2005.

123. Kleindienst, N., Severus, W. E., Moller, H. J., and Greil, W. Is polarity of recurrence related to serum lithium level in patients with bipolar disorder? Eur. Arch. Psychiat. Clin. Neurosci., *255*:72–74, 2005.

124. Kohn, R., Saxena, S., Levav, I., and Saraceno, B. The treatment gap in mental health care. Bull. World Health Org., *82*:858–866, 2004.

125. Kotlyar, M., Dysken, M., and Adson, D. E. Update on drug-induced depression in the elderly. Am. J. Geriat. Psychiat., *3*:288–300, 2005.

126. Kraepelin, E. *Manic Depressive Insanity and Paranoia*. Edinburgh: E.S. Livingstone, 1921.

127. Kuehner, C. Gender differences in unipolar depression: an update of epidemiological findings and possible explanations. Acta Psychiat. Scand., 108:163–174, 2003.

128. Kwon, S. M., and Oei, T. P. Cognitive change processes in a group cognitive behavior therapy of depression. J. Behav. Ther. Exp. Psychiat., 34:73–85, 2003.

129. Lara, M. E., and Klein, D. N. Psychosocial processes underlying the maintenance and persistence of depression: implications for understanding chronic depression. Clin. Psychol. Rev., 19:553–570, 1999.

130. Lenze, E. L., Miller, A., Munir, Z., Pornoppadol, C., and North, C. S. Psychiatric symptoms endorsed by somatization disorder patients in a psychiatric clinic. Ann. Clin. Psychiat., 11:73–79, 1999.

131. Leonhard, K., Korff, I., and Shulz, H. Die Temperamente in den Familien der monopolaren und bipolaren phasichen. Psychosen. Psychiat. Neurol., 143:416–434, 1962.

132. Leverich, G. S., Altshuler, L. L., Frye, M. A., Suppes, T., McElroy, S. L., Keck, P. E., Jr., Kupka, R. W., Denicoff, K. D., Nolen, W. A., Grunze, H., Martinez, M. I., and Post, R. M. Risk of switch in mood polarity to hypomania or mania in patients with bipolar depression during acute and continuation trials of venlafaxine, sertraline, and bupropion as adjuncts to mood stabilizers. Am. J. Psychiat., 163:232–239, 2006.

133. Lewis, A. Melancholia: a historical review. In *The State of Psychiatry: Essays and Addresses.* New York: Science House, 1967, pp. 71–110.

134. Lichtenthal, W. G., Cruess, D. G., and Prigerson, H. G. A case for establishing complicated grief as a distinct mental disorder in DSM-V. Clin. Psychol. Rev., 24:637–662, 2004.

135. Lin, P. I., McInnis, M. G., Potash, J. B., Willour, V., MacKinnon, D. F., DePaulo, J. R., and Zandi, P. P. Clinical correlates and familial aggregation of age at onset in bipolar disorder. Am. J. Psychiat., 163:240–246, 2006.

136. Loo, C. K., and Mitchell, P. B. A review of the efficacy of transcranial magnetic stimulation (TMS) treatment for depression, and current and future strategies to optimize efficacy. J. Affect. Disord., 88:255–267, 2005.

137. MacQueen, G. M., Campbell, S., McEwen, B. S., Macdonald, K., Amano, S., Joffe, R. T., Nahmias, C., and Young, L. T. Course of illness, hippocampal function, and hippocampal volume in major depression. Proc. Natl. Acad. Sci. USA, 100:1387–1392, 2003.

138. MacQueen, G. M., Hajek, T., and Alda, M. The phenotypes of bipolar disorder: relevance for genetic investigations. Mol. Psychiat., 10:811–826, 2005.

139. Maier, W., Hofgen, B., Zobel, A., and Rietschel, M. Genetic models of schizophrenia and bipolar disorder: overlapping inheritance or discrete genotypes? Eur. Arch. Psychiat. Clin. Neurosci., 255:159–166, 2005.

140. Maletzky, B. M. The first-line use of electroconvulsive therapy in major affective disorders. J. ECT, 20:112–117, 2004.

141. Mann, J. J. The medical management of depression. N. Engl. J. Med., 353:1819–1834, 2005.

142. Markowitz, J. C. Developments in interpersonal psychotherapy. Can. J. Psychiat., 44:556–561, 1999.

143. Martinez-Aran, A., Vieta, E., Colom, F., Reinares, M., Benabarre, A., Gasto, C., and Salamero, M. Cognitive dysfunctions in bipolar disorder: evidence of neuropsychological disturbances. Psychother. Psychosom., 69:2–18, 2000.

144. Martinez-Aran, A., Vieta, E., Colom, F., Torrent, C., Sanchez-Moreno, J., Reinares, M., Benabarre, A., Goikolea, J. M., Brugue, E., Daban, C., and Salamero, M. Cognitive impairment in euthymic bipolar patients: implications for clinical and functional outcome. Bipolar Disord., 6:224–232, 2004.

145. Martinez-Aran, A., Vieta, E., Reinares, M., Colom, F., Torrent, C., Sanchez-Moreno, J., Benabarre, A., Goikolea, J. M., Comes, M., and Salamero, M. Cognitive function across manic or hypomanic, depressed, and euthymic states in bipolar disorder. Am. J. Psychiat., 161:262–270, 2004.

146. Marvel, C. L., and Paradiso, S. Cognitive and neurological impairment in mood disorders. Psychiat. Clin. N. Am., 27:19–36, vii–viii, 2004.

147. Mathew, S. J., Keegan, K., and Smith, L. Glutamate modulators as novel interventions for mood disorders. Rev. Bras. Psiquiatr., 27:243–248, 2005.

148. McGuffin, P., Rijsdijk, F., Andrew, M., Sham, P., Katz, R., and Cardno, A. The heritability of bipolar affective disorder and the genetic relationship to unipolar depression. Arch. Gen. Psychiat., 60:497–502, 2003.

149. McIntyre, R. S., Mancini, D. A., Parikh, S., and Kennedy, S. H. Lithium revisited. Can. J. Psychiat., 46:322–327, 2001.

150. Meilman, P. W., Manley, C., Gaylor, M. S., and Turco, J. H. Medical withdrawals from college for mental health reasons and their relation to academic performance. J. Am. Coll. Health, 40:217–223, 1992.

151. Melartin, T. K., Rytsala, H. J., Leskela, U. S., Lestela-Mielonen, P. S., Sokero, T. P., and Isometsa, E. T. Severity and comorbidity predict episode duration and recurrence of DSM-IV major depressive disorder. J. Clin. Psychiat., 65:810–819, 2004.

152. Mendelwicz, J., Souery, D., and Rivelli, S. K. Short-term and long-term treatment for bipolar patients: beyond the guidelines. J. Affect. Dis., 55:79–85, 1999.

153. Merikangas, K. R., and Low, N. C. The epidemiology of mood disorders. Curr. Psychiat. Rep., 6:411–421, 2004.

154. Mialet, J. P., Pope, H. G., and Yurgelun-Todd, D. Impaired attention in depressive states: a non-specific deficit? Psychol. Med., 26:1009–1020, 1996.

155. Mitchell, P. B., and Malhi, G. S. Bipolar depression: phenomenological overview and clinical characteristics. Bipolar Disord., 6:530–539, 2004.

156. Moller, H. J., and Nasrallah, H. A. Treatment of bipolar disorder. J. Clin. Psychiat., 64 Suppl 6:9–17, 2003.

157. Mondimore, F. M. Unipolar depression/bipolar depression: connections and controversies. Int. Rev. Psychiat., 17:39–47, 2005.

158. Moretti, A., Gorini, A., and Villa, R. F. Affective disorders, antidepressant drugs and brain metabolism. Mol. Psychiat., 8:773–785, 2003.

159. Müller-Oerlinghausen, B. Arguments for the specificity of the antisuicidal effect of lithium. Eur. Arch. Psychiat. Clin. Neurosci., 251 Suppl 2:II72–II75, 2001.

160. Mundo, E., Cattaneo, E., Russo, M., and Altamura, A. C. Clinical variables related to antidepressant-induced mania in bipolar disorder. J. Affect. Disord., 92:227–230, 2006.

161. Munro, A. The classification of delusional disorders. Psychiat. Clin. N. Am., 18:199–212, 1995.

162. Myers, J. K., Weissman, M. M., Tischler, G. L., Holzer III, C. E., Leaf, P. J., Orvaschel, H., Anthony, J. C., Boyd, J. H., Burke Jr, J. D., Kramer, M., and Stoltzman, R. Six-month prevalence of psychiatric disorders in three communities. Arch. Gen. Psychiat., 41:959–967, 1984.

163. Nahas, Z., Teneback, C., Chae, J. H., Mu, Q., Molnar, C., Kozel, F. A., Walker, J., Anderson, B., Koola, J., Kose, S., Lomarev, M., Bohning, D. E., and George, M. S. Serial vagus nerve stimulation functional MRI in treatment-resistant depression. Neuropsychopharmacol., 32:1649–1660, 2007.

164. Nemeroff, C. B., Bremner, J. D., Foa, E. B., Mayberg, H. S., North, C. S., and Stein, M. B. Posttraumatic stress disorder: a state-of-the-science review. J. Psychiat. Res., 40:1–21, 2006.

165. Nierenberg, A. A. An analysis of the efficacy of treatments for bipolar depression. J. Clin. Psychiat., 69 Suppl 5:4–8, 2008.

166. Nierenberg, A. A. Effective agents in treating bipolar depression. J. Clin. Psychiat, 69:e29, 2008.

167. Nussbaum, P. D. Pseudodementia: a slow death. Neuropsychol. Rev., 4:71–90, 1994.

168. O'Leary, D. The endogenous subtype and naturalistic course in depression. J. Affect. Disord., 41:117–123, 1996.

169. O'Leary, D., Paykel, E., Todd, C., and Vardulaki, K. Suicide in primary affective disorders revisited: a systematic review by treatment era. J. Clin. Psychiat., 62:804–811, 2001.

170. Oswald, P., Souery, D., and Mendlewicz, J. Molecular genetics of affective disorders. Prog. Neuropsychopharmacol. Biol. Psychiat., 28:865–877, 2004.

171. Owens, D., Horrocks, J., and House, A. Fatal and non-fatal repetition of self-harm. Systematic review. Br. J. Psychiat., 181:193–199, 2002.

172. Pampallona, S., Bollini, P., Tibaldi, G., Kupelnick, B., and Munizza, C. Combined pharmacotherapy and psychological treatment for depression: a systematic review. Arch. Gen. Psychiat., 61:714–719, 2004.

173. Pascual-Leone, A., Rubio, B., Pallardo, F., and Catala, M. D. Rapid-rate transcranial magnetic stimulation of left dorsolateral prefrontal cortex in drug-resistant depression. Lancet, 348:233–237, 1996.

174. Patten, S. B., and Barbui, C. Drug-induced depression: a systematic review to inform clinical practice. Psychother. Psychosom., 73:207–215, 2004.

175. Payne, J. L., Potash, J. B., and DePaulo, J. R., Jr. Recent findings on the genetic basis of bipolar disorder. Psychiat. Clin. N. Am., 28:481–498, 2005.

176. Perris, C. The importance of Karl Leonhard's classification of endogenous psychoses. Psychopathol., 23:282–290, 1990.

177. Post, R. M., Denicoff, K. D., Leverich, G. S., Altshuler, L. L., Frye, M. A., Suppes, T. M., Rush, A. J., Keck, P. E., Jr., McElroy, S. L., Luckenbaugh, D. A., Pollio, C., Kupka, R., and Nolen, W. A. Morbidity in 258 bipolar outpatients followed for 1 year with daily prospective ratings on the NIMH life chart method. J. Clin. Psychiat., 64:680–690, 2003.

178. Price, J. S. Chronic depressive illness. Br. Med. J., 1:1200–1201, 1979.

179. Quraishi, S., and Frangou, S. Neuropsychology of bipolar disorder: a review. J. Affect. Disord., 72:209–226, 2002.

180. Rapaport, M. H. Prevalence, recognition, and treatment of comorbid depression and anxiety. J. Clin. Psychiat., 62 Suppl 24:6–10, 2001.

181. Räsänen, P., Tiihonen, J., and Hakko, H. The incidence and onset-age of hospitalized bipolar affective disorder in Finland. J. Affect. Disord., 48:63–68, 1998.

182. Reich, J. The effect of Axis II disorders on the outcome of treatment of anxiety and unipolar depressive disorders: a review. J. Personal. Disord., 17:387–405, 2003.

183. Rey, J. M., and Walter, G. Half a century of ECT use in young people. Am. J. Psychiat., 154:595–602, 1997.

184. Rihmer, Z., and Kiss, K. Bipolar disorders and suicidal behaviour. Bipolar Disord., 4 Suppl 1:21–25, 2002.

185. Robinson, D. S., and Amsterdam, J. D. The selegiline transdermal system in major depressive disorder: A systematic review of safety and tolerability. J. Affect. Disord., 105:15–23, 2007.

186. Rosentha, N. E., Sack, D. A., Gillin, J. C., Lewy, A. J., Goodwin, F. K., Davenport, Y., Mueller, P. S., Newsome, D. A., and Wehr, T. A. Seasonal affective disorder: a description of the syndrome and preliminary findings with light therapy. Arch. Gen. Psychiat., 41:72–80, 1995.

187. Roy, A., Nielsen, D., Rylander, G., Sarchiapone, M., and Segal, N. Genetics of suicide in depression. J. Clin. Psychiat., 60 Suppl 2:12–17, 1999.

188. Roy-Byrne, P. P., Stang, P., Wittchen, H. U., Ustun, B., Walters, E. E., and Kessler, R. C. Lifetime panic-depression comorbidity in the National Comorbidity Survey. Association with symptoms, impairment, course and help-seeking. Br. J. Psychiat., 176:229–235, 2000.

189. Santarelli, L., Saxe, M., Gross, C., Surget, A., Battaglia, F., Dulawa, S., Weisstaub, N., Lee, J., Duman, R., Arancio, O., Belzung, C., and Hen, R. Requirement of hippocampal neurogenesis for the behavioral effects of antidepressants. Science, 301:805–809, 2003.

190. Schaffer, A., Cairney, J., Cheung, A., Veldhuizen, S., and Levitt, A. Community survey of bipolar disorder in Canada: lifetime prevalence and illness character-istics. Can. J. Psychiat., 51:9–16, 2006.

191. Schechter, L. E., Ring, R. H., Beyer, C. E., Hughes, Z. A., Khawaja, X., Malberg, J. E., and Rosenzweig-Lipson, S. Innovative approaches for the development of antidepressant drugs: current and future strategies. NeuroRx, 2:590–611, 2005.

192. Segurado, R., Detera-Wadleigh, S. D., Levinson, D. F., Lewis, C. M., Gill, M., Nurnberger, J. I., Jr., Craddock, N., DePaulo, J. R., Baron, M., Gershon, E. S.,

Ekholm, J., Cichon, S., Turecki, G., Claes, S., Kelsoe, J. R., Schofield, P. R., Badenhop, R. F., Morissette, J., Coon, H., Blackwood, D., McInnes, L. A., Foroud, T., Edenberg, H. J., Reich, T., Rice, J. P., Goate, A., McInnis, M. G., McMahon, F. J., Badner, J. A., Goldin, L. R., Bennett, P., Willour, V. L., Zandi, P. P., Liu, J., Gilliam, C., Juo, S. H., Berrettini, W. H., Yoshikawa, T., Peltonen, L., Lonnqvist, J., Nothen, M. M., Schumacher, J., Windemuth, C., Rietschel, M., Propping, P., Maier, W., Alda, M., Grof, P., Rouleau, G. A., Del Favero, J., Van Broeckhoven, C., Mendlewicz, J., Adolfsson, R., Spence, M. A., Luebbert, H., Adams, L. J., Donald, J. A., Mitchell, P. B., Barden, N., Shink, E., Byerley, W., Muir, W., Visscher, P. M., Macgregor, S., Gurling, H., Kalsi, G., McQuillin, A., Escamilla, M. A., Reus, V. I., Leon, P., Freimer, N. B., Ewald, H., Kruse, T. A., Mors, O., Radhakrishna, U., Blouin, J. L., Antonarakis, S. E., and Akarsu, N. Genome scan meta-analysis of schizophrenia and bipolar disorder, part III: Bipolar disorder. Am. J. Hum. Genet., 73:49–62, 2003.

193. Shih, R. A., Belmonte, P. L., and Zandi, P. P. A review of the evidence from family, twin and adoption studies for a genetic contribution to adult psychiatric disorders. Int. Rev. Psychiat., 16:260–283, 2004.

194. Sim, M. G., Hulse, G., and Khong, E. Alcohol and other drug use in later life. Aust. Fam. Physician, 33:820–824, 2004.

195. Sloan, D. M., and Mizes, J. S. Foundations of behavior therapy in the contemporary healthcare context. Clin. Psychol. Rev., 19:255–274, 1999.

196. Smoller, J. W., and Finn, C. T. Family, twin, and adoption studies of bipolar disorder. Am. J. Med. Genet. C Semin. Med. Genet., 123:48–58, 2003.

197. Soares, J. C., and Gershon, S. The lithium ion: a foundation for psychopharmacological specificity. Neuropsychopharmacol., 19:167–182, 1998.

198. Soares, M. B., Moreno, R. A., and Moreno, D. H. Electroconvulsive therapy in treatment-resistant mania: case reports. Rev. Hosp. Clin. Fac. Med. Sao Paulo, 57:31–38, 2002.

199. Solomon, D. S., Keitner, G. I., Ryan, C. E., and Miller, I. W. Lithium plus valproate as maintenance polypharmacy for patients with bipolar I disorder: a review. J. Clin. Psychopharmacol., 18:38–49, 1998.

200. Son, S. E., and Kirchner, J. T. Depression in children and adolescents. Am. Fam. Physician, 62:2297–2312, 2000.

201. Sporn, J., and Sachs, G. The anticonvulsant lamotrigine in treatment-refractory manic-depressive illness. J. Clin. Psychopharmacol., 17:185–189, 1997.

202. Sugahara, H., Akamine, M., Kondo, T., Fujisawa, K., Yoshimasu, K., Tokunaga, S., and Kubo, C. Somatic symptoms most often associated with depression in an urban hospital medical setting in Japan. Psychiat. Res., 126:151–158, 2004.

203. Sullivan, L. E., Fiellin, D. A., and O'Connor, P. G. The prevalence and impact of alcohol problems in major depression: a systematic review. Am. J. Med., 118:330–341, 2005.

204. Taieb, O., Flament, M. F., Chevret, S., Jeammet, P., Allilaire, J. F., Mazet, P., and Cohen, D. Clinical relevance of electroconvulsive therapy (ECT) in

adolescents with severe mood disorder: evidence from a follow-up study. Eur. Psychiat., *17*:206–212, 2002.

205. Tanaka, E. Toxicological interactions involving psychiatric drugs and alcohol: an update. J. Clin. Pharm. Ther., *28*:81–95, 2003.

206. Taylor, L., Faraone, S. V., and Tsuang, M. T. Family, twin, and adoption studies of bipolar disease. Curr. Psychiat. Rep., *4*:130–133, 2002.

207. Taylor, M. A., and Fink, M. Catatonia in psychiatric classification: a home of its own. Am. J. Psychiat., *160*:1233–1241, 2003.

208. Tejedor, M. C., Diaz, A., Castillon, J. J., and Pericay, J. M. Attempted suicide: repetition and survival–findings of a follow-up study. Acta Psychiat. Scand., *100*:205–211, 1999.

209. Terman, M., and Terman, J. S. Light therapy for seasonal and nonseasonal depression: efficacy, protocol, safety, and side effects. CNS Spectr., *10*:647–663, 2005.

210. Thacher, J. A., Morey, E., and Craighead, W. E. Using patient characteristics and attitudinal data to identify depression treatment preference groups: a latent-class model. Depress. Anxiety, *21*:47–54, 2005.

211. Thase, M. E., Salloum, I. M., and Cornelius, J. D. Comorbid alcoholism and depression: treatment issues. J. Clin. Psychiat., *62 Suppl 20*:32–41, 2001.

212. Tomita, T., and Kitamura, T. Clinical and research measures of grief: a reconsideration. Compr. Psychiat., *43*:95–102, 2002.

213. Tondo, L., Baldessarini, R. J., and Floris, G. Long-term clinical effectiveness of lithium maintenance treatment in types I and II bipolar disorders. Br. J. Psychiat., *178*:S184–S190, 2001.

214. Tondo, L., Baldessarini, R. J., Hennen, J., Minnai, G. P., Salis, P., Scamonatti, L., Masia, M., Ghiani, C., and Mannu, P. Suicide attempts in major affective disorder patients with comorbid substance use disorders. J. Clin. Psychiat., *60 Suppl 2*:63–69, 1999.

215. Tondo, L., Hennen, J., and Baldessarini, R. J. Lower suicide risk with long-term lithium treatment in major affective illness: a meta-analysis. Acta Psychiat. Scand., *104*:163–172, 2001.

216. Tsuno, N., Besset, A., and Ritchie, K. Sleep and depression. J. Clin. Psychiat., *66*:1254–1269, 2005.

217. Verdoux, H., and Bourgeois, M. Social class in unipolar and bipolar probands and relatives. J. Affect. Disord., *33*:181–187, 1995.

218. Waraich, P., Goldner, E. M., Somers, J. M., and Hsu, L. Prevalence and incidence studies of mood disorders: a systematic review of the literature. Can. J. Psychiat., *49*:124–138, 2004.

219. Weissman, M. M., Bland, R. C., Canino, G. J., Faravelli, C., Greenwald, S., Hwu, H. G., Joyce, P. R., Karam, E. G., Lee, C. K., Lellouch, J., Lepine, J. P., Newman, S. C., Rubio-Stipec, M., Wells, J. E., Wickramaratne, P. J., Wittchen, H., and Yeh, E. K. Cross-national epidemiology of major depression and bipolar disorder. JAMA, *276*:293–299, 1996.

220. Weissman, M. M., Bruce, M. L., Leaf, P. J., Florio, L. P., and Holzer, I. C. Affective disorders. In *Psychiatric Disorders in America: The Epidemiologic Catchment Area Study*, Robins, L. N., Regier, D. A. (eds.). New York: The Free Press, pp. 53–80, 1991.

221. Winokur, G. Types of depressive illness. Br. J. Psychiat., *120*:265–266, 1972.

222. Winokur, G., Coryell, W., Keller, M., Endicott, J., and Akiskal, H. A prospective follow-up of patients with bipolar and primary unipolar affective disorder. Arch. Gen. Psychiat., *50*:457–465, 1993.

223. Winokur, G., Coryell, W., Keller, M., Endicott, J., and Leon, A. A family study of manic-depressive (bipolar I) disease. Is it a distinct illness separable from primary unipolar depression? Arch. Gen. Psychiat., *52*:367–373, 1995.

224. Wittchen, H. U., Beesdo, K., Bittner, A., and Goodwin, R. D. Depressive episodes– evidence for a causal role of primary anxiety disorders? Eur. Psychiat., *18*:384–393, 2003.

225. Woodruff, R. A., Robins, L. N., Winokur, G., and Reich, T. Manic depressive illness and social achievement. Acta Psychiat. Scand., *47*:237–249, 1971.

226. Wurtman, R. J. Genes, stress, and depression. Metabolism, *54*:16–19, 2005.

227. Yatham, L. N., Kusumakar, V., Calabrese, J. R., Rao, R., Scarrow, G., and Kroeker, G. Third generation anticonvulsants in bipolar disorder: a review of efficacy and summary of clinical recommendations. J. Clin. Psychiat., *63*:275–283, 2002.

228. Yatham, L. N., Srisurapanont, M., Zis, A. P., and Kusumakar, V. Comparative studies of the biological distinction between unipolar and bipolar depressions. Life Sci., *61*:1445–1455, 1997.

229. Youdim, M. B., Edmondson, D., and Tipton, K. F. The therapeutic potential of monoamine oxidase inhibitors. Nat. Rev. Neurosci., *7*:295–309, 2006.

230. Zapotoczky, H. G. Problems of differential diagnosis between depressive pseu- dodementia and Alzheimer's disease. J. Neural Transm. Suppl., *53*:91–95, 1998.

231. Zauszniewski, J. A., and Rong, J. R. Depressive cognitions and psychosocial functioning: a test of Beck's cognitive theory. Arch. Psychiat. Nurs., *13*:286–293, 1999.

232. Zilberman, M. L., Tavares, H., Blume, S. B., and el Guebaly, N. Substance use disorders: sex differences and psychiatric comorbidities. Can. J. Psychiat., *48*:5–13, 2003.

233. Zimmerman, M., and Mattia, J. I. Principal and additional DSM-IV disorders for which outpatients seek treatment. Psychiat. Serv., *51*:1299–1304, 2000.

234. American Psychiatric Association, *Diagnostic and Statistical Manual of Mental Disorders*, 4th edition, text revision. Washington, DC: Author, 2000.

3

Schizophrenic Disorders

Hallucinations and delusions are widely considered to be hallmarks of mental disorder and thus are of great interest to psychiatrists. These symptoms may be seen in a wide variety of illnesses, including mood disorders, brain syndromes, alcohol and drug dependence, and a group of conditions that may be called the "schizophrenic disorders." Many investigators believe that schizophrenic disorders comprise a number of different conditions, but efforts to divide them into valid subgroups have not been entirely successful, and inconsistent usage has made the nomenclature confusing. Extensive work, however, has indicated that the schizophrenic disorders may be divided into two major categories: one with a relatively poor prognosis, the other with a relatively good prognosis (109, 153). Various terms historically applied to the poor-prognosis cases are chronic schizophrenia, process schizophrenia, nuclear schizophrenia, and nonremitting schizophrenia; the good-prognosis cases have been called schizophreniform disorder, acute schizophrenia, reactive schizophrenia, schizoaffective disorder, and remitting schizophrenia (136).

A cardinal feature of schizophrenia is the occurrence of delusions and hallucinations in a clear sensorium. Other noteworthy features are a blunted, shallow, or strikingly inappropriate affect; odd, sometimes bizarre, motor behavior (termed "catatonic"); and disordered thinking in which goal directedness and normal associations between ideas are markedly distorted (loosening of associations and tangential thinking).

Recent research has demonstrated that schizophrenic conditions actually have considerable variability in outcome, and consistent predictors of outcomes have been identified (67, 70). Patients with more favorable prognosis are those whose previous general adjustment has been good, and their illness presents episodically with intervening periods of remission (150). Many of these patients show striking mood symptoms during the acute psychotic illness (110). They may seem perplexed and bewildered and may be mildly disoriented. Subsequent episodes may be less pronounced and may sometimes resemble mood disorders (182, 183).

Historical Background

In now-classic studies, Emil Kraepelin (1856–1926), a German psychiatrist, built upon the work of his countrymen Kahlbaum (1828–1899) and Hecker (1843–1909), who described "catatonia" and "hebephrenia," respectively, to lay the groundwork for present views of schizophrenia (89). After careful follow-up of hospitalized patients, Kraepelin separated "manic depressive psychosis" from "dementia praecox." The latter term referred to the disorder now called chronic schizophrenia. Even though Kraepelin believed dementia praecox to be a chronic disorder that frequently ended in marked deterioration of the personality, he recognized that a small number of patients recovered completely. His "narrow" view of schizophrenia has been followed by most European psychiatrists, particularly those in the Scandinavian countries and Great Britain.

A broader approach to schizophrenia (and the name itself) was offered by Eugene Bleuler (1857–1939), a Swiss psychiatrist, who realized that he might be dealing with a group of disorders (12). His diagnostic criteria were not based on their ability to predict course and outcome, but on conformance to his hypothesis concerning the basic defect, namely, the "splitting" of psychic functions. By this he meant inconsistency, inappropriateness, and disorganization of affect, thought, and action, in the absence of obvious brain disease. Despite his less-strict approach to diagnosis and the variable course that his patients experienced, Bleuler believed that patients with schizophrenia never recovered completely, never returned to their premorbid state (*restituo ad integrum*). Because his "fundamental" symptoms included autistic thinking (defined by Bleuler as "divorce from reality"), blunted or inappropriate affect, ambivalence, and disturbed association of thought—all often difficult to define and specify—Bleuler's work set the stage for the very broad concepts of schizophrenia developed by psychoanalysts and adopted for years by many American psychiatrists.

Psychoanalysts viewed schizophrenia primarily as a manifestation of a "weak ego." Unable to cope with the problems of life and unable to use effectively the "defenses of the ego" to handle instinctual forces and anxiety, patients "regress" to a primitive level of functioning ("primary process") manifested by thought disorder, affective poverty, disorganization, and inability to conform to the demands of "reality" (13). In this psychoanalytic view of schizophrenia, all evidence of weak ego (including a wide range of personality handicaps and abnormalities) or of "primary process" (such as hallucinations, delusions, poor reality-testing, tangential thinking, and ambivalence) may be a manifestation of schizophrenia. It is not surprising, therefore, that the diagnosis was used in a wide range of clinical situations.

In the late 1930s, a number of European and American investigators began again to approach the problem of the schizophrenias in terms of predicting course, response to treatment, and long-term outcome. They recognized that proper evaluation of treatment requires a knowledge of the natural history of the disorder being treated, especially the factors associated with different clinical courses and outcomes. Such factors can be identified only by follow-up studies such as those carried out by the above investigators. Thus, current clinical and research approaches to the schizophrenic disorders are based on extensive follow-up studies supplemented by family studies (136).

Differences between European and American psychiatrists in conceptualizing schizophrenic disorders were largely resolved after the introduction of systematic diagnostic criteria in *DSM-III* in 1980. Most psychiatrists around the world came to accept the narrower approach to schizophrenia now referred to as "neo-Kraepelinian" (135). To a considerable degree, this consensus is based on empirical and systematic studies indicating that the narrower approach produces more consistent findings with regard to course, response to treatment, long-term outcome, and familial illness patterns. Many of these studies are discussed below.

Epidemiology

Chronic schizophrenia occurs in somewhat less than 1% of the population, but because of its early onset, chronicity, and associated disability, it is one of the most important psychiatric illnesses. A significant percentage of all hospitalized psychiatric patients suffer from this condition. Historically, epidemiologic studies have typically neither distinguished between good- and poor-prognosis forms of schizophrenia nor considered the possibility that some of the good-prognosis cases may represent other disorders. Available evidence suggests that the good-prognosis cases may be relatively common (135, 142, 162). The combined prevalence of both good- and poor-prognosis disorders is probably between 1% and 2%.

Schizophrenic disorders are found in all cultures. A number of studies have indicated that they are more prevalent among people from lower socioeconomic backgrounds. For some investigators, this has meant that poverty, limited education, and associated handicaps predispose to schizophrenic illness. Studies have shown, however, that the association between schizophrenic illness and low socioeconomic status can be explained by "downward drift," a term that refers to the effect of an illness on the patient's socioeconomic status (5, 97). If a disorder interferes with education and work performance, so that individuals are not able to complete advanced schooling or hold positions of responsibility, their socioeconomic status—characteristically defined by income, educational achievement, and job prestige—cannot be high.

Studies of schizophrenia in England (54), Denmark (189), Finland (6), and the United States (36) have shown that the distribution of socioeconomic class among the fathers of children with the illness is the same as in the general population, indicating that the lower socioeconomic status of patients with schizophrenic illness is at least partially the result of downward drift. Studies of ethnic minorities in Europe, however, have identified high psychosis rates, especially among African-Caribbean and other black-African immigrants whose low social status cannot be entirely explained by selective downward social drift (27, 148). Migrants generally appear to have higher rates of schizophrenia than native-born groups, possibly reflecting effects of environmental stressors in the development of the illness (148). Schizophrenia is less prevalent in migrants of undeveloped countries compared to those of emerging and developed countries (144).

In hundreds of studies, dating as far back as 1929, researchers have consistently identified an excess of births during the late winter and early spring months among individuals who develop schizophrenia in the Northern Hemisphere (21), and in the summer and fall months in the Southern Hemisphere (21). The seasonal effect may be nonspecific: A similar association has been found with bipolar affective disorder (21, 176). Though most births in schizophrenia do not occur during these months and the effect size is small, the importance of these findings is a suggestion that something associated with such births (e.g., increased exposure to perinatal influenza) may predispose to schizophrenic illness. This line of research is supported by studies documenting a seven-fold increase in risk for schizophrenia among children with maternal serologic evidence of first-trimester exposure to influenza (126). Other research has shown convincing evidence of increased rates of schizophrenia among individuals with prenatal exposure to maternal starvation during famines (73, 101, 158).

Schizophrenia appears to have a male preponderance (86, 169). A recent meta-analysis found a 1.4-fold increase of the disorder among males (102). Males also seem to experience earlier onset, more severe clinical manifestations, and a more chronic course (145, 190).

Clinical Picture

Common delusions in schizophrenia are those of persecution and control in which patients believe others are spying on them, spreading false rumors about them, planning to harm them, trying to control their thoughts or actions, or reading their minds (Table 3.1). For instance, a young woman complained bitterly that her brother was sending special mysterious messages to her by means of television in order to make her do things that would

TABLE 3.1 Diagnostic Criteria for Schizophrenia

A. *Characteristic symptoms:* Two (or more) of the following, each present for a significant portion of time during a 1-month period (or less if successfully treated):

  (1) Delusions
  (2) Hallucinations
  (3) Disorganized speech (e.g., frequent derailment or incoherence)
  (4) Grossly disorganized or catatonic behavior
  (5) Negative symptoms (i.e., affective flattening, alogia, or avolition)

Note: Only one Criterion A symptom is required if delusions are bizarre or hallucinations consist of a voice keeping up a running commentary on the person's behavior or thoughts, or two or more voices conversing with each other.

B. *Social/occupational dysfunction:* For a significant portion of the time since the onset of the disturbance, one or more major areas of functioning such as work, interpersonal relations, or self-care are markedly below the level achieved prior to the onset (or when the onset is in childhood or adolescence, failure to achieve expected level of interpersonal, academic, or occupational achievement).

C. *Duration:* Continuous signs of the disturbance persist for at least 6 months. This 6-month period must include at least 1 month of symptoms (or less if successfully treated) that meet Criterion A (i.e., active-phase symptoms) and may include periods of prodromal or residual symptoms. During these prodromal or residual periods, the signs of the disturbance may be manifested by only negative symptoms or two or more symptoms listed in Criterion A present in an attenuated form (e.g., odd beliefs, unusual perceptual experiences).

D. *Schizoaffective and mood disorder exclusion:* Schizoaffective disorder and mood disorder with psychotic features have been ruled out because either (1) no major depressive, manic, or mixed episodes have occurred concurrently with the active-phase symptoms; or (2) if mood episodes have occurred during active-phase symptoms, their total duration has been brief relative to the duration of the active and residual periods.

E. *Substance/general medical condition exclusion:* The disturbance is not due to the direct physiological effects of a substance (e.g., a drug of abuse, a medication) or a general medical condition.

F. *Relationship to a pervasive developmental disorder:* If there is a history of autistic disorder or another pervasive developmental disorder, the additional diagnosis of Schizophrenia is made only if prominent delusions or hallucinations are also present for at least a month (or less if successfully treated).

Adapted from diagnostic criteria in the *DSM-IV-TR* (196).

call attention to her and lead to trouble with the police. A young man was convinced that he was being followed and observed on the streets and in various buildings, but he concluded that this was being directed by his psychiatrist as a way to monitor the patient's progress. Patients may express the belief that they are the victims of conspiracies by neighbors, aliens, the FBI, al Qaeda, and so on. Delusions of depersonalization are also common. These may be feelings that bizarre bodily changes are taking place, sometimes as a result of the deliberate but obscure actions of others. "My insides are rotting because they are poisoning my food. It's because they know I'm wise to them and have reported them to the police."

The most common hallucinations are auditory. They may involve solitary or multiple voices. The patient may or may not recognize the voices or talk back to them. The voices may seem to come from within the patient's body or from outside sources such as radios or walls. The voices may criticize, ridicule, or threaten; often they urge the patient to do something she or he believes is wrong.

Visual hallucinations may not be as prevalent in schizophrenia as in bipolar disorder, but neither are they unusual (7). These hallucinations may vary from frightening vague forms to images of dead or absent relatives to scenes of violence or hell. Olfactory hallucinations, which are infrequent, usually consist of unpleasant smells arising from the patient's own body. Tactile (haptic) hallucinations, also infrequent, may consist of feelings that one's genitals are being manipulated, that there are animals inside one's body, or that there is "grit" on one's skin that cannot be washed off.

Though the so-called "typical" flat schizophrenic affect is highly characteristic when it is severe, its diagnostic value is limited because it frequently is subtle, leading to disagreement about its presence. Even when clearly present, it is not easy to describe. Patients seem emotionally unresponsive, without warmth or empathy. They can talk about frightening or shocking thoughts without seeming to experience their usual emotional impact ("inappropriate" affect). It is often difficult to feel compassion and sympathy for the patient or to believe that he or she can empathize with others.

Recurrent posturing, grimacing, prolonged immobility, and "waxy flexibility" are dramatic examples of catatonic behavior. These may be independent symptoms or responses to auditory hallucinations.

The impaired goal directedness of schizophrenic thought and speech may take various forms, all likely to occur in the same patient: blocking, in which the patient's thought and speech stop for periods of time only to begin again with an apparently different subject; tangential associations, in which connections between thoughts are difficult or impossible to follow; neologisms, in which the patient makes up new words; or "word salad," in which the patient's speech consists of words without any understandable sequence or meaning.

Delusions, hallucinations, bizarre and disorganized behavior, and formal thought disorder in schizophrenia have been collectively termed "positive" symptoms; blunted affect, social withdrawal, amotivation, apathy, anhedonia, and social and occupational deficits are considered "negative" symptoms (190). The positive symptoms may fluctuate during the course of the illness and the negative symptoms tend to be more constant. The negative symptoms have consistently been shown to be associated with a poorer prognosis (31, 132, 165). "Deficit" schizophrenia refers to the most severe form of the illness with enduring negative symptoms and cognitive problems (104). Positive and negative symptom groupings, however, have not offered enduring utility for subtyping forms of schizophrenia based on them. Recognition of the positive/negative symptom distinction, however, stimulated clinicians to pay more attention to the full spectrum of clinical features of schizophrenia (10) and spurred the development of novel medications to target the negative symptoms that had been largely unresponsive to the earlier antipsychotic medications.

From the time of Kraepelin's application of the name *dementia praecox* to the schizophrenias, the associated cognitive deficits have been recognized as a central feature of the illness. Most research into these cognitive deficits has focused on attention and memory, specifically abnormalities in sustained and selective attention, defective perceptual and cognitive processing resulting in slowed reaction times, and impaired encoding and retrieval processes manifesting as poor memory performance (40, 190). Impaired executive function is also an important cognitive deficit (190).

Following Kraepelin and Bleuler (12, 89), many psychiatrists have grouped the schizophrenias into paranoid, catatonic, hebephrenic, and simple types, depending on whether the predominant symptoms are delusions, bizarre motor behavior, disturbances in affect and associations, or social withdrawal and inadequacy. In practice, however, symptoms vary with time, so a patient may seem to fit several of the subclassifications during the course of his or her illness (13, 82). Attempts to identify delusions or hallucinations characteristic of good- or poor-prognosis cases have not been consistently successful (55).

Patients with schizophrenic disorders may display prominent alterations of mood, usually depression but sometimes euphoria, during the course of illness (133). Other affective symptoms—such as insomnia, anorexia, weight loss, alterations in interest and energy, impairment of mental concentration, guilt, and suicidal preoccupation—may also be present. In fact, a substantial proportion of patients with schizophrenia experience episodes of depression that symptomatically resemble those seen in primary major depression (3). Because the first-degree relatives of such patients do not appear to have an increased prevalence of affective disorders, their depression may be regarded as symptomatic of schizophrenia rather than the manifestation of a second illness.

The criteria for diagnosing schizophrenia according to *DSM-IV-TR* are presented in Table 3.1. Other criteria have been proposed (160) that overlap *DSM-IV-TR* in many ways but at the same time identify somewhat different populations of patients. This does not mean, however, that the situation is chaotic. Most patients identified by one set of criteria but not by another would be diagnosed as having "possible" or "suspected" schizophrenia by nearly all clinicians and investigators. Variations among different sets of criteria reflect differences in relative importance assigned to particular features with regard to differential diagnosis. In time further research should clarify these issues.

Biological Findings

Although schizophrenia is now generally accepted to be a "brain-based" illness, the exact etiology remains uncertain (40 65). The likelihood that the schizo-phrenias represent a collection of syndromes representing the end state of different biological pathways only complicates the scientific search for the source of the disorder (65, 190). Although neuropathology, neurochemistry, neuroimaging, and neurocognitive studies have demonstrated consistent types of brain abnormalities in schizophrenia, there is yet no laboratory test for schizophrenia (65). Despite demonstration of group differences for patients with schizophrenia compared to controls on many biologic measures, such differences are nonspecific, representing substantial overlap among other diagnostic groups and normal controls that preclude use of these abnormalities for clinical applications (65, 190).

Modern neuropathological methods have facilitated the investigation of brain pathology in schizophrenia (65). Postmortem brains of patients with schizophrenia show subtle macroscopic and microscopic differences from nonschizophrenic brains. Brain abnormalities most consistently demonstrated in schizophrenia are low brain weight and decreased cortical volume. The most remarkable reductions of brain tissue are found in the temporal lobe and its structures, the superior temporal gyrus, the hippocampus, the parahippo-campal gyrus, and the amygdala (65). These changes are more pronounced in gray matter than in white matter, and especially in the left hemisphere (65). A corresponding increased volume is found in the lateral and third ventricles, especially the right temporal horn of the lateral ventricle (65, 190). The amount of temporal volume reduction does not appear to correlate with increased ventricular size (187). Additionally, cortical and hippocampal neurons are small in size, neurons in prefrontal cortex and mediodorsal thalamus are reduced in number, and the density of Purkinje cells in the cerebellar vermis is diminished (65, 178, 190). Some, but not all, histopathology studies have described neurons in the hippocampus and entorhinal cortex to be relatively sparse and in disarray (57, 65, 66, 186). Gliosis is not a consistent brain finding in schizophrenia, suggesting, but not proving, a neurodevelopmental rather than degenerative hypothesis (65). A major methodological limitation of neuropathological studies is that first-episode and medication-naïve patients have generally not been included. Thus, some brain findings may represent artifacts of antipsychotic medication, illness chronicity, medical comorbidity, or smoking (66).

Brain imaging techniques—computerized tomography (CT), magnetic resonance imaging (MRI), positron emission tomography (PET), single photon emission computed tomography (SPECT), functional magnetic resonance imaging (fMRI), and magnetic resonance spectroscopy (MRS)—have opened new vistas into brain structure and function in schizophrenia. Brain imaging studes have confirmed the structural abnormalities identified in neuropathological studies and also demonstrated enlargement of the lateral and third ventricles, increased lateral ventricle-to-brain tissue ratio (VBR), and widened cortical sulci (35). Functional brain imaging techniques have identified "hypofrontality," or failure to activate the prefrontal dorsolateral cortex, during tasks of executive performance and working memory in schizophrenia (53, 190). Brain imaging studies have also found reduced thalamic volume and abnormalities in structure and function of the corpus callosum (15, 44, 103) and basal ganglia in schizophrenia (84, 170). Abnormalities also documented in the cerebellum in schizophrenia (74, 118) may contribute to disruptions in networks mediating communications between the cortex and cerebellum that are relayed through the thalamus (the cortico-cerebellar-thalalmic-cortical circuit) (4).

The increased ventricular size and hypofunctional frontal cortex identified in schizophrenia appear to be correlated with negative symptoms (blunted affect, amotivation, apathy, and anhedonia), poor prognosis, and cognitive impairment as demonstrated on standard neuropsychological tests (50, 141, 191). Positive symptoms such as thought disorder and auditory hallucinations are found to be selectively associated with reduced gray matter volume of the left posterior superior temporal gyrus and decreased metabolism in lateral temporal language areas (35, 65, 190). PET studies conducted in patients experiencing active auditory hallucinations have demonstrated increased cerebral blood flow to the Broca area of the left inferior frontal cortex, the anterior cingulate and medial temporal cortex, hippocampus and parahippocampal cortex, thalamus, inferior colliculus, and striatum; these are the brain areas involved in speech and auditory processing (106, 190).

Considerable evidence has accumulated implicating abnormalities in three neurotransmitter systems—the dopaminergic, serotonergic, and glutamatergic systems—in schizophrenia. Historically, the main neurochemical theory has been the "dopamine hypothesis" postulating hyperactivity of dopamine D_2 receptors in the mesencephalic projections to the limbic striatum (106). Both postmortem and PET studies have demonstrated increased dopamine D_2 levels in the brain in schizophrenia, especially in subcortical structures such as the striatum. Recent claims of a heritable abnormality in the catechol-O-methyl transferase (COMT) enzyme involved in dopamine metabolism in schizophrenia (69, 106) have not panned out in other research, as indicated by a recent meta-analysis (114). Accumulating research has revealed the dopamine hypothesis to be insufficiently comprehensive, and models of pathogenesis in schizophrenia have subsequently evolved into more diversified systems of complex circuitries involving several neurotransmitters (20, 87).

A "serotonin hypothesis" of schizophrenia is based on findings of abnormalities in cortical serotonin receptors, impairment of their activation in prefrontal cortex, and polymorphisms of serotonin receptor genes associated with schizophrenia (106). The evidence for a primary role of the serotonin syndrome in schizophrenia is not as strong as the evidence implicating the dopamine system (190). Because serotonergic and dopaminergic systems appear to be interdependent in the brain, it is not unexpected that studies would also find abnormal serotonergic function in schizophrenia.

A "glutamate hypothesis" of schizophrenia was suggested from evidence that antagonists at the N-methyl-D-aspartate (NMDA) receptor, such as phencyclidine and ketamine, can precipitate or increase psychotic symptoms (123, 124, 190). Excitatory effects at the NMDA receptor may be linked to damage to hippocampal and cortical neurons. Glutamate is the primary excitatory neurotransmitter in the brain, acting at the NMDA receptor. The glutamate system likely interacts with the dopamine system. Abnormal pruning of glutaminergic systems during neurodevelopmental periods is a hypothesized mechanism in the development of schizophrenia (32).

The possibility of a viral etiology for some cases of schizophrenia, based on findings of elevated antibody titers and reverse transcriptase in cerebrospinal fluid marking the presence of retrovirus, has attracted interest (95, 175, 193), but has not been proven.

Eye tracking dysfunction has been reported in 50%–80% of patients with schizophrenia and in 25%–40% of their unaffected relatives (100). Both smooth pursuit and anti-saccade functions are abnormal and appear to be interrelated. Eye tracking dysfunction is associated with frontal lobe dysfunction in schizophrenia, in both patients and unaffected relatives (194). Eye tracking dysfunction involves complex processes in many of the cortical and subcortical brain areas affected in schizophrenia, and it may represent an important component of the spectrum of manifestations associated with schizophrenia, including dysfunction in effortful cognitive processing (194).

Neurophysiology studies using event-related potentials and magnetoencephalographic fields have contributed to the understanding of temporally related aspects of cognition in schizophrenia. The amplitude of the auditory P300 component of event-related potentials—considered one of the most consistent biological markers of schizophrenia—is reduced in patients with the disorder (45, 80, 121). This abnormality of the auditory P300 appears to represent both a state and a trait marker, being associated not only with current symptom severity but also with indicators of disease progression and poor prognosis: gray matter volume deficits, negative symptoms, and cognitive impairment (45, 80). The P50 wave (generated from primary auditory cortex) and mismatch negativity (generated in prefrontal and superior temporal cortex) represent electrical indicators of early information processing and stimulus gating; consistently diminished amplitudes are seen in these measures in schizophrenia (80). Amplitudes of inhibitory event-related potentials indicating suppression of task-irrelevant auditory information are also reduced in schizophrenia (80).

It might be argued that specific brain abnormalities documented in schizophrenia may represent effects of chronic neuroleptic medication exposure. It is especially interesting that findings of ventricular enlargement (35, 188), hypofrontality (107, 154, 190), reduced hippocampal (35) and cerebellar vermis (74) volumes, excessive blood flow in the left globus pallidus, and increased subcortical D_2 dopamine receptors (69) have been demonstrated in young, first-episode, or never-medicated patients with the illness and are not associated with age, illness chronicity, duration of neuroleptic treatment, length of previous hospitalization, or the use of electroconvulsive therapy (35, 74). The evidence of brain abnormalities found early in the course of schizophrenia, without change over time, and unassociated with treatment, supports a primary disease process and negates concerns relating to a potential central role of long-term effects of antipsychotic medications and other treatments. The role of antipsychotic drug exposure in association with the increased caudate volume observed in schizophrenia is less clear, however. In never-medicated patients with schizophrenia, caudate volume was demonstrated to be decreased (35).

The biologic studies of the brain in schizophrenia reviewed here collectively indicate that the disorder is unlikely to be explained by any lesion in a single structure. Rather, widespread abnormalities in structures throughout the brain supporting many different cognitive and emotional processes appear to be involved (35). The primary disturbance appears to involve networks and communications involving many brain areas—prefrontal and temporal cortex, limbic regions, and basal ganglia (33, 65)—connections that ordinarily work together to enable cognitive processing and emotional and behavioral regulation.

Natural History

As chronic schizophrenia typically begins insidiously, it is often hard to determine when the disorder started. In retrospect, the majority of patients, but clearly not all, show certain prepsychotic personality abnormalities: excessive shyness, social awkwardness, withdrawal from personal relationships, and inability to form close relationships (the so-called "schizoid personality"). A parent put it this way: "He was always afraid to make friends and felt that other people wouldn't like him. He couldn't be comfortable with girls, never knew what to say. I'd try to help him but it was very hard to change him. He'd cry and say it made him too uncomfortable to be with others." These traits may be present from early adolescence; often they are of concern to the patient's family for months or years before delusions or hallucinations become manifest.

A number of studies have revealed an increased frequency of pregnancy and birth complications in the records of individuals who later developed schizophrenia (30, 52, 77, 126). In childhood and adolescence, long before the diagnostic symptoms of schizophrenia are evident, signs of neurodevelopmental problems may be evident among individuals who later develop schizophrenia. Prospective studies have provided considerable evidence that individuals at risk for schizophrenia or who are destined to develop the illness manifest early abnormalities. Compared to siblings and other controls, they evidence more neuromotor developmental delays in infancy, delayed speech milestones, difficulties in reading and spelling, problems with sustaining attention, academic difficulties, poor premorbid adjustment and abnormal social interactions, and schizophrenia spectrum traits in childhood and early adolescence (28, 35, 37, 38, 76, 115, 184). In studies of videotapes made long before the onset of schizophrenia, raters blind to the diagnosis of schizophrenia in the children identified more negative emotional expressions, thought dis-order, and negative symptoms in the children destined to develop schizo-phrenia than in their unaffected siblings (127, 185). Some authors consider neurocognitive difficulties to constitute core deficits that may be manifest early in the course of the illness (29, 90).

The peak period of onset of clinical problems that may be diagnosed as schizophrenia is in late adolescence and early adulthood. Delusions, hallucina-tions, and strange behavior usually become apparent in the late teens or 20s. At first, these aberrations may be brief and vague, leaving families uncertain of their significance. Gradually the symptoms become more obvious and dis-turbing, usually leading to psychiatric consultation. Onset before age 12 is uncommon; the early childhood-onset type appears to represent the same disorder seen in adults, although with a more severe course.

Schizophrenia infrequently begins after age 40. The illness generally has a fluctuating course. One or more psychiatric hospitalizations commonly occur. Some patients spend most of their lives in psychiatric hospitals, although this is far less common than in previous eras. Even when not hospitalized, people with this illness lead disturbed lives: They usually fail to form satisfactory personal relationships, marry less often than their contemporaries, have poor job his-tories, and seldom achieve positions of responsibility. They may become neigh-borhood eccentrics or socially isolated residents of inner cities, doing irregular unskilled work or being supported by welfare. Those who lack insight into their illness and who have comorbid substance abuse are particularly vulnerable to homelessness. Studies in large urban areas have found schizophrenia to be overrepresented among the homeless population, in the range of 5%–15% (43).

In recent years, clinicians and investigators have noted an increased fre-quency of drug and alcohol abuse and dependence, now evident in a significant proportion of their patients with schizophrenia (1). While self-medication may be a compelling explanation for the associated substance abuse, there is con-siderable evidence that people with schizophrenia use substances for the same reason and in the same manner as the general population (1). Not surprisingly, comorbid substance abuse makes the care of such patients much more difficult (34, 62). Integrated treatment is the standard of care for patients with comorbid schizophrenia and substance abuse (45, 195).

Two historic developments have dramatically altered the general clinical course in the treatment of schizophrenia: the introduction of antipsychotics and the shift away from prolonged hospitalization. With antipsychotics, sig-nificant control of hallucinations, delusions, and bizarre behavior is possible in a substantial number of cases. As a result, and because of the policy of early discharge, many patients spend far less time in psychiatric hospitals than was the case in earlier years, though rehospitalization for relatively brief periods is common. The more recent advent of the atypical antipsychotic medications, beginning with clozapine, targeted negative symptoms not substantially affected by traditional antipsychotics, allowing many patients with previously incapacitating functional deficits based on amotivation and apathy to achieve new levels of occupational and social functioning.

Good-prognosis cases generally begin more abruptly than poor-prognosis cases, without a history of long-standing personality abnormalities. Although poor- and good-prognosis cases may differ somewhat clinically, the most important difference relates to outcome (8, 78). When patients are seen for the first time, it may be difficult to predict what the course and prognosis will be. Several studies have identified criteria associated with the difference in prognosis among the schizophrenic disorders. Table 3.2 summarizes the data from these studies. When most of the criteria are present, the prognosis associated with the criteria will be accurate in the majority of cases. These criteria appear to be more predictive when the diagnosis of schizophrenia includes a broader range of disorders than are contained in established diagnostic criteria, however (64). This may indicate only that the criteria help distinguish true schizophrenia from other disorders—such as psychotic affective illness and acute intoxications—that can mimic schizophrenia.

Some patients presenting with an acute schizophrenic picture lose their psychotic features during hospitalization and their symptoms then take on a depressive appearance; others recover from the psychotic episode and then after a prolonged remission present with typical depression (146). These observations are of great theoretical interest. Some have interpreted them to suggest

TABLE 3.2 Predictors of Good- and Poor-Prognosis Cases

	Good Prognosis	Poor Prognosis
Mode of onset	Acute	Insidious
Precipitating events	Frequently reported	Usually not reported
Prepsychotic history	Good	Poor; frequent history of "schizoid" traits (aloofness, social isolation)
Confusion	Often present	Usually absent
Affective symptoms	Often present and prominent	Often absent or minimal; affective responses usually "blunted" or "flat"
Marital status	Usually married	Often single, especially males
Family history of affective disorder	Often present	May be present but less likely
Family history of schizophrenia	Absent or rare	Increased

that the distinction between schizophrenic and mood disorders may be too arbitrary (146); others, emphasizing the familial prevalence of mood disorders in the overlapping cases, have argued that such cases are more appropriately classified as mood disorders (163, 180).

In the past, an apparent absence of rheumatoid arthritis in patients suffering from schizophrenia has been noted. This observation was based on long psychiatric hospitalizations and clinical records often extending over many decades. Recently, this question has received renewed attention in the hope that it may lead to new ideas about the etiology or pathogenesis of schizophrenia (122, 177).

Complications

In no illness is it more difficult to distinguish between the typical clinical picture and the complications than in chronic schizophrenia. For example, difficulties in school or at work are common features of schizophrenia. Yet it is usually hard to tell whether these problems arise because of the patient's disordered thinking or loss of motivation, or whether they result from the reactions of teachers, fellow students and workers, or supervisors to the patient's abnormal behavior.

Suspicious, fearful, and deluded individuals may not perform well in school or at work because of preoccupation with abnormal thoughts; at the same time, withdrawn, preoccupied, and unresponsive students may draw criticism and other adverse responses from teachers and supervisors. These, in turn, will reinforce the individuals' pathological behaviors. The definition of the disorder encompasses its natural history and at the same time specifies the complications. These include impaired education, poor work history and job achievement, celibacy, and prolonged psychiatric hospitalization. Increased risk of suicide among young patients also appears to be a complication.

Because chronic schizophrenia typically begins early in life and is characterized by recurrent or persistent manifestations, the patient's schooling and education suffer. Early school difficulties have been noted, but even among those who do well in elementary school, difficulties may arise in high school or college. Social withdrawal and loss of interest in studies may become evident. These changes coupled with the need to leave school at the onset of more dramatic symptoms eventually lead to dropping out of school in many cases. If the illness peaks after the completion of formal education, the same clinical features may lead to marked reduction of effectiveness at work, demotions, being fired, frequent job changes, and financial dependency. Men with schizophrenia are less likely to marry, presumably because male initiative is more important than female initiative in getting married. Thus, schizophrenia in a man might reduce his success in courtship, whereas schizophrenia in a woman might not keep her from attracting a suitor. With the advent of modern drug treatment and the reduction in prolonged psychiatric hospitalization, marriage and childbearing rates in schizophrenia have approached those of the general population, though the sex differences persist (116, 117).

Despite the great reduction in chronic psychiatric hospitalization of patients with schizophrenia, no other illness results in more time spent in psychiatric hospitals. Hospitalization is usually for repeated, relatively brief periods, but a few patients spend many years in hospitals.

A common fear regarding deluded patients with schizophrenia is that they are likely to act on their delusions and commit crimes. Available data suggest, however, that there is only a modestly increased risk of significant crimes committed by individuals with this illness (119). They may be arrested for vagrancy, disturbing the peace, or similar misdemeanors, but only rarely are they involved in serious or violent felonies.

Approximately 1 out of 20 people with schizophrenia will eventually commit suicide (130). The most vulnerable time is during proximity to illness onset, often following discharge from a hospital inpatient stay. A recent systematic review found that suicide risk in schizophrenia is related less to the core psychotic symptoms of the illness and more to depressive symptoms, agitation, motor restlessness, and awareness of effects of the illness on cognitive functioning (68). Additionally, previous suicide attempts, recent loss, poor adherence to treatment, and drug misuse were identified as risk factors. Presence of hallucinations was actually associated with decreased risk of suicide, and command hallucinations did not confer increased risk. Social support, positive coping skills, life satisfaction, and cooperation with treatment appear to be protective against the potential for suicide in schizophrenia (111).

Family and Genetic Studies

Schizophrenia has increased prevalence among the close relatives of patients with schizophrenia (87). Most studies have indicated a prevalence of about 5%–10% among first-degree relatives of index cases compared with a general population figure of just less than 1%. Prevalence of schizophrenia increases with closeness of relationship to a family member with schizophrenia (58).

A series of twin studies reported over a 70-year period (Table 3.3) provides overwhelming evidence of significantly higher concordance rates for

TABLE 3.3 Schizophrenia Concordance Rates in Twins

	MZ Twins		DZ Twins (Same Sex)	
Investigator(s)	"Strict" Schizophrenia (%)	Including "Borderline" cases (%)	"Strict" Schizophrenia (%)	Including "Borderline" cases (%)
Luxenberger, 1928 (Germany) (98)	50	71	0	0
Rosanoff et al., 1934 (USA) (138)	44	61	9	13
Essen-Möller, 1941 (Sweden) (39)	14	71	8	17
Kallmann, 1941 (USA) (79)		69		17
Slater and Shields, 1953 (UK) (152)		65		14
Inouye, 1963 (Japan) (75)		60		18
Tienari, 1963 (Finland) (172)	6	31	5	5
Kringlen, 1964 (Norway) (91)	25		16	
Kringlen, 1966 (Norway) (92)	28	38	6	14
Gottesman and Shields, 1966 (UK) (60)	42	54	9	18
Kringlen, 1968 (Norway) (93)	25	38	4	10
Fischer et al., 1969 (Denmark) (42)	24	40	10	19
Allen et al., 1972 (USA) (2)		27		5
Tienari, 1975 (Finland) (171)				
pairwise method	15		7	
proband method	33		14	
Kendler and Robinette, 1983 (USA) (83)		31		7
Onstad et al., 1991 (Norway) (125)	33		1	
pairwise method	48		4	
proband method				

continued

TABLE 3.3 (Continued)

Investigator(s)	MZ Twins		DZ Twins (Same Sex)	
	"Strict" Schizophrenia (%)	Including "Borderline" cases (%)	"Strict" Schizophrenia (%)	Including "Borderline" cases (%)
Tsujita et al., 1992 (181)		50		14
Kläning, 1996 (Denmark) (88)	44		11	
Cannon et al., 1998 (Finland) (16)		46		9
Franzek and Beckman, 1998 (Germany) (49)	46		17	
pairwise method	61		24	
proband method				
Cardno et al., 1999 (England) (19)	39		5	

Adapted from Fischer et al. (42), Allen et al. (2), Sullivan (164), Kringlen (94), and Cardno and Gottesman (18).

schizophrenia among monozygotic twins than among dizygotic twins of the same sex (2, 16, 19, 39, 42, 49, 60, 61, 75, 79, 83, 88, 91–93, 98, 125, 138, 152, 171, 172, 181). The prevalence of schizophrenia among dizygotic twins is only slightly higher than the prevalence among ordinary siblings of the same sex (94). Although the actual concordance rates varied from study to study, probably depending on methods of ascertainment (18, 94, 164), the rate for monozygotic twins was generally three to six times that of dizygotic twins. The heritability of schizophrenia, the proportion of variance in risk explained by genetic effects, has consistently been found in a fairly narrow range of 80%–86% (18, 87, 129, 164, 179).

The failure to find complete concordance in monozygotic twins has naturally led to the conclusion that there must be important environmental factors in the etiology of schizophrenia (94). A recent review of twin studies of genetic and environmental contributors to schizophrenia found consistent evidence of joint or shared environmental influences on liability to schizophrenia, estimated at 11% (164). Often such environmental factors are assumed to be of a social or psychological nature. However, environmental factors may include a variety of profoundly biological processes, such as insults to the developing brain, particularly during fetal development or birth, teratogens and other intrauterine factors, toxins, and nutritional factors (30, 52, 77, 126, 164).

Because the environments of twins are most similar during gestation and infancy and then tend to diverge with time resulting in the largest differences by the time of adulthood, this suggests that the environmental influences in liability to schizophrenia most likely occur early in life (164). Further, evidence from twin studies indicates that differences in social environment of monozygotic twins are more representative of a consequence rather than a cause of their behavioral differences (94). The observation that as discordant monozygotic twins are followed, many pairs become concordant (9) suggests that the age of onset may in some cases be affected by nongenetic factors.

Adoption studies provide more specific evidence untangling genetic from environmental factors (63). The first adoption study of schizophrenia, an American study, examined children separated early in life from parents with schizophrenia and raised by unrelated adoptive parents. Schizophrenia was found in 5 of 47 children of hospitalized schizophrenic mothers and no cases were found in 50 control children (71). In a second study, carried out in Denmark, 32% of the children of schizophrenic parents received a diagnosis in the "schizophrenia spectrum," compared to 18% of controls (139). It is unclear how many would be considered schizophrenic in the "narrow" sense. "Schizophrenia spectrum" refers to a range of disorders, including schizophrenia, affective and atypical psychoses, and personality disorders that appear to cluster in certain families. The most recent study comparing adopted-away children of biological parents with and without schizophrenia found 13 cases of schizophrenia among 144 adopted-away children of biological parents with schizophrenia, but only 2 cases of schizophrenia among 178 adopted-away children of biological matched control parents without schizophrenia (173). In 1968, Kety conducted adoption studies of schizophrenia in Copenhagen by starting with schizophrenic adoptees and examining the prevalence of schizophrenia in their biological relatives in comparison with biological relatives of control adoptees. Chronic schizophrenia was observed in 6% of the relatives of adoptees with schizophrenia but only in 1% of relatives of controls; a schizophrenia-like "latent schizophrenia" condition was observed in 15% of biological relatives of adoptees with schizophrenia and only 1% of biological relatives of controls. Replication of this work in 1994 yielded similar findings (85).

Another Danish study approached the problem of hereditary predisposition to schizophrenia in a different way. Monozygotic twin pairs were identified in which one twin was schizophrenic and the other was not. The children of these discordant twins were studied. It was found that the frequency of schizophrenia was the same in children of nonaffected discordant schizophrenic twins as in children of affected members of discordant twin pairs (41). A follow-up study of this same cohort 18 years later by Gottesman and

Bertelsen (59) confirmed the original study's findings, detecting schizophrenia in 17% of offspring of both affected and nonaffected twins at follow-up. The findings were strikingly different in the offspring of dizygotic twin pairs discordant for schizophrenia: 17% of the offspring of the affected twins had schizophrenia compared to only 2% of the offspring of the unaffected twins. The authors concluded that a schizophrenic genotype or diathesis may not be expressed unless it is accompanied by critical nonfamilial, environmental factors. The results of all these investigations point to the likelihood of a hereditary predisposition to at least some schizophrenic illnesses.

A frequent problem in studies of the familial distribution of psychiatric disorders is the failure to examine both parents of index cases. As a result, puzzling familial associations between different disorders may be observed. For example, in the adoption studies of schizophrenia described earlier, anti-social personality disorders have been found to be associated with schizo-phrenia. This could possibly indicate that antisocial behavior can be one of the manifestations of schizophrenia, but an equally likely explanation is a tendency for some individuals with schizophrenia to mate with individuals manifesting other psychiatric disorders, especially antisocial personality (46–48, 131, 159).

Family studies have investigated the concept of a familial schizophrenia spectrum, which dates to observations by Kraepelin that many family members of patients with schizophrenia who do not have schizophrenia appear to have long-standing, schizophrenia-like characteristics (18). Studies examining co-aggregation and comorbidity in families have suggested a relationship between schizophrenia and other psychotic disorders and certain personality disorders, such as schizotypal personality disorder, among biological relatives (18, 81, 94). Several studies have shown a familial and even a genetic relation-ship between schizophrenia and schizotypal personality, thus supporting the validity of a familial schizophrenia-spectrum concept (105, 166, 174). Schizotypal personality, described in *DSM-IV-TR*, includes many of the chronic personality features seen in schizophrenia but does not include delusions or hallucinations.

From time to time, case reports have been published describing both schizophrenia and bipolar affective disorder in the same family (134, 134). The significance of these observations is uncertain because of the possibility of the two conditions occurring together by chance alone. Prior research suggests that the prevalence of mood disorders is increased in close relatives of good-prognosis cases. One interpretation given these data is that at least some good-prognosis cases are atypical forms of mood disorders (136). Recent reviews have described a growing literature suggesting partial overlap in family susceptibility for schizophrenia and bipolar disorder (11, 99, 108). Research excluding patients with schizoaffective disorder, however, has demonstrated familial independence of schizophrenia and bipolar disorder (155), and inadvertent misclassification of affective illness as schizophrenia in relatives may contribute to appearance of familial co-segregation (113).

The recognition that schizophrenic disorders are familial and that they probably result in part from hereditary factors has focused attention on identifying at an early age those individuals within a vulnerable family who are at greatest risk of developing the clinical disorders. Such "high-risk" studies have been ongoing in many countries (17, 63, 72, 105, 128). One of the first studies, conducted in Denmark (147), found the risk of schizophrenia during a 10-year follow-up of 10- to 20-year-old children of mothers with schizophrenia to be about eight times greater than in matched control children. Other high-risk studies have identified more attention problems, delinquency, intellectual functioning and memory impairment, affective deficits, delinquency, and social underdevelopment among high-risk children compared to controls (63).

The search for genetic markers cosegregating with schizophrenia has produced numerous genetic linkage scans. The findings of these studies have implicated regions on more than half of the 23 chromosomes. Replication of these findings has not come easily (63), but a recent meta-analysis concluded "with considerable confidence" (p. 44) that schizophrenia susceptibility loci likely exist in most of these chromosomal regions (96). The strongest evidence for linkage to susceptibility loci lies within chromosomes 6p, 8p, 10p, and 22q; other areas of interest have been identified on 5q, 13q, and 18p (63). The most convincing susceptibility gene candidate for schizophrenia to date maps to chromosome 6p, with a total of eight published replication studies for this entity (120). Combined family and genetic evidence to date, however, suggests that no single gene or gene locus will account for the illness in a substantial proportion of cases, and that genetic liability to schizophrenia is likely polygenic (99).

Differential Diagnosis

A small number of patients hospitalized for depression will, at follow-up, be found to be suffering from chronic schizophrenia (137). This is much more likely to be the case when the depression is accompanied by striking delusions or hallucinations. Some patients who present with the symptoms of somatization disorder will show at follow-up the full clinical picture of chronic schizophrenia (192), but this too is infrequent.

Obsessional disorder, early in its course, occasionally is difficult to distinguish from schizophrenia. If the obsessions are bizarre or if the patient clearly does not have insight into the abnormal nature of his or her thoughts and impulses, it may not be possible to make a confident diagnosis. The risk of schizophrenia in patients with obsessional disorder is small after the first year or two of illness and when the obsessions are classical (56).

A clinical picture resembling schizophrenia has been described in association with complex partial seizure disorder (14). This clinical picture may be indistinguishable from typical schizophrenia in individual cases, but the absence of a higher prevalence of schizophrenia in their close relatives suggests that it is a separate entity. Other features of the clinical presentation, such as soft or hard neurological signs, history of seizures, olfactory and somatosensory hallucinations, absence episodes, automatisms, EEG focal abnormalities especially on the left side, and MRI evidence of temporal-limbic lesions, are suggestive of complex partial seizure disorder.

Although many good-prognosis cases of schizophrenia are probably manifestations of affective illness, the question of differential diagnosis is often one of diagnostic conventions or style. Certain delusions (those of poverty, sinfulness, disease) are common in depression, and others (those of overconfidence and unusual powers) in mania. Delusions of control, persecution, and depersonalization are more likely to present as part of illness eventually to be declared as schizophrenia.

The differential diagnosis of good-prognosis illness and brain syndrome may also at times be a matter of convention. If disorientation and memory impairment are transient and less striking than the delusions, hallucinations, and bizarre behavior, a diagnosis of schizophrenia may be made. Patients with systemic medical illnesses affecting the brain such as lupus erythematosus may develop psychiatric symptoms that vary over time from those of depression to those of a brain syndrome, with a schizophrenic picture in between. Most patients with brain syndromes, however, present no problem in differential diagnosis. Even when striking delusions and hallucinations are present, the persistent disorientation and memory impairment point to the correct diagnosis.

Persistent alcoholic hallucinosis is a syndrome of striking hallucinations, chiefly auditory, with a clear sensorium, following alcohol withdrawal. It may occur either after other withdrawal symptoms have subsided or in the absence of other manifestations of withdrawal. Alcoholic hallucinosis usually subsides within a couple of weeks. Occasionally, it persists and becomes chronic, resembling schizophrenia. Family studies of alcoholic hallucinosis have attempted to determine whether the prevalence of schizophrenia in close relatives is increased (suggesting that the alcoholism precipitated or was superimposed on typical schizophrenia) or the same (suggesting that, like epilepsy, alco-holism may produce a "symptomatic schizophrenia"). The findings are contra-dictory and the issue remains unresolved (156).

Amphetamines and cocaine, taken chronically in large quantities, can cause a schizophrenia-like illness (22, 23, 157), and they are responsible for a substantial percentage of cases of acute psychosis seen in emergency depart-ments or admitted to psychiatric hospitals. This psychotic state almost always subsides within 10–14 days after the drug is discontinued. In rare chronic cases, the situation is similar to that seen in chronic alcoholic hallucinosis, in which it is uncertain which came first—the drug abuse or the schizophrenic disorder (149).

Other psychotomimetic drugs such as LSD and PCP can cause acute psy-chotic states that may be indistinguishable from naturally occurring schizophrenia on initial assessment (112, 140). Patients with chronic schizophrenia may also suffer acute intensification of the illness as the result of using these drugs.

Clinical Management

Antipsychotic medication has become the keystone of standard treatment for schizophrenia. A policy of early discharge from psychiatric hospitals was made possible in part by antipsychotic medications, beginning with chlorpromazine in the 1950s. The first-generation medications, such as haloperidol and thior-idazine, dramatically helped reduce positive symptoms of schizophrenia such as delusions, hallucinations, and bizarre behavior, but they were not particu-larly effective for negative symptoms such as amotivation and emotional and social withdrawal. These antipsychotic medications are classified in relation to their potency, and the prescribed doses are inversely proportional to potency. The high-potency medications are most likely to cause extrapyramidal side effects such as rigidity, dystonic reactions, akathisia, and tremor, and the low-potency medications are associated with more sedation and autonomic side effects. Anticholinergic effects of some of these medications as well as antic-holinergic medications used to remedy extrapyramidal side effects may further contribute to cognitive problems in schizophrenia (26, 151).

The advent of newer "atypical" or second-generation antipsychotic medica-tion beginning with clozapine in the 1990s further improved treatment of schizophrenia and for the first time targeted negative symptoms as well as being equally effective for positive symptoms. These medications (e.g., risper-idone, olanzapine, and quetiapine) are "atypical" because they act at serotonin as well as dopamine D_2 receptors, and as a result are less likely to produce extrapyramidal side effects (26, 143). Unwelcome side effects may occur with these agents, such as sedation, hypotension, seizures, weight gain, and hyperglycemia and other features of metabolic syndrome (26, 151).

Patients vary considerably in their metabolism of these medications, and therefore individualization of dosage is indicated. Larger doses are usually needed during acute exacerbations but may be reduced as the patient's symptoms abate. Clozapine may be particularly effective for refractory illness and for suicidal ideation (151). Long-acting depot formulations of some of these medications have helped the problem of unsatisfactory treatment adherence that can result from lack of insight into the illness that is often present in schizophrenia (51). Some patients may also benefit from the use of the calming properties of benzodiazepines in addition to neuroleptics (161). Occasionally, the combination of antipsychotics and electroconvulsive treatments produces better results than antipsychotics alone (24, 25, 167, 168). There is no evidence that any psychosocial intervention is effective in the absence of pharmacologic treatment (151).

Antipsychotic drugs do not control all schizophrenic symptoms. Patients continue to suffer from intermittent delusions and hallucinations, personality changes, and general social impairment. Many experienced clinicians believe, though, that the reduction in chronic hospitalization and the greater efforts at rehabilitation resulting from increased optimism about more effective treatment prevent some personality deterioration. The return of patients with chronic schizophrenia to the community is not without problems. Many, if not most, of these patients are not able to support themselves financially and require family or community help. Although patients may improve with drug treatment, most continue to experience symptoms and their adjustment to family life is difficult and stressful. Patients may be severely burdensome to their families. Case management programs can reduce the family burden and have been shown to enhance standard treatment effectiveness.

REFERENCES

1. Akerele, E. O., and Levin, F. R. Substance abuse among patients with schizophrenia. J. Psychiat. Pract., 8:70–80, 2002.
2. Allen, M. G., Cohen, S., and Pollin, W. Schizophrenia in veteran twins: a diagnostic review. Am. J. Psychiat., 128:939–945, 1972.
3. an der Heiden, W., Konnecke, R., Maurer, K., Ropeter, D., and Hafner, H. Depression in the long-term course of schizophrenia. Eur. Arch. Psychiat. Clin. Neurosci., 255:174–184, 2005.

4. Andreasen, N. C. A unitary model of schizophrenia: Bleuler's "fragmented phrene" as schizencephaly. Arch. Gen. Psychiat., 56:781–787, 1999.

5. Aro, S., Aro, H., and Keskimaki, I. Socio-economic mobility among patients with schizophrenia or major affective disorder. A 17-year retrospective follow-up. Br. J. Psychiat., 166:759–767, 1995.

6. Aslokangas, R. R. K. Social class of the parents of schizophrenic patients. Proceedings of the 18th Nordic Psychiatric Congress. Acta Psychiat. Scand., 54:30, 1976.

7. Baethge, C., Baldessarini, R. J., Freudenthal, K., Streeruwitz, A., Bauer, M., and Bschor, T. Hallucinations in bipolar disorder: characteristics and comparison to unipolar depression and schizophrenia. Bipolar Disord., 7:136–145, 2005.

8. Bailer, J., Brauer, W., and Rey, E. R. Premorbid adjustment as predictor of outcome in schizophrenia: results of a prospective study. Acta Psychiat. Scand., 93:368–377, 1996.

9. Belmaker, R., Pollin, W., Wyatt, R. J., and Cohen, S. A follow-up of monozygotic twins discordant for schizophrenia. Arch. Gen. Psychiat., 30:219–222, 1974.

10. Berman, I., Viegner, B., Merson, A., Allan, E., Pappas, D., and Green, A. I. Differential relationships between positive and negative symptoms and neuropsychological deficits in schizophrenia. Schizophr. Res., 25:1–10, 1997.

11. Berrettini, W. Evidence for shared susceptibility in bipolar disorder and schizophrenia. Am. J. Med. Genet. C Semin. Med. Genet., 123:59–64, 2003.

12. Bleuler, E. *Dementia Praecox or the Group of Schizophrenias*, Zinkin, J. trans. New York: International Universities Press, 1950.

13. Brenner, D. *Elementary Textbook of Psychoanalysis*. New York: International Universities Press, 1955.

14. Brewerton, T. D. The phenomenology of psychosis associated with complex partial seizure disorder. Ann. Clin. Psychiat., 9:31–51, 1997.

15. Busatto, G. F., and Kerwin, R. W. Schizophrenia, psychosis, and the basal ganglia. Psychiat. Clin. N. Am., 20:897–910, 1997.

16. Cannon, T. D., Kaprio, J., Lonnqvist, J., Huttunen, M., and Koskenvuo, M. The genetic epidemiology of schizophrenia in a Finnish twin cohort. A population-based modeling study. Arch. Gen. Psychiat., 55:67–74, 1998.

17. Cannon, T. D., and Mednick, S. A. The schizophrenia high-risk project in Copenhagen: three decades of progress. Acta Psychiat. Scand. Suppl., 370:33–47, 1993.

18. Cardno, A. G., and Gottesman, I. I. Twin studies of schizophrenia: from bow-and-arrow concordances to star wars Mx and functional genomics. Am. J. Med. Genet., 97:12–17, 2000.

19. Cardno, A. G., Marshall, E. J., Coid, B., Macdonald, A. M., Ribchester, T. R., Davies, N. J., Venturi, P., Jones, L. A., Lewis, S. W., Sham, P. C., Gottesman, I. I., Farmer, A. E., McGuffin, P., Reveley, A. M., and Murray, R. M. Heritability estimates for psychotic disorders: the Maudsley twin psychosis series. Arch. Gen. Psychiat., 56:162–168, 1999.

20. Carlsson, A., Hansson, L. O., Waters, N., and Carlsson, M. L. A glutamatergic deficiency model of schizophrenia. Br. J. Psychiat. Suppl., 37:2–6, 1999.

21. Castrogiovanni, P., Iapichino, S., Pacchierotti, C., and Pieraccini, F. Season of birth in psychiatry. A review. Neuropsychobiol., 37:175–181, 1998.

22. Caton, C. L., Drake, R. E., Hasin, D. S., Dominguez, B., Shrout, P. E., Samet, S., and Schanzer, B. Differences between early-phase primary psychotic disorders with concurrent substance use and substance-induced psychoses. Arch. Gen. Psychiat., 62:137–145, 2005.

23. Caton, C. L., Samet, S., and Hasin, D. S. When acute-stage psychosis and substance use co-occur: differentiating substance-induced and primary psychotic disorders. J. Psychiat. Pract., 6:256–266, 2000.

24. Chanpattana, W. Maintenance ECT in treatment-resistant schizophrenia. J. Med. Assoc. Thai., 83:657–662, 2000.

25. Chanpattana, W., Chakrabhand, M. L., Kongsakon, R., Techakasem, P., and Buppanharun, W. Short-term effect of combined ECT and neuroleptic therapy in treatment-resistant schizophrenia. J. ECT, 15:129–139, 1999.

26. Citrome, L., and Volavka, J. The promise of atypical antipsychotics: fewer side effects mean enhanced compliance and improved functioning. Postgrad. Med., 116:49–63, 2004.

27. Cooper, B. Schizophrenia, social class and immigrant status: the epidemiological evidence. Epidemiol. Psichiatr. Soc., 14:137–144, 2005.

28. Cornblatt, B., Obuchowski, M., Roberts, S., Pollack, S., and Erlenmeyer-Kimling, L. Cognitive and behavioral precursors of schizophrenia. Dev. Psychopathol., 11:487–508, 1999.

29. Crawford, J. R., Besson, J. A., Bremner, M., Ebmeier, K. P., Cochrane, R. H., and Kirkwood, K. Estimation of premorbid intelligence in schizophrenia. Br. J. Psychiat., 161:69–74, 1992.

30. Dalman, C., Allebeck, P., Cullberg, J., Grunewald, C., and Koster, M. Obstetric complications and the risk of schizophrenia: a longitudinal study of a national birth cohort. Arch. Gen. Psychiat., 56:234–240, 1999.

31. Davidson, L., and McGlashan, T. H. The varied outcomes of schizophrenia. Can. J. Psychiat., 42:34–43, 1997.

32. Deakin, J. F., and Simpson, M. D. A two-process theory of schizophrenia: evidence from studies in post-mortem brain. J. Psychiat. Res., 31:277–295, 1997.

33. Dean, B. Understanding the pathology of schizophrenia: recent advances from the study of the molecular architecture of postmortem CNS tissue. Postgrad. Med. J., 78:142–148, 2002.

34. Drake, R. E., Osher, F. C., Noordsy, D. L., Hurlbut, S. C., Teague, G. B., and Beaudett, M. S. Diagnosis of alcohol use disorders in schizophrenia. Schizophr. Bull., 16:57–67, 1990.

35. Drevets, W. C., Botteron, K., and Barch, D. M. Neuroimaging in psychiatry. In *Adult Psychiatry*, 2nd edition, Rubin, E. H., Zorumski, C. F. (eds.). Malden, MA: Blackwell, pp. 45–75, 2005.

36. Dunham, H. W. *Community and Schizophrenia*. Detroit: Wayne State University Press, 1965.

37. Ellison, Z., van Os, J., and Murray, R. Special feature: childhood personality characteristics of schizophrenia: manifestations of, or risk factors for, the disorder? J. Personal. Disord., 12:247–261, 1998.

38. Erlenmeyer-Kimling, L., Rock, D., Roberts, S. A., Janal, M., Kestenbaum, C., Cornblatt, B., Adamo, U. H., and Gottesman, I. I. Attention, memory, and motor skills as childhood predictors of schizophrenia-related psychoses: the New York High-Risk Project. Am. J. Psychiat., 157:1416–1422, 2000.

39. Essen-Möller, E. *Psychiatrische Untersuchungen an einer Serie von Zwillingen.* Copenhagen: Ejnar Munksgaard, 1941.

40. Fioravanti, M., Carlone, O., Vitale, B., Cinti, M. E., and Clare, L. A meta-analysis of cognitive deficits in adults with a diagnosis of schizophrenia. Neuropsychol. Rev., 15:73–95, 2005.

41. Fischer, M. Psychoses in the offspring of schizophrenic monozygotic twins and their normal co-twins. Br. J. Psychiat., 118:43–52, 1971.

42. Fischer, M., Harvald, B., and Hauge, M. A Danish twin study of schizophrenia. Br. J. Psychiat., 115:981–990, 1969.

43. Folsom, D., and Jeste, D. V. Schizophrenia in homeless persons: a systematic review of the literature. Acta Psychiat. Scand., 105:404–413, 2002.

44. Foong, J., Maier, M., Clark, C. A., Barker, G. J., Miller, D. H., and Ron, M. A. Neuropathological abnormalities of the corpus callosum in schizophrenia: a diffusion tensor imaging study. J. Neurol. Neurosurg. Psychiat., 68:242–244, 2000.

45. Ford, J. M. Schizophrenia: the broken P300 and beyond. Psychophysiol., 36:667–682, 1999.

46. Fowler, R. C., and Tsuang, M. T. Spouses of schizophrenics: a blind comparative study. Compr. Psychiat., 16:339–342, 1975.

47. Fowler, R. C., Tsuang, M. T., and Cadoret, R. J. Parental psychiatric illness associated with schizophrenia in the siblings of schizophrenics. Compr. Psychiat., 18:271–275, 1977.

48. Fowler, R. C., Tsuang, M. T., and Cadoret, R. J. Psychiatric illness in the offspring of schizophrenics. Compr. Psychiat., 18:127–134, 1977.

49. Franzek, E., and Beckmann, H. Different genetic background of schizophrenia spectrum psychoses: a twin study. Am. J. Psychiat., 155:76–83, 1998.

50. Frodl, T., Meisenzahl, E. M., Muller, D., Greiner, J., Juckel, G., Leinsinger, G., Hahn, H., Moller, H. J., and Hegerl, U. Corpus callosum and P300 in schizophrenia. Schizophr. Res., 49:107–119, 2001.

51. Gaebel, W., Janssen, B., and Riesbeck, M. Modern treatment concepts in schizophrenia. Pharmacopsychiat., 36 Suppl 3:S168–S175, 2003.

52. Geddes, J. R., Verdoux, H., Takei, N., Lawrie, S. M., Bovet, P., Eagles, J. M., Heun, R., McCreadie, R. G., McNeil, T. F., O'Callaghan, E., Stober, G., Willinger, U., and Murray, R. M. Schizophrenia and complications of pregnancy and labor: an individual patient data meta-analysis. Schizophr. Bull., 25:413–423, 1999.

53. Glahn, D. C., Ragland, J. D., Abramoff, A., Barrett, J., Laird, A. R., Bearden, C. E., and Velligan, D. I. Beyond hypofrontality: a quantitative meta-analysis of

functional neuroimaging studies of working memory in schizophrenia. Hum. Brain Mapp., 25:60–69, 2005.

54. Goldberg, E. M., and Morrison, S. L. Schizophrenia and social class. Br. J. Psychiat., 109:785–802, 1963.

55. Goodwin, D. W., Alderson, P., and Rosenthal, R. Clinical significance of hallucinations in psychiatric disorders. Arch. Gen. Psychiat., 24:76–80, 1971.

56. Goodwin, D. W., Guze, S. B., and Robins, E. Follow-up studies in obsessional neurosis. Arch. Gen. Psychiat., 20:182–187, 1969.

57. Gothelf, D., Soreni, N., Nachman, R. P., Tyano, S., Hiss, Y., Reiner, O., and Weizman, A. Evidence for the involvement of the hippocampus in the pathophysiology of schizophrenia. Eur. Neuropsychopharmacol., 10:389–395, 2000.

58. Gottesman, I. I. *Schizophrenia Genesis: The Origins of Madness.* New York: Freeman, 1991.

59. Gottesman, I. I., and Bertelsen, A. Confirming unexpressed genotypes for schizophrenia. Risks in the offspring of Fischer's Danish identical and fraternal discordant twins. Arch. Gen. Psychiat., 46:867–872, 1989.

60. Gottesman, I. I., and Shields, J. Contributions of twin studies to perspectives in schizophrenia. Vol. 3. In *Progress in Experimental Personality Research*, Maher, B. A. (ed.). New York: Academic Press, pp. 1–84, 1966.

61. Gottesman, I. I., and Shields, J. *Schizophrenia: The Epigenetic Puzzle.* Cambridge: Cambridge University Press, 1982.

62. Haddock, G., Barrowclough, C., Tarrier, N., Moring, J., O'Brien, R., Schofield, N., Quinn, J., Palmer, S., Davies, L., Lowens, I., McGovern, J., and Lewis, S. Cognitive-behavioural therapy and motivational intervention for schizophrenia and substance misuse. 18-month outcomes of a randomised controlled trial. Br. J. Psychiat., 183:418–426, 2003.

63. Hallmayer, J. The epidemiology of the genetic liability for schizophrenia. Aust. N. Z. J. Psychiat., 34 Suppl:S47–S55, 2000.

64. Hanson, D. R., Gottesman, I. I., and Heston, L. L. Some possible childhood indicators of adult schizophrenia inferred from children of schizophrenics. Br. J. Psychiat., 129:142–154, 1976.

65. Harrison, P. J. The neuropathology of schizophrenia. A critical review of the data and their interpretation. Brain, 122:593–624, 1999.

66. Harrison, P. J. The hippocampus in schizophrenia: a review of the neuropathological evidence and its pathophysiological implications. Psychopharmacol. (Berl)., 174:151–162, 2004.

67. Harrow, M., and Jobe, T. H. Factors involved in outcome and recovery in schizophrenia patients not on antipsychotic medications: a 15-year multifollow-up study. J. Nerv. Ment. Dis., 195:406–414, 2007.

68. Hawton, K., Sutton, L., Haw, C., Sinclair, J., and Deeks, J. J. Schizophrenia and suicide: systematic review of risk factors. Br. J. Psychiat., 187:9–20, 2005.

69. Heinz, A., Romero, B., Gallinat, J., Juckel, G., and Weinberger, D. R. Molecular brain imaging and the neurobiology and genetics of schizophrenia. Pharmacopsychiat., 36 Suppl 3:S152–S157, 2003.

70. Helldin, L., Kane, J. M., Karilampi, U., Norlander, T., and Archer, T. Remission in prognosis of functional outcome: a new dimension in the treatment of patients with psychotic disorders. Schizophr. Res., 93:160–168, 2007.

71. Heston, L. L. Psychiatric disorders in foster home reared children of schizophrenic mothers. Br. J. Psychiat., 112:819–825, 1966.

72. Hodges, A., Byrne, M., Grant, E., and Johnstone, E. People at risk of schizophrenia. Sample characteristics of the first 100 cases in the Edinburgh High-Risk Study. Br. J. Psychiat., 174:547–553, 1999.

73. Hulshoff Pol, H. E., Hoek, H. W., Susser, E., Brown, A. S., Dingemans, A., Schnack, H. G., van Haren, N. E., Pereira Ramos, L. M., Gispen-de Wied, C. C., and Kahn, R. S. Prenatal exposure to famine and brain morphology in schizophrenia. Am. J. Psychiat., 157:1170–1172, 2000.

74. Ichimaya, T., Okubo, Y., Suhara, T., and Sudo, Y. Reduced volume of the cerebellar vermis in neuroleptic-naive schizophrenia. Biol. Psychiat., 49:20–27, 2001.

75. Inouye, E. Similarity and dissimilarity of schizophrenia in twins. Proceedings of the 3rd World Congress on Psychiatry. Montreal: University of Toronto Press, 1963.

76. Isohanni, M., Murray, G. K., Jokelainen, J., Croudace, T., and Jones, P. B. The persistence of developmental markers in childhood and adolescence and risk for schizophrenic psychoses in adult life. A 34-year follow-up of the Northern Finland 1966 birth cohort. Schizophr. Res., 71:213–225, 2004.

77. Jones, P. B., Rantakallio, P., Hartikainen, A. L., Isohanni, M., and Sipila, P. Schizophrenia as a long-term outcome of pregnancy, delivery, and perinatal complications: a 28-year follow-up of the 1966 north Finland general population birth cohort. Am. J. Psychiat., 155:355–364, 1998.

78. Jonsson, H., and Nyman, A. K. Predicting long-term outcome in schizophrenia. Acta Psychiat. Scand., 83:342–346, 1991.

79. Kallman, F. J. The genetic theory of schizophrenia. An analysis of 691 twin index families. Am. J. Psychiat., 103:309–322, 1941.

80. Kasai, K., Iwanami, A., Yamasue, H., Kuroki, N., Nakagome, K., and Fukuda, M. Neuroanatomy and neurophysiology in schizophrenia. Neurosci. Res., 43:93–110, 2002.

81. Kendler, K. S., and Gardner, C. O. The risk for psychiatric disorders in relatives of schizophrenic and control probands: a comparison of three independent studies. Psychol. Med., 27:411–419, 1997.

82. Kendler, K. S., Gruenberg, A. M., and Tsuang, M. T. Subtype stability in schizophrenia. Am. J. Psychiat., 142:827–832, 1985.

83. Kendler, K. S., and Robinette, C. D. Schizophrenia in the National Academy of Sciences-National Research Council Twin Registry: a 16-year update. Am. J. Psychiat., 140:1551–1563, 1983.

84. Keshavan, M. S., Diwadkar, V. A., Harenski, K., Rosenberg, D. R., Sweeney, J. A., and Pettegrew, J. W. Abnormalities of the corpus callosum in first episode, treatment naive schizophrenia. J. Neurol. Neurosurg. Psychiat., 72:757–760, 2002.

85. Kety, S. S., Wender, P. H., Jacobsen, B., Ingraham, L. J., Jansson, L., Faber, B., and Kinney, D. K. Mental illness in the biological and adoptive relatives of

schizophrenic adoptees. Replication of the Copenhagen Study in the rest of Denmark. Arch. Gen. Psychiat., *51*:442–455, 1994.

86. Kirkbride, J. B., Fearon, P., Morgan, C., Dazzan, P., Morgan, K., Tarrant, J., Lloyd, T., Holloway, J., Hutchinson, G., Leff, J. P., Mallett, R. M., Harrison, G. L., Murray, R. M., and Jones, P. B. Heterogeneity in incidence rates of schizophrenia and other psychotic syndromes: findings from the 3-center AeSOP study. Arch. Gen. Psychiat., *63*:250–258, 2006.

87. Kirov, G., O'Donovan, M. C., and Owen, M. J. Finding schizophrenia genes. J. Clin. Invest., *115*:1440–1448, 2005.

88. Kläning, U. Schizophrenia in twins: incidence and risk factors. Unpublished doctoral dissertation, University of Aarhus, Denmark, 1996.

89. Kraepelin, E. *Dementia Praecox and Paraphrenia* (Barclay, R. M.; Robertson, G. M., trans.). Edinburgh: E. & S. Livingstone, 1919.

90. Kremen, W. S., Seidman, L. J., Faraone, S. V., and Tsuang, M. T. Intelligence quotient and neuropsychological profiles in patients with schizophrenia and in normal volunteers. Biol. Psychiat., *50*:453–462, 2001.

91. Kringlen, E. Schizophrenia in male monozygotic twins. Acta Psychiat. Scand., *40 Suppl*:1–76, 1964.

92. Kringlen, E. Schizophrenia in twins. An epidemiological-clinical study. Psychiat., *29*:172–184, 1966.

93. Kringlen, E. *Heredity and Environment in the Functional Psychoses: an Epidemiological-Clinical Twin Study, Vol. I and II (Case Histories)*. London: William Heinemann, 1968.

94. Kringlen, E. Twin studies in schizophrenia with special emphasis on concordance figures. Am. J. Med. Genet., *97*:4–11, 2000.

95. Leweke, F. M., Gerth, C. W., Koethe, D., Klosterkotter, J., Ruslanova, I., Krivogorsky, B., Torrey, E. F., and Yolken, R. H. Antibodies to infectious agents in individuals with recent onset schizophrenia. Eur. Arch. Psychiat. Clin. Neurosci., *254*:4–8, 2004.

96. Lewis, C. M., Levinson, D. F., Wise, L. H., DeLisi, L. E., Straub, R. E., Hovatta, I., Williams, N. M., Schwab, S. G., Pulver, A. E., Faraone, S. V., Brzustowicz, L. M., Kaufmann, C. A., Garver, D. L., Gurling, H. M., Lindholm, E., Coon, H., Moises, H. W., Byerley, W., Shaw, S. H., Mesen, A., Sherrington, R., O'Neill, F. A., Walsh, D., Kendler, K. S., Ekelund, J., Paunio, T., Lonnqvist, J., Peltonen, L., O'Donovan, M. C., Owen, M. J., Wildenauer, D. B., Maier, W., Nestadt, G., Blouin, J. L., Antonarakis, S. E., Mowry, B. J., Silverman, J. M., Crowe, R. R., Cloninger, C. R., Tsuang, M. T., Malaspina, D., Harkavy-Friedman, J. M., Svrakic, D. M., Bassett, A. S., Holcomb, J., Kalsi, G., McQuillin, A., Brynjolfson, J., Sigmundsson, T., Petursson, H., Jazin, E., Zoega, T., and Helgason, T. Genome scan meta-analysis of schizophrenia and bipolar disorder, part II: Schizophrenia. Am. J. Hum. Genet., *73*:34–48, 2003.

97. Löffler, W., and Häfner, H. Ecological pattern of first admitted schizophrenics in two German cities over 25 years. Soc. Sci. Med., *49*:93–108, 1999.

98. Luxenburger, H. Bericht uber psychiatrischen Serieuntersuchungen an Zwillingen. Z. Ges. Neurol. Psychiat., *176*:297–326, 1928.

99. Maier, W., Hofgen, B., Zobel, A., and Rietschel, M. Genetic models of schizophrenia and bipolar disorder: overlapping inheritance or discrete genotypes? Eur. Arch. Psychiat. Clin. Neurosci., 255:159–166, 2005.

100. Matthysse, S., Holzman, P. S., Gusella, J. F., Levy, D. L., Harte, C. B., Jorgensen, A., Moller, L., and Parnas, J. Linkage of eye movement dysfunction to chromosome 6p in schizophrenia: additional evidence. Am. J. Med. Genet. B Neuropsychiat. Genet., 128:30–36, 2004.

101. McClellan, J. M., Susser, E., and King, M. C. Maternal famine, de novo mutations, and schizophrenia. JAMA, 296:582–584, 2006.

102. McGrath, J., Saha, S., Welham, J., El Saadi, O., MacCauley, C., and Chant, D. A systematic review of the incidence of schizophrenia: the distribution of rates and the influence of sex, urbanicity, migrant status and methodology. BMC Med., 2:13, 2004.

103. Menon, V., Anagnoson, R. T., Glover, G. H., and Pfefferbaum, A. Functional magnetic resonance imaging evidence for disrupted basal ganglia function in schizophrenia. Am. J. Psychiat., 158:646–649, 2001.

104. Messias, E., Kirkpatrick, B., Bromet, E., Ross, D., Buchanan, R. W., Carpenter, W. T., Jr., Tek, C., Kendler, K. S., Walsh, D., and Dollfus, S. Summer birth and deficit schizophrenia: a pooled analysis from 6 countries. Arch. Gen. Psychiat., 61:985–989, 2004.

105. Miller, P., Byrne, M., Hodges, A., Lawrie, S. M., Owens, D. G., and Johnstone, E. C. Schizotypal components in people at high risk of developing schizophrenia: early findings from the Edinburgh High-Risk Study. Br. J. Psychiat., 180:179–184, 2002.

106. Miyamoto, S., LaMantia, A. S., Duncan, G. E., Sullivan, P., Gilmore, J. H., and Lieberman, J. A. Recent advances in the neurobiology of schizophrenia. Mol. Interv., 3:27–39, 2003.

107. Molina, V., Sanz, J., Reig, S., Martinez, R., Sarramea, F., Luque, R., Benito, C., Gispert, J. D., Pascau, J., and Desco, M. Hypofrontality in men with first-episode psychosis. Br. J. Psychiat., 186:203–208, 2005.

108. Moller, H. J. Bipolar disorder and schizophrenia: distinct illnesses or a continuum? J. Clin. Psychiat., 64 Suppl 6:23–27, 2003.

109. Moller, H. J., Bottlender, R., Gross, A., Hoff, P., Wittmann, J., Wegner, U., and Strauss, A. The Kraepelinian dichotomy: preliminary results of a 15-year follow-up study on functional psychoses: focus on negative symptoms. Schizophr. Res., 56:87–94, 2002.

110. Moller, H. J., Bottlender, R., Wegner, U., Wittmann, J., and Strauss, A. Long-term course of schizophrenic, affective and schizoaffective psychosis: focus on negative symptoms and their impact on global indicators of outcome. Acta Psychiat. Scand. Suppl., 407:54–57, 2000.

111. Montross, L. P., Zisook, S., and Kasckow, J. Suicide among patients with schizophrenia: a consideration of risk and protective factors. Ann. Clin. Psychiat., 17:173–182, 2005.

112. Morris, B. J., Cochran, S. M., and Pratt, J. A. PCP: from pharmacology to modelling schizophrenia. Curr. Opin. Pharmacol., 5:101–106, 2005.

113. Mortensen, P. B., Pedersen, C. B., Melbye, M., Mors, O., and Ewald, H. Individual and familial risk factors for bipolar affective disorders in Denmark. Arch. Gen. Psychiat., 60:1209–1215, 2003.

114. Munafo, M. R., Bowes, L., Clark, T. G., and Flint, J. Lack of association of the COMT (Val158/108 Met) gene and schizophrenia: a meta-analysis of case-control studies. Mol. Psychiat., 10:765–770, 2005.

115. Murray, G. K., Jones, P. B., Moilanen, K., Veijola, J., Miettunen, J., Cannon, T. D., and Isohanni, M. Infant motor development and adult cognitive functions in schizophrenia. Schizophr. Res., 81:65–74, 2006.

116. Nimgaonkar, V. L. Reduced fertility in schizophrenia: here to stay? Acta Psychiat. Scand., 98:348–353, 1998.

117. Nimgaonkar, V. L., Ward, S. E., Agarde, H., Weston, N., and Ganguli, R. Fertility in schizophrenia: results from a contemporary US cohort. Acta Psychiat. Scand., 95:364–369, 1997.

118. Nopoulos, P. C., Ceilley, J. W., Gailis, E. A., and Andreasen, N. C. An MRI study of cerebellar vermis morphology in patients with schizophrenia: evidence in support of the cognitive dysmetria concept. Biol. Psychiat., 46:703–711, 1999.

119. Nordstrom, A., Kullgren, G., and Dahlgren, L. Schizophrenia and violent crime: the experience of parents. Int. J. Law Psychiat., 29:57–67, 2006.

120. Norton, N., Williams, H. J., and Owen, M. J. An update on the genetics of schizophrenia. Curr. Opin. Psychiat., 19:158–164, 2006.

121. O'Donnell, B. F., McCarley, R. W., Potts, G. F., Salisbury, D. F., Nestor, P. G., Hirayasu, Y., Niznikiewicz, M. A., Barnard, J., Shen, Z. J., Weinstein, D. M., Bookstein, F. L., and Shenton, M. E. Identification of neural circuits under-lying P300 abnormalities in schizophrenia. Psychophysiol., 36:388–398, 1999.

122. Oken, R. J., and Schulzer, M. At issue: schizophrenia and rheumatoid arthritis: the negative association revisited. Schizophr. Bull., 25:625–638, 1999.

123. Olney, J. W., and Farber, N. B. Glutamate receptor dysfunction and schizo-phrenia. Arch. Gen. Psychiat., 52:998–1007, 1995.

124. Olney, J. W., Newcomer, J. W., and Farber, N. B. NMDA receptor hypofunction model of schizophrenia. J. Psychiat. Res., 33:523–533, 1999.

125. Onstad, S., Skre, I., Torgersen, S., and Kringlen, E. Twin concordance for DSM-III-R schizophrenia. Acta Psychiat. Scand., 83:395–401, 1991.

126. Opler, M. G., and Susser, E. S. Fetal environment and schizophrenia. Environ. Health Perspect., 113:1239–1242, 2005.

127. Ott, S. L., Allen, J., and Erlenmeyer-Kimling, L. The New York High-Risk Project: observations on the rating of early manifestations of schizophrenia. Am. J. Med. Genet., 105:25–27, 2001.

128. Ott, S. L., Allen, J., and Erlenmeyer-Kimling, L. The New York High-Risk Project: observations on the rating of early manifestations of schizophrenia. Am. J. Med. Genet., 105:25–27, 2001.

129. Owen, M. J., Craddock, N., and O'Donovan, M. C. Schizophrenia: genes at last? Trends Genet., 21:518–525, 2005.

130. Palmer, B. A., Pankratz, V. S., and Bostwick, J. M. The lifetime risk of suicide in schizophrenia: a reexamination. Arch. Gen. Psychiat., 62:247–253, 2005.

131. Parnas, J. Assortative mating in schizophrenia: results from the Copenhagen High-Risk Study. Psychiat., 51:58–64, 1988.

132. Peralta, V., Cuesta, M. J., and de Leon, J. Positive and negative symptoms/syndromes in schizophrenia: reliability and validity of different diagnostic systems. Psychol. Med., 25:43–50, 1995.

133. Planansky, K., and Johnston, R. Depressive syndrome in schizophrenia. Acta Psychiat. Scand. Suppl., 57:207–218, 1978.

134. Pope, H. G., Jr., and Yurgelun-Todd, D. Schizophrenic individuals with bipolar first-degree relatives: analysis of two pedigrees. J. Clin. Psychiat., 51:97–101, 1990.

135. Riecher-Rössler, A., and Rössler, W. The course of schizophrenic psychoses: what do we really know? A selective review from an epidemiological perspective. Eur. Arch. Psychiat. Clin. Neurosci., 248:189–202, 1998.

136. Robins, E., and Guze, S. B. Establishment of diagnostic validity in psychiatric illness: its application to schizophrenia. Am. J. Psychiat., 126:983–987, 1970.

137. Robins, E., and Guze, S. B. Classification of affective disorders: the primary-secondary, the endogenous-reactive, and the neurotic-psychotic concepts. In *Recent Advances in Psychobiology of the Depressive Illnesses,* Proceedings of a Workshop Sponsored by the NIMH, Williams, T. A., Katz, M. M., Shield, J. A. (eds.). Washington, DC: National Institutes of Mental Health and Department of Health, Education, and Welfare, pp. 283–293, 1972.

138. Rosanoff, A. J., Handy, I. M., Plesset, I. R., and Brush, S. The etiology of so-called schizophrenic psychoses. With special reference to their occurrence in twins. Am. J. Psychiat., 81:247–286, 1934.

139. Rosenthal, D., Wender, P. H., Kety, S. S., Welner, J., and Schulsinger, F. The adopted-away offspring of schizophrenics. Am. J. Psychiat., 128:307–311, 1971.

140. Rosse, R. B., Collins, J. P., Jr., Fay-McCarthy, M., Alim, T. N., Wyatt, R. J., and Deutsch, S. I. Phenomenologic comparison of the idiopathic psychosis of schizophrenia and drug-induced cocaine and phencyclidine psychoses: a retrospective study. Clin. Neuropharmacol., 17:359–369, 1994.

141. Rubin, P. Neurobiological findings in first admission patients with schizophrenia or schizophreniform disorder. Dan. Med. Bull., 44:140–154, 1997.

142. Ruggeri, M., Lasalvia, A., Tansella, M., Bonetto, C., Abate, M., Thornicroft, G., Allevi, L., and Ognibene, P. Heterogeneity of outcomes in schizophrenia. 3-year follow-up of treated prevalent cases. Br. J. Psychiat., 184:48–57, 2004.

143. Rummel, C., Hamann, J., Kissling, W., and Leucht, S. New generation antipsychotics for first episode schizophrenia. Cochrane Database Syst. Rev.:CD004410, 2003.

144. Saha, S., Chant, D., Welham, J., and McGrath, J. A systematic review of the prevalence of schizophrenia. PLoS Med., 2:e141, 2005.

145. Salem, J. E., and Kring, A. M. The role of gender differences in the reduction of etiologic heterogeneity in schizophrenia. Clin. Psychol. Rev., 18:795–819, 1998.

146. Sands, J. R., and Harrow, M. Depression during the longitudinal course of schizophrenia. Schizophr. Bull., 25:157–171, 1999.

147. Schulsinger, H. A ten-year follow-up of children of schizophrenic mothers. Clinical assessment. Acta Psychiat. Scand., 53:371–386, 1976.

148. Selten, J. P., Cantor-Graae, E., and Kahn, R. S. Migration and schizophrenia. Curr. Opin. Psychiat., 20:111–115, 2007.

149. Shaner, A., Roberts, L. J., Eckman, T. A., Racenstein, J. M., Tucker, D. E., Tsuang, J. W., and Mintz, J. Sources of diagnostic uncertainty for chronically psychotic cocaine abusers. Psychiat. Serv., 49:684–690, 1998.

150. Simonsen, E., Friis, S., Haahr, U., Johannessen, J. O., Larsen, T. K., Melle, I., Opjordsmoen, S., Rund, B. R., Vaglum, P., and McGlashan, T. Clinical epidemiologic first-episode psychosis: 1-year outcome and predictors. Acta Psychiat. Scand., 116:54–61, 2007.

151. Singh, B. Recognition and optimal management of schizophrenia and related psychoses. Intern. Med. J., 35:413–418, 2005.

152. Slater, E., and Shields, J. *Psychotic and Neurotic Illnesses in Twins.* London: Her Majesty's Stationery Office, 1953.

153. Slopen, N. B., and Corrigan, P. W. Recovery in schizophrenia: reality or mere slogan. Curr. Psychiat. Rep., 7:316–320, 2005.

154. Snitz, B. E., MacDonald, A., III, Cohen, J. D., Cho, R. Y., Becker, T., and Carter, C. S. Lateral and medial hypofrontality in first-episode schizophrenia: functional activity in a medication-naive state and effects of short-term atypical antipsychotic treatment. Am. J. Psychiat., 162:2322–2329, 2005.

155. Somnath, C. P., Janardhan Reddy, Y. C., and Jain, S. Is there a familial overlap between schizophrenia and bipolar disorder? J. Affect. Disord., 72:243–247, 2002.

156. Soyka, M. Alcohol dependence and schizophrenia: what are the interrelationships? Alcohol Alcohol. Suppl., 2:473–478, 1994.

157. Srisurapanont, M., Kittiratanapaiboon, P., and Jarusuraisin, N. Treatment for amphetamine psychosis. Cochrane Database Syst. Rev. CD003026, 2001.

158. St Clair, D., Xu, M., Wang, P., Yu, Y., Fang, Y., Zhang, F., Zheng, X., Gu, N., Feng, G., Sham, P., and He, L. Rates of adult schizophrenia following prenatal exposure to the Chinese famine of 1959–1961. JAMA, 294:557–562, 2005.

159. Stephens, D. A., Atkinson, M. W., Kay, D. W., Roth, M., and Garside, R. F. Psychiatric morbidity in parents and sibs of schizophrenics and non-schizophrenics. Br. J. Psychiat., 127:97–108, 1975.

160. Stephens, J. H., Astrup, C., Carpenter, W. T., Jr., Shaffer, J. W., and Goldberg, J. A comparison of nine systems to diagnose schizophrenia. Psychiat. Res., 6:127–143, 1982.

161. Stimmel, G. L. Benzodiazepines in schizophrenia. Pharmacother., 16:148S–151S, 1996.

162. Strous, R. D., Pollack, S., Robinson, D., Sheitman, B., and Lieberman, J. A. Seasonal admission patterns in first episode psychosis, chronic schizophrenia, and nonschizophrenic psychoses. J. Nerv. Ment. Dis., 189:642–644, 2001.

163. Subotnik, K. L., Nuechterlein, K. H., Asarnow, R. F., Fogelson, D. L., Goldstein, M. J., and Talovic, S. A. Depressive symptoms in the early course of schizophrenia: relationship to familial psychiatric illness. Am. J. Psychiat., 154:1551–1556, 1997.

164. Sullivan, P. F., Kendler, K. S., and Neale, M. C. Schizophrenia as a complex trait: evidence from a meta-analysis of twin studies. Arch. Gen. Psychiat., 60:1187–1192, 2003.

165. Tamminga, C. A., Buchanan, R. W., and Gold, J. M. The role of negative symptoms and cognitive dysfunction in schizophrenia outcome. Int. Clin. Psychopharmacol., 13 Suppl 3:S21–S26, 1998.

166. Thaker, G. K., Cassady, S., Adami, H., Moran, M., and Ross, D. E. Eye movements in spectrum personality disorders: comparison of community subjects and relatives of schizophrenic patients. Am. J. Psychiat., 153:362–368, 1996.

167. Tharyan, P. Electroconvulsive therapy for schizophrenia. Cochrane Database Syst. Rev. CD000076, 2000.

168. Tharyan, P., and Adams, C. E. Electroconvulsive therapy for schizophrenia (Cochrane Review). Cochrane Database Syst. Rev. CD000076, 2002.

169. Thorup, A., Waltoft, B. L., Pedersen, C. B., Mortensen, P. B., and Nordentoft, M. Young males have a higher risk of developing schizophrenia: a Danish register study. Psychol. Med., 37:479–484, 2007.

170. Tibbo, P., Nopoulos, P., Arndt, S., and Andreasen, N. C. Corpus callosum shape and size in male patients with schizophrenia. Biol. Psychiat., 44:405–412, 1998.

171. Tienari, E. Schizophrenia in Finnish male twins. In Studies of Schizophrenia. British Journal of Psychiatry, Special Publication No. 10, Lader, M. H. (ed.), pp. 29–35, 1975.

172. Tienari, P. Psychiatric illnesses in identical twins. Acta Psychiat. Scand., 39:1–195, 1963.

173. Tienari, P. Interaction between genetic vulnerability and family environment: the Finnish adoptive family study of schizophrenia. Acta Psychiat. Scand., 84:460–465, 1991.

174. Torgersen, S., Edvardsen, J., Oien, P. A., Onstad, S., Skre, I., Lygren, S., and Kringlen, E. Schizotypal personality disorder inside and outside the schizophrenic spectrum. Schizophr. Res., 54:33–38, 2002.

175. Torrey, E. F. Stalking the schizovirus. Schizophr. Bull., 14:223–229, 1988.

176. Torrey, E. F., Rawlings, R. R., Ennis, J. M., Merrill, D. D., and Flores, D. S. Birth seasonality in bipolar disorder, schizophrenia, schizoaffective disorder and stillbirths. Schizophr. Res., 21:141–149, 1996.

177. Torrey, E. F., and Yolken, R. H. The schizophrenia-rheumatoid arthritis connection: infectious, immune, or both? Brain Behav. Immun., 15:401–410, 2001.

178. Tran, K. D., Smutzer, G. S., Doty, R. L., and Arnold, S. E. Reduced Purkinje cell size in the cerebellar vermis of elderly patients with schizophrenia. Am. J. Psychiat., 155:1288–1290, 1998.

179. Tsuang, M. Schizophrenia: genes and environment. Biol. Psychiat., 47:210–220, 2000.

180. Tsuang, M. T., Dempsey, G. M., Dvoredsky, A., and Struss, A. A family history study of schizo-affective disorder. Biol. Psychiat., 12:331–338, 1977.

181. Tsujita, T., Okazaki, Y., Fujimaru, K., Minami, Y., Mutoh, Y., Maeda, H., Fukazawa, T., Yamashita, H., and Nakane, Y. Twin concordance rate of DSM-III-R schizophrenia in a new Japanese sample. Abstracts of the Seventh International Congress on Twin Studies, Tokyo, Japan, 1992.

182. Vaillant, G. E. The prediction of recovery in schizophrenia. Int. J. Psychiat. Clin. Prac., 2:617–627, 1962.

183. Vaillant, G. E. Prospective prediction of schizophrenic remission. Arch. Gen. Psychiat., 11:509–518, 1964.

184. Vourdas, A., Pipe, R., Corrigall, R., and Frangou, S. Increased developmental deviance and premorbid dysfunction in early onset schizophrenia. Schizophr. Res., 62:13–22, 2003.

185. Walker, E. F., Grimes, K. E., Davis, D. M., and Smith, A. J. Childhood precursors of schizophrenia: facial expressions of emotion. Am. J. Psychiat., 150:1654–1660, 1993.

186. Walker, M. A., Highley, J. R., Esiri, M. M., McDonald, B., Roberts, H. C., Evans, S. P., and Crow, T. J. Estimated neuronal populations and volumes of the hippo-campus and its subfields in schizophrenia. Am. J. Psychiat., 159:821–828, 2002.

187. Ward, K. E., Friedman, L., Wise, A., and Schulz, S. C. Meta-analysis of brain and cranial size in schizophrenia. Schizophr. Res., 22:197–213, 1996.

188. Waring, E. M. The psychobiology of first-episode schizophrenia. Can. J. Psychiat., 40:S33–S37, 1995.

189. Wender, P. H., Rosenthal, D., Kety, S. S., Schulsinger, F., and Welner, J. Social class and psychopathology in adoptees. Arch. Gen. Psychiat., 2:318–325, 1973.

190. Wong, A. H., and Van Tol, H. H. Schizophrenia: from phenomenology to neurobiology. Neurosci. Biobehav. Rev., 27:269–306, 2003.

191. Woodruff, P. W., Phillips, M. L., Rushe, T., Wright, I. C., Murray, R. M., and David, A. S. Corpus callosum size and inter-hemispheric function in schizophrenia. Schizophr. Res., 23:189–196, 1997.

192. Woodruff, R. A., Clayton, P. J., and Guze, S. B. Hysteria: studies of diagnosis, outcome, and prevalence. JAMA, 215:425–428, 1971.

193. Yolken, R. Viruses and schizophrenia: a focus on herpes simplex virus. Herpes, 11 Suppl 2:83A–88A, 2004.

194. Zanelli, J., Simon, H., Rabe-Hesketh, S., Walshe, M., McDonald, C., Murray, R. M., and Maccabe, J. H. Eye tracking in schizophrenia: does the antisaccade task measure anything that the smooth pursuit task does not? Psychiat. Res., 136:181–188, 2005.

195. Ziedonis, D. M., Smelson, D., Rosenthal, R. N., Batki, S. L., Green, A. I., Henry, R. J., Montoya, I., Parks, J., and Weiss, R. D. Improving the care of individuals with schizophrenia and substance use disorders: consensus recommendations. J. Psychiat. Pract., 11:315–339, 2005.

196. American Psychiatric Association, *Diagnostic and Statistical Manual of Mental Disorders,* 4th edition, text revision. Washington, DC: Author, 2000.

4

Panic Disorder and Phobias

In current diagnostic nomenclature, panic disorder is defined in relation to a type of phobia (panic disorder with or without agoraphobia), and agoraphobia is defined in relation to panic disorder (agoraphobia without panic disorder) (5). This chapter will cover both panic and phobic disorders.

Panic disorder is a chronic illness characterized by recurrent, acute panic attacks. Panic attacks are discrete episodes of anxiety or fearfulness with definite onset, rapid increase, and spontaneous termination. During attacks patients may have overwhelming feelings of impending doom. The attacks are accompanied by symptoms associated with the autonomic nervous system: palpitations, tachycardia, rapid or shallow breathing, dizziness, and tremor. Between attacks, patients may be relatively asymptomatic though some experience fatigue, headache, and symptoms of anxiety attacks that persist. A panic attack is a symptom rather than a syndrome, and panic attacks can be part of the course of any psychiatric illness. When panic attacks occur together, independent of other significant psychiatric symptoms, the diagnosis of panic disorder is made.

Panic is distinguished from ordinary fear by the lack of an appropriate stimulus precipitating the emotions. Sometimes, however, patients experience panic attacks in response to a fear-provoking situation such as facing an angry employer or giving a public speech. In these cases the clinician must decide whether the anxiety is grossly out of proportion to the fear-provoking stimulus, as well as make a diagnosis based on the complete history. Most patients with panic disorder report some panic attacks without any fear-provoking stimulus, but on other occasions they overreact to situations that would produce some degree of apprehension in individuals without the disorder.

A phobic disorder is a chronic condition dominated by one or more phobias. A phobia is an intense, recurrent, unreasonable fear of a specific object, activity, or situation that results in a compelling desire to avoid the dreaded object, activity, or situation. *DSM-IV-TR* subdivides phobias into specific phobias (e.g., fear of animals), social phobias (e.g., fear of public speaking), and agoraphobia. The last is often characterized by multiple phobias involving a fear of being in places where help might not be available in the event of an anxiety attack.

Historical Background

My cheek is cold and white, alas!
O lift me from the grass!
I die! I faint! I fall!
. . .

My cheek is cold and white, alas!
My heart beats loud and fast.
Percy Bysshe Shelley,
The Indian Serenade

It has been suggested that Shelley was having a panic attack when he wrote these lines. If so, he probably would have called it something else. In the nineteenth century, "anxiety reactions" referring to fainting—which was fashionable among women of that era—were called "vapors." Modern patients with panic disorder also sometimes faint—probably from hyperventilating. In Victorian times the prototype of a refined young woman was a "swooner, pale and trembling, who responded to unpleasant or unusual social situations by taking to the floor in a graceful and delicious maneuver, in no way resembling the crash of the epileptic" (29). A Jane Austen heroine found one social situation "too pathetic for the feelings of Sophie and myself. We fainted alternately on a sofa." Overly tight corsets may have been responsible for some of the fainting. A nineteenth-century physician, Dr. John Brown, cured fainting by "cutting the stay laces, which ran before the knife and cracked like a bow string" (29).

One of the first medical terms to describe anxiety disorders was "neurasthenia," defined by an American physician, G. M. Beard, in 1869 (10).

Neurasthenia broadly included patients with hysteria, obsessional illness, and anxiety disorders, as well as hypochondriacs and swooners (23). The term "anxiety neurosis" was first used by Freud in 1895. It was not until 1980 that the concept of neurosis was dropped from American Psychiatric Association general nomenclature, and the term "panic disorder" replaced the older term "anxiety neurosis" as the disorder's official name (2). Panic disorder was later subdivided into two types, with and without agoraphobia (3), a distinction that still holds today.

The term *phobia* originates from the name of a Greek god, Phobos, whose likeness was painted on masks and shields for the purpose of frightening the enemy (84). The word *phobia* first appeared in medical terminology in Rome 2,000 years ago, when hydrophobia was used to describe a symptom of rabies. Hippocrates also described cases of phobic fears.

During the nineteenth century, the term *phobia* appeared increasingly in descriptions of morbid fears, beginning with syphilophobia, defined in a medical dictionary published in 1848 as "a morbid dread of syphilis giving rise to fancied symptoms of the disease." Later authorities compiled long lists of phobias, naming each in Greek or Latin terms after the object or situation feared. Thus, as Nemiah pointed out, "the patient who was spared the pangs of taphaphobia (fear of being buried alive) or ailurophobia (fear of cats) might yet fall prey to belonophobia (fear of needles), siderodromophobia (fear of railways), or triskaidekaphobia (fear of thirteen at table), and pantaphobia was the diagnostic fate of that unfortunate soul who feared them all" (94).

The term *phobia* was not applied in a psychiatric sense until the nineteenth century. In 1871, Westphal described three men who feared public places and labeled the condition agoraphobia, *agora* derived from the Greek word for place of assembly or marketplace (135). Westphal recommended companionship, alcohol, or the use of a cane to treat the condition. Numerous theories were advanced to explain phobias, including poor upbringing (72).

Phobias and panic attacks have long been known to occur in a variety of psychiatric conditions. Controversy has continued since the late nineteenth century over the relationship of phobias and panic to other psychiatric disorders such as obsessional and mood disorders, substance abuse, and personality disorders (7, 63, 84, 120, 123, 148).

Epidemiology

Panic and phobic disorders are among the most common psychiatric syndromes. As many as 2%–4% of the adult population may have panic disorder at some time in their lifetimes (35, 64, 111), and women have at least twice the prevalence of men (36, 64). Disparities in reported rates of panic disorder may relate to whether agoraphobia is considered separate from or a part of panic disorder: one-third to one-half of general population panic disorder cases are associated with agoraphobia, and this proportion is greater, 80% or more, in clinical samples (19, 36, 58).

Two population studies using structured diagnostic interviews have provided lifetime prevalence rates of phobic disorders. In the 1980s, the Epidemiologic Catchment Area (ECA) study (112) examined over 19,000 representative members of the U.S. population with the National Institutes of Mental Health (NIMH) Diagnostic Interview Schedule. In the 1990s, the National Comorbidity Study (NCS) interviewed over 8,000 representative U.S. population members with the World Health Organization (WHO) Composite International Diagnostic Interview (CIDI) (64). These systematic studies found higher lifetime prevalence of phobic disorders than in previous studies, 14% in the ECA study and 22% in the NCS. Specific diagnosis rates in the NCS were 13% for social phobia, 11% for specific phobia, and 5% for agoraphobia without panic disorder. Despite the higher overall prevalence of phobic disorders in these studies, the findings challenged prevailing notions of the ubiquitous nature of specific phobias, such as fear of snakes and heights, especially in childhood and among women.

The prevalence of phobic disorders varies according to the sample surveyed, the interview employed, and the choice of diagnostic criteria (41, 138). A possible explanation for the higher prevalence of phobias in these population studies compared to earlier studies is that respondents were shown lists of feared objects and situations, unlike many previous studies that may have depended on people to remember phobic fears more spontaneously. Because inconsistency in methods between studies is a common problem in psychiatric epidemiology, findings often must be considered only tentative. Because future studies will undoubtedly test different diagnostic criteria and use different instruments for measurement, close replication of the findings is unlikely. In clinical samples, discrepancy in prevalence data concerning phobias may also be attributed to inclusion by some physicians in their statistics of what others consider normal fears to and to embarrassment about revealing phobias. It is not unusual in psychiatric practice to see patients for years before they describe, almost in passing, a phobia that has bothered them for a long time.

In both the ECA and NCS studies, the prevalence of phobic disorders in the 12 months preceding the interview was lower than the lifetime prevalence, by about half, suggesting that phobic disorders are either episodic or temporary. This finding contradicts previous clinical observations and studies characterizing phobias as chronic conditions. Because few phobic individuals ever receive treatment for their phobias, most of the difference between lifetime and 12-month rates cannot be attributed to medications or psychotherapy.

Both the ECA study and the NCS found phobias to be more prevalent among women than men, but the NCS contradicted the ECA study and other studies reporting that phobias are more prevalent among African Americans than whites (55). People with phobic disorders have lower socioeconomic status than other people and are more likely to be unmarried (55). The NCS, ECA, and other studies all found an association of alcoholism with phobias (71, 108).

In contrast to findings from phobic disorder research, panic disorder research has been inconsistent regarding the association of low educational level and socioeconomic status (36, 133). Childhood experiences of bereavement, birth order, and history of violence between parents do not appear to predispose to panic disorder (50, 106, 141). Panic disorder in early adulthood was found to be associated with self-report of childhood abuse history, but the association was modest, most of it explained by other childhood and family factors (44).

Many people with panic disorder experience a mild form and, like those with phobic disorders, do not seek medical care for their symptoms (89). Many others consult family practitioners or internists rather than psychiatrists. Panic disorder patients who see psychiatrists may represent a small group with a high prevalence of comorbid mood disorder (119).

Clinical Picture

Panic attacks are the hallmark of panic disorder. The attacks usually begin suddenly, sometimes in a public place or at a social gathering, or even at home. There is a sense of foreboding, fear, and apprehension; a sense that one had suddenly become seriously ill; and a feeling that one's life may be threatened by such illness. Some patients, especially those with agoraphobia, describe a disturbing sense of their body changing or becoming distorted (depersonalization) (22). These feelings are hard to define and appear to be an unpleasant, scary sense of being unreal, strange, and disembodied, cut off from one's surroundings. Feelings of alien change may extend to the surrounding world (derealization). Symptoms of labored breathing, smothering, palpitation, blurred vision, tremulousness, and weakness usually accompany the apprehension and foreboding. Patients examined during such an attack manifest signs of distress: tachycardia, sweating, tachypnea, tremor, hyperactive deep tendon reflexes, and dilated pupils. The criteria for panic disorder are provided in Table 4.1.

TABLE 4.1 Diagnostic Criteria for Panic Disorder

A. Both (1) and (2):

  (1) Recurrent unexpected panic attacks (manifested by four or more of the following symptoms):
      (a) Palpitations, pounding heart, or accelerated heart rate
      (b) Sweating
      (c) Trembling or shaking
      (d) Sensations of shortness of breath or smothering
      (e) Feeling of choking
      (f) Chest pain or discomfort
      (g) Nausea or abdominal distress
      (h) Feeling dizzy, unsteady, lightheaded, or faint
      (i) Derealization (feelings of unreality) or depersonalization (being detached from oneself)
      (j) Fear of losing control or going crazy
      (k) Fear of dying
      (l) Paresthesias (numbness or tingling sensations)
      (m) Chills or hot flushes
  (2) At least one of the attacks has been followed by 1 month (or more) of one (or more) of the
      following:
      (a) Persistent concern about having additional attacks
      (b) Worry about the implications of the attack or its consequences (e.g., losing control,
          having a heart attack, "going crazy")
      (c) A significant change in behavior related to the attacks
B. Agoraphobia may or may not be present. Agoraphobia also may exist in the absence of panic
    attacks.
C. The panic attacks are not due to the direct physiological effects of a substance (e.g., a drug of
    abuse, a medication) or a general medical condition (e.g., hyperthyroidism).
D. The panic attacks are not better accounted for by another mental disorder, such as social phobia
    (e.g., occurring on exposure to feared social situations), specific phobia (e.g., on exposure to a
    specific phobic situation), obsessive-compulsive disorder (e.g., on exposure to dirt in someone
    with an obsession about contamination), posttraumatic stress disorder (e.g., in response to
    stimuli associated with a severe stressor), or separation anxiety disorder (e.g., in response to
    being away from home or close relative).

Adapted from diagnostic criteria in the *DSM-IV-TR* (151).

Panic attacks vary in frequency among patients. Some experience them on
a daily basis; others have them only once or twice a year. Other symptoms may
occur between attacks. Table 4.2 lists these symptoms and their frequency as
reported in a classic study of this disorder. Again, the symptoms can occur in
practically any pattern.

Cardiorespiratory symptoms are the most frequent chief complaints that
panic disorder patients report to physicians: "I have heart spells," "I think I'll
smother," or "There is no way for me to get enough air." The chief complaint is
occasionally psychological, but more often it indicates that the patient considers
the disorder medical, and frequently fears it may be very serious.

TABLE 4.2 Symptoms of Panic Disorder

Symptoms	60 Patients (%)	102 Controls* (%)
Palpitation	97	9
Tires easily	93	19
Breathlessness	90	13
Nervousness	88	27
Chest pain	85	10
Sighing	79	16
Dizziness	78	16
Faintness	70	12
Apprehensiveness	61	3
Headache	58	26
Paresthesias	58	7
Weakness	56	3
Trembling	54	17
Breathing unsatisfactory	53	4
Insomnia	53	4
Unhappiness	50	2
Shakiness	47	16
Fatigued all the time	45	6
Sweating	42	33
Fear of death	42	2
Smothering	40	3
Syncope	37	11
Nervous chill	24	0
Urinary frequency	18	2
Vomiting and diarrhea	14	0
Anorexia	12	3
Paralysis	0	0
Blindness	0	0

*Healthy controls consisted of 50 men and 11 women from a large industrial plant and 41 healthy postpartum women from the Boston Lying-In Hospital.

Adapted from Cohen and White (25).

A 51-year-old electrical engineer was brought to an emergency room by ambulance, complaining of severe left anterior chest pain. His breathing was labored and he complained of numbness and tingling in his lips and fingers. His pulse rate was 110. He was perspiring heavily and visibly frightened. However, the electrocardiogram was normal, and blood enzymes were within normal limits. He was observed over the next 24 hours and then discharged asymptomatic.

The history revealed that the patient had first experienced severe chest pain at the age of 21 while watching a movie. He had many subsequent episodes of chest pain accompanied by dyspnea and anxiety and had been taken to an emergency room on at least 10 previous occasions. Although the examinations were always normal, he had undergone a variety of cardiovascular procedures, including cardiac catheterization. He had never been seen by a psychiatrist and at no time had been told that he very likely suffered from a common psychiatric disorder characterized by panic attacks.

Symptoms may become associated with specific situations that patients will try to avoid. For example, they may choose aisle seats in theaters, preferably close to exits, so that if an attack occurs, they will not be confined. Or patients may avoid social situations in which an attack would be both frightening and embarrassing.

Phobias are common in patients with panic disorder. Some clinicians, in fact, do not distinguish between panic disorder and phobic disorders. By definition, panic disorder is diagnosed when panic symptoms predominate; phobic disorder is the diagnosis when phobias predominate.

Phobias can be distinguished from "normal" fears by their intensity, duration, irrationality, and the disablement resulting from avoidance of the feared situation. *DSM-IV-TR* divides phobic disorders into three types: specific, social, and agoraphobia (see Tables 4.3, 4.4, and 4.5).

A *specific phobia* (formerly called *simple phobia*) is an isolated fear of a single object or situation, leading to avoidance of the object or situation. The fear is irrational and excessive but not always disabling because the object or situation can sometimes be easily avoided (e.g., snakes, if you are a city dweller). Impairment may be considerable if the phobic object is common and cannot be avoided, such as a fear of elevators in someone who must use elevators at work.

Specific phobias almost always involve a single isolated phobia. People with specific phobias typically are no more (or less) anxious than anyone else until exposed to the phobic object or situation. Then they become overwhelmingly uncomfortable and fearful, sometimes having symptoms associated with a panic attack (palpitations, sweating, dizziness, difficulty breathing). The phobic person also fears the possibility of confronting the phobic stimulus. Called "anticipatory anxiety," this leads to avoidance of situations in which the stimulus might be present.

Some common specific phobias are fear of animals, heights, closed spaces, wind, storms, lightning, loud noises, driving a car, flying in airplanes, riding in subways, hypodermic needles, and blood. Less common ones include fear of running water and of going to the hairdresser. There is even the case of the tennis player who wore gloves because he was afraid of fuzz, and tennis balls are fuzzy. Phobias can develop toward almost any object or situation.

Animal phobias are perhaps the most common specific phobias or at least the most commonly studied. They occur often in childhood and are usually

TABLE 4.3 Diagnostic Criteria for Specific Phobia

A. Marked and persistent fear that is excessive or unreasonable, cued by the presence or anticipation of a specific object or situation (e.g., flying, heights, animals, receiving an injection, seeing blood)

B. Exposure to the phobic stimulus almost invariably provokes an immediate anxiety response, which may take the form of a situationally bound or situationally predisposed panic attack. Note: In children, the anxiety may be expressed by crying, tantrums, freezing, or clinging.

C. The person recognizes that the fear is excessive or unreasonable. Note: In children, this feature may be absent.

D. The phobic situation(s) is avoided or else is endured with intense anxiety or distress.

E. The avoidance, anxious anticipation, or distress in the feared situation(s) interferes significantly with the person's normal routine, occupational (or academic) functioning, or social activities or relationships, or there is marked distress about having the phobia.

F. In individuals under age 18 years, the duration is at least 6 months.

G. The anxiety, panic attacks, or phobic avoidance associated with the specific object or situation is not better accounted for by another mental disorder, such as obsessive-compulsive disorder (e.g., fear of dirt in someone with an obsession about contamination), posttraumatic stress disorder (e.g., avoidance of stimuli associated with a severe stressor), separation anxiety disorder (e.g., avoidance of school), social phobia (e.g., avoidance of social situations because of fear of embarrassment), panic disorder with agoraphobia, or agoraphobia without history of panic disorder.

Specify type:

Animal type: if the fear is cued by animals or insects. This subtype generally has a childhood onset.

Natural environment type: if the fear is cued by objects in the natural environment, such as storms, heights, or water. This subtype generally has a childhood onset.

Blood-injection-injury type: if the fear is cued by seeing blood or an injury or by receiving an injection or other invasive medical procedure. This subtype is highly familial and is often characterized by a strong vasovagal response.

Situational type: if the fear is cued by a specific situation such as public transportation, tunnels, bridges, elevators, flying, driving, or enclosed places. This subtype has a bimodal age-at-onset distribution, with one peak in childhood and another peak in the mid-20s. This subtype appears to be similar to panic disorder with agoraphobia in its characteristic sex ratios, familial aggregation pattern, and age at onset.

Other type: if the fear is cued by other stimuli. These stimuli might include the fear or avoidance of situations that might lead to choking, vomiting, or contracting an illness; "space" phobia (i.e., the individual is afraid of falling down if away from walls or other means of physical support); and children's fears of loud sounds or costumed characters.

Adapted from diagnostic criteria in the *DSM-IV-TR* (151).

transient. Among adults, women are subject to animal phobias more often than men. The phobia usually involves only one kind of animal but may lead to frequent distress with mild social disablement if the animals are domestic, such as dogs or cats (43).

Fear of heights is another common phobia. The fear may be totally unrealistic. The person may be close enough to the ground so that a fall would not cause injury. Some people with phobias will not walk down a flight of stairs if

TABLE 4.4 Diagnostic Criteria for Social Phobia

A. A marked and persistent fear of one or more social or performance situations in which the person is exposed to unfamiliar people or to possible scrutiny by others. The individual fears that he or she will act in a way (or show anxiety symptoms) that will be humiliating or embarrassing. Note: In children, there must be evidence of the capacity for age-appropriate social relationships with familiar people and the anxiety must occur in peer settings, not just in interactions with adults.

B. Exposure to the feared social situation almost invariably provokes anxiety, which may take the form of a situationally bound or situationally predisposed panic attack. Note: In children, the anxiety may be expressed by crying, tantrums, freezing, or shrinking from social situations with unfamiliar people.

C. The person recognizes that the fear is excessive or unreasonable. Note: In children, this feature may be absent.

D. The feared social or performance situations are avoided or else are endured with intense anxiety or distress.

E. The avoidance, anxious anticipation, or distress in the feared social or performance situation(s) interferes significantly with the person's normal routine, occupational (academic) functioning, or social activities or relationships, or there is marked distress about having the phobia.

F. In individuals under age 18 years, the duration is at least 6 months.

G. The fear or avoidance is not due to the direct physiological effects of a substance (e.g., a drug of abuse, a medication) or a general medical condition and is not better accounted for by another mental disorder (e.g., panic disorder with or without agoraphobia, separation anxiety disorder, body dysmorphic disorder, a pervasive developmental disorder, or schizoid personality disorder).

H. If a general medical condition or another mental disorder is present, the fear in criterion A is unrelated to it, for example, the fear is not of stuttering, trembling in Parkinson disease, or exhibiting abnormal eating behavior in anorexia nervosa or bulimia nervosa.

Specify if:

Generalized: if the fears include most social situations (e.g., initiating or maintaining conversations, participating in small groups, dating, speaking to authority figures, attending parties). Note: Also consider the additional diagnosis of avoidant personality disorder.

Adapted from diagnostic criteria in the *DSM-IV-TR* (151).

they see the open stairwell. Some will not look out a window from the second floor or above, particularly if the window goes from floor to ceiling. Others will not cross a bridge on foot, though they may go by car.

Social phobias are another form of isolated phobia that generally lead to only mild forms of impairment. These include fears of eating in public, public speaking, receiving criticism from superiors, urinating in the presence of others, practicing musical instruments because the neighbors will hear mistakes, and swimming or undressing in front of others because of shame at one's appearance. Social phobias often involve two or more phobias. Social phobias do not generally lead to total avoidance of the situations, but occasionally, severe handicap may result.

TABLE 4.5 Diagnostic Criteria for Agoraphobia

A. Anxiety about being in places or situations from which escape might be difficult (or embarrassing) or in which help may not be available in the event of having an unexpected or situationally predisposed panic attack or panic-like symptoms. Agoraphobic fears typically involve characteristic clusters of situations that include being outside the home alone; being in a crowd or standing in a line; being on a bridge; and traveling in a bus, train, or automobile.

B. The situations are avoided (e.g., travel is restricted) or else are endured with marked distress or with anxiety about having a panic attack or panic-like symptoms, or require the presence of a companion.

C. The anxiety or phobic avoidance is not better accounted for by another mental disorder, such as social phobia (e.g., avoidance limited to social situation because of fear of embarrassment), specific phobia (e.g., avoidance limited to a single situation like elevators), obsessive-compulsive disorder (e.g., avoidance of dirt in someone with an obsession about contamination), posttraumatic stress disorder (e.g., avoidance of stimuli associated with a severe stressor), or separation anxiety disorder (e.g., avoidance of leaving home or relatives).

Adapted from diagnostic criteria in the *DSM-IV-TR* (151).

The young wife of a business executive refused to entertain associates of her husband with a dinner party or attend dinner parties in restaurants or someone else's home. Her husband made excuses for her but felt his career was being damaged by their lack of social life. At first her explanation for refusing to join in dinner parties was that it was a waste of time or too much trouble. Later she confessed, tearfully and with much embarrassment, that she was afraid of being unable to eat if strangers were watching. Questioned by her concerned husband, she said she was afraid that once food was in her mouth she would be unable to swallow it and then find herself in the embarrassing situation of not knowing where to dispose of the food. She was also afraid that she would gag on the food and possibly vomit. She could eat in front of her husband with no difficulty until she told him about the phobia and then became concerned that he was watching her eat and expecting her to gag or vomit. From then on she ate alone in the kitchen. The marriage survived, but barely (43).

Unlike specific and social phobias, *agoraphobia* has a complex clinical picture involving various combinations of phobic fears, including the following:

1. *Public transportation*: trains, buses, subways, airplanes. When crowded, these vehicles may be intolerable to people with agoraphobia. Waiting in line is almost as bad, whether for a bus or a movie.

2. *Other confining places*: tunnels, bridges, elevators, the hairdresser or barber's chair, and the dentist's chair. These fears belong to the category

of claustrophobia, but most people with claustrophobia have only a single phobia and do not actually have agoraphobia. Paradoxically, people with agoraphobia may also be fearful of open spaces, such as empty parking lots.

3. *Being home alone.* Some people with agoraphobia require constant companionship, to the despair of friends, neighbors, and family.

4. *Being away from home* or another "safe" place where help cannot be readily obtained if needed. The agoraphobia sufferer is sometimes comforted just knowing there is a police officer or a doctor somewhere nearby.

Depending on which symptoms predominate—the panic attacks or phobias—agoraphobia may fall in one of three categories: Panic Disorder with Agoraphobia, Panic Disorder without Agoraphobia, and Agoraphobia without History of Panic Disorder. Agoraphobia is not a psychiatric disorder apart from consideration of panic disorder. It is diagnosed only as part of Panic Disorder with Agoraphobia or as Agoraphobia without History of Panic Disorder.

Klein and associates observed that most agoraphobia patients give a history of panic attacks preceding the onset of phobias, and anticipatory anxiety about another panic attack leads to phobic avoidance of places where panic attacks might occur (68). Thus, a bridge phobia may not involve a fear of bridges per se, but may develop from a fear of experiencing panic on a bridge. Phobias about buses, trains, or airplanes may arise from concern that a panic attack might occur in a vehicle from which escape is impossible or embarrassing. Adopting Klein's conceptualization, *DSM-III-R* reconsidered agoraphobia within the context of panic disorder.

Biological Findings

Over the last two centuries, many theories of the origin of anxiety syndromes and anxiety disorders have evolved, from constitutional weakness of the nervous system to social and psychological factors and more recent biological hypotheses. Although the cause of panic disorder remains unknown, discovery of physiologic abnormalities associated with panic disorder and advances in understanding of the neural circuitry of anxiety states have led to the elaboration of plausible theoretical models of anxiety disorders.

Physiologic findings are well documented in anxiety disorders. People with panic disorder have greater cardiac and respiratory reactivity than healthy subjects during sleep (69, 88). In people with panic or phobic disorders, sodium lactate infusion and breathing carbon dioxide induce respiratory alkalosis and exaggerated elevations in brain lactate and may elicit panic attacks as well (28, 45, 47, 79). Elevated levels of lactate or carbon dioxide may trigger an inborn survival mechanism to warn the body of impending suffocation or danger. Researchers speculate that in panic disorder, this "suffocation alarm" feedback system may be dysregulated (67).

Much attention has been focused on the locus ceruleus, a nucleus that serves as a relay center for the body's alarm system. The locus ceruleus, representing a major part of the noradrenergic system, projects to the limbic system and cortex. Dysregulated activation of the locus ceruleus may produce subjective fear responses and inefficient compensatory mechanisms, primarily of respiratory rate (6, 101). Drugs that increase the firing rate of locus ceruleus neurons increase anxiety levels, whereas drugs that block the firing of these neurons apparently have opposite effects. Several medications used to relieve anxiety and prevent spontaneous panic attacks also reduce anxiety symptoms produced by carbon dioxide inhalation and block lactate-induced panic attacks among patients with panic disorder: beta blockers such as propranolol, benzodiazepines such as alprazolam, tricyclic antidepressants such as amitriptyline, and serotonin-selective reuptake inhibitor (SSRI) antidepressants such as paroxetine, sertraline, fluvoxamine, and citalopram (15, 95, 117).

Evidence that panic disorder involves changes in brain activity has come from studies using positron emission tomography (PET) (17, 105, 109, 110). Patients with panic disorder who are vulnerable to lactate-induced anxiety attacks have strikingly abnormal hemispheric asymmetries of parahippocampal blood flow, blood volume, and oxygen metabolism. Shedding further light on neural circuitry of panic and fear states, brain imaging studies have demonstrated increased glucose metabolism, implicating amygdala, hypothalamus, and prefrontal cortex (95) as well as a fear network involving the nucleus of the solitary tract (providing viscerosensory input), the thalamus (providing sensory and auditory input), and the hippocampus (providing fear-related memories) (116).

Dopamine receptors may be involved in conditioned anxiety by increasing excitability in the amygdala and enhancing declarative memory associations in the hippocampus. Dopamine receptors in the prefrontal cortex may also be involved in avoidance conditioning (95). Other brain imaging studies point to dysregulation of the serotonin neurotransmitter system in panic disorder, with demonstrably decreased serotonin transporter (5-HTT) binding in the midbrain, temporal lobes, and thalamus. The magnitude of these abnormalities reflects symptom severity. With symptom remission, only midbrain and temporal 5-HTT binding normalize, however, suggesting that the reduced 5-HTT binding in thalamus may represent anticipatory anxiety or underlying trait differences (86).

Natural History

Panic disorder most often begins in the third decade of life, and most cases begin between the ages of 18 and 35 (35, 36). A study of 38 families with transgenerational occurrence of the disorder found the age of onset to be earlier in subsequent generations (mean age 23 in younger generations compared to 37 in the older generation) (9). Panic disorder may begin acutely with a discrete anxiety attack, but it also may begin insidiously with feelings of tenseness, nervousness, fatigue, or dizziness for years before the first anxiety attack. Some patients may remember the exact time and circumstances of the first attack, such as a time of stress (e.g., while making a speech in class).

In patients with panic disorder uncomplicated by comorbid conditions, symptoms characteristically wax and wane in an irregular pattern ranging from mild and remitting to severe and unrelenting (145). The symptom fluctuations may or may not be associated with events and circumstances interpreted by the patient as stressful.

The initial medical contacts of panic disorder patients are not always helpful. Patients commonly present to physicians complaining of cardiorespiratory symptoms, fearful of heart disease. Physicians unacquainted with the natural history of panic disorder may reinforce these patients' fears by referring them to a specialist and warning them to limit exertion.

Somatic symptoms among panic disorder patients are not confined to the cardiorespiratory system. Some patients present with symptoms of "irritable colon" or irritable bowel (56, 76, 77). Such patients usually consult a gastroenterologist. Among their most common presenting symptoms are abdominal cramping, diarrhea, constipation, nausea, belching, flatus, and sometimes dysphagia without objective findings of structural bowel disease. Panic disorder is not the only psychiatric disorder associated with such complaints, however, as major depressive disorder and somatization disorder may also present similarly (90, 96). Panic disorder patients also have many nongastrointestinal symptoms, including musculoskeletal complaints, dizziness, fatigue, and pain (56, 77), and may receive diagnoses without identified pathology (often called "functional" disorders) in other body systems such as fibromyalgia, chronic fatigue syndrome, migraine, and irritable bowel syndrome (53, 76, 93, 124, 128).

Although panic disorder has long been considered to be a chronic disorder, recent longitudinal studies have not demonstrated it to be a uniformly chronic and progressive disorder (58). A follow-up study of 423 panic disorder patients an average of 4 years later found 31% to have fully remitted and remained well, 19% having a severe chronic course, and 25% with an episodic course with panic-free intervals (58). A longer follow-up study, of 77 panic disorder patients over 8 years, found that more than two-thirds of patients with panic disorder only and more than one-third of patients with panic disorder and agoraphobia had remitted from the disorder (146). A study with even longer follow-up, 12 years, compared the course of 50 panic disorder patients without agoraphobia and 244 panic disorder patients with agoraphobia. Recovery from the index episode was achieved by 82% of the panic disorder patients without agora-phobia and 48% of those with agoraphobia (19). Slightly over half of the patients who had recovered from their disorder experienced a relapse during the follow-up period, with similar relapse rates for the group with panic disorder only and the group with panic disorder and agoraphobia.

Agoraphobia usually develops in the middle or late 20s, and almost never before 18 or after 35 (59). The first anxiety attack often occurs against a back-ground of worry and unhappiness: job dissatisfaction, domestic crisis, serious medical illness, a death in the family. Nevertheless, people with agoraphobia do not associate the first anxiety attack with a specific stress that would justify panic. Isaac Marks quotes a patient as saying (83):

> I was standing at the bus stop wondering what to cook for dinner when suddenly I felt panicky and sweaty, my knees felt like jelly, and I had to hold on to the lamppost and I was afraid I would die. I got on the bus and was terribly nervous, but just managed to totter home. Since then I haven't liked to go out on the street and have never been on a bus again.

Specific and social phobias have an earlier onset than agoraphobia. The onset of specific phobias most often occurs in childhood (64). Most social phobias first occur in adolescence or the early 20s. They rarely begin before puberty or after age 35 (138). Unlike specific phobias and agoraphobia, which affect many more women than men, social phobias affect both sexes more equally (138). Most social phobias develop over several months, beginning without any apparent precipitating event, and stabilizing after a period of years with a gradual diminution of severity in middle life.

Specific phobias beginning in childhood and early adolescence tend to improve and eventually disappear, approximately half of them disappearing within 5 years (1). Phobias beginning after adolescence persist longer and gradually worsen in about one-third of patients. Specific phobias that persist into adulthood have only about a 20% likelihood of remission (4). Follow-up studies of social phobia demonstrate a more chronic course: only about one-third of patients are in remission after 5–8 years (87, 146). Early-onset social phobia appears to be more severe and persistent than later-onset social phobia (62).

Outcomes of panic and phobic disorders may vary according to psychiatric comorbidities. Among panic disorder patients, comorbidity with major depressive disorder reduces the recovery rates by approximately half and approximately doubles the likelihood of relapse (19). Personality disorder, observed in more than one-third of 141 patients with social phobia but in only one-fifth of 386 patients with panic disorder, was associated with a more chronic course in social phobia but not in panic disorder over a 1–5 year follow-up period (87). Men and women fare about equally well (or poorly) in outcomes of panic and phobic disorders (145).

Complications

Depression is the most common complication of panic disorder. Half of panic disorder patients experience comorbidity with major depressive disorder (12). There is no predilection for either disorder to precede the other in initial onset (34, 120).

Because of the frequent comorbidity of major depression with panic disorder, there has been speculation that panic disorder is a variant or an epiphenomenon of major depressive disorder (34). Both conditions are relieved by antidepressant medications. Arguments against the illnesses being identical are as follows: *(1)* panic disorder has an earlier age of onset than major depressive disorder; *(2)* panic attacks can usually be precipitated in people with a history of spontaneous panic attacks by the intravenous infusion of sodium lactate, and this rarely happens in depressed controls (103); and *(3)* failure of suppression in the dexamethasone suppression test occurs in about half of patients with major depressive disorder but is rare in individuals with spontaneous panic attacks (21).

Psychiatric comorbidity is to be expected in people with social phobia, occurring in 80%. Major depressive disorder, panic disorder, and substance use disorders commonly accompany social phobia (75). In contrast, specific phobias are far less likely to have associated psychiatric comorbidities (59).

Accumulating evidence from epidemiologic research has documented a definite overabundance of alcohol problems among people with panic or phobic disorders, and, conversely, increased prevalence of panic and phobic disorders among individuals with alcohol use disorders (27, 92, 127). There are three possible causal interpretations of these associations: *(1)* anxiety symptoms might lead to problems with alcohol, potentially through a hypothesized process of "self-medication" of anxiety symptoms with alcohol; *(2)* anxiety might result from neurological changes induced by alcohol use or withdrawal (as many alcoholics are observed to have panic attacks, particularly when hung over); or *(3)* there may be no direct causal relationship but rather an indirect connection between alcohol and anxiety problems through associations with other causal factors such as common genetic vulnerabilities (27).

Causal directionality is theoretically not possible if temporality of onset is inconsistent with it (92). In other words, if the onset of the alcohol disorder regularly preceded the anxiety disorder, then the alcohol disorder cannot regularly be a result of the anxiety disorder. Research studies have documented the onset of phobic disorders to precede the onset of alcohol use disorders most of the time (75, 92, 127). Studies of relative onset of panic disorder and alcohol use disorders have been less consistent, although panic precedes alcohol problems slightly more often than the opposite pattern (27). Temporal directionality does not necessarily imply causality, however. It has also been pointed out that while the causal hypotheses regarding the association of alcohol and panic disorder may seem diametrically opposed, they may not necessarily be mutually exclusive: When the panic disorder precedes the alcohol disorder, panic may promote alcohol problems, and when the alcohol problem comes first it may promote panic (27). Drug abuse may occur as a complication of panic disorder, the occasional result of overzealous prescription of habit-forming medication by well-meaning physicians.

Panic disorder is associated with reduced longevity. Men with panic disorder have twice the expected death rates, largely from cardiovascular disease and suicide (26, 46). Reduced heart rate variability, documented among patients with panic disorder (143), is considered an indicator of elevated cardiac sympathetic activity and may contribute to risk for cardiac mortality in these individuals (143, 144). Research has not determined, however, whether the panic disorder itself or something else increases the risk for cardiovascular death (40, 74). Panic disorder is also associated with another cardiac risk factor, elevated cholesterol levels, but the causal directionalities in this relationship are unclear. Cholesterol levels are not associated with panic symptom severity and do not change with remission of panic disorder (142). Although an association between panic disorder and suicidality has often been described (65), controversy has long surrounded this finding. Recent work has clarified that apparent associations between suicidality and panic disorder can be explained by the presence of comorbid psychiatric disorders such as major depression (33). Suicide does not appear to be a complication of phobic disorders in patients without psychiatric comorbidity such as major depressive and alcohol use disorders (75).

Although many people with panic disorder are able to function and experience a satisfactory quality of life, the disorder can be associated with varying degrees of disability. In a study of 72 outpatients with panic disorder and agoraphobia, 15% reported that they were completely unable to work and another 46% described significantly impaired work functioning (73). Those with avoidance behavior had the most impairment in work functioning. Rubin and colleagues (115) found that panic disorder patients lost the equivalent of 39 functional days per year, similar to patients with non-insulin-dependent diabetes. In general population data, a diagnosis of panic disorder increased the likelihood of starting to receive disability benefits by a factor of 5.2 (70). Among 85 panic disorder patients studied by Carpiniello and colleagues (20), 60% reported a significant difficulty in performing daily activities and 40% expressed dissatisfaction in their quality of life. The patients with comorbid agoraphobia had more disability than those with panic disorder only. Curiously, symptom severity was not associated with level of disability. Other work has demonstrated that psychiatric comorbidity, personality abnormalities, increasing age, and lack of education are associated with greater impairment in functioning in panic disorder patients (52).

With the passage of years, functional disability related to panic disorder may diminish. In an 11-year follow-up study of panic disorder patients, Swoboda and colleagues (130) found that 33% were in remission from the disorder and 90% had only mild or no disability in family or work life. Two-thirds, however, described significant social disabilities, suggesting important effects on the patients' quality of life despite intact functioning in workplace and home settings.

Social phobia is associated with limited educational attainment and with increased likelihood of teenage childbearing and exposure to marital violence (62). Sexual maladjustments, such as inability to experience orgasm, are also known complications of agoraphobia and social phobia (16). Oddly, the sexual difficulties often antedate the phobic symptoms. In isolated phobias, the disability tends to be mild and is limited to responses to the phobic object or situation. About 20% of patients with specific phobia find that the problem impairs their work or social functioning.

Agoraphobia is considered the most disabling of the phobic disorders. When severe, it can be as crippling as severe schizophrenia, but chronic hospitalization is not required. These patients are sometimes unable to leave home for months or years at a time. In extreme cases, patients may confine themselves to a single room or spend most of their time in bed. Even milder cases involve restrictions in social functioning such as inability to visit friends and neighbors or to go on family outings. Agoraphobic individuals recruit other people to do their shopping and take their children to school. They postpone seeing the dentist and may cut their own hair. Fortunately, available treatments—behavioral and pharmacological—provide relief for many (see section "Clinical Management").

Family and Genetic Studies

Panic disorder is a strikingly familial condition (38, 42, 122). Relatives of individuals with panic disorder have a 3%–17% higher likelihood of developing panic disorder, compared to the general population (38). Twin studies find a much higher concordance of panic disorder among monozygotic twins than in dyzygotic twins (38, 102). These findings support a genetic predisposition.

Studies addressing the question of whether phobias are heritable have also provided evidence of familial aggregation (51, 59, 81, 122). Numerous twin studies have addressed the nature–nurture issue of phobias, and the largest, in which more than 2,000 twins were interviewed, showed varying degrees of heritability for the different phobias (59). Agoraphobia demonstrated the greatest genetic heritability and specific phobias the least heritability of the phobic disorders. Social phobia was intermediate between agoraphobia and specific phobias in genetic heritability.

Smoller and Tsuang (122) reviewed research on the relationship between panic disorder and agoraphobia in family members of patients with these disorders. Relatives of probands with panic disorder show increased risk of panic disorder, although inconsistent risk for agoraphobia. Relatives of probands with agoraphobia appear to have increased risk of both agoraphobia and panic disorder. These findings do not support conceptualization of agoraphobia as a subtype of panic disorder.

Panic disorder and major depression appear to overlap in family transmission (60, 80). This might suggest a common diathesis. Patients with primary major depression alone, however, have increased rates of major depressive disorder but not panic disorder among their relatives; conversely, patients with primary panic disorder and secondary depression have increased rates of panic disorder but not major depressive disorder among family members (34, 134). These findings contradict notions that panic disorder and major depression may represent an epiphenomenon or a complication of one another or that comorbid major depression and panic disorder may constitute a distinct syndrome transmitted in families.

Patients with panic disorder and agoraphobia have higher rates of alcoholism among their first-degree family members compared to first-degree family members of controls (49, 118).

Differential Diagnosis

The diagnosis of panic disorder obviously requires the exclusion of medical conditions that give rise to similar symptoms. Medical illnesses that produce symptoms resembling those of panic disorder include cardiac arrhythmias (especially paroxysmal atrial tachycardia), angina, chronic obstructive pulmonary disease, asthma, hyperthyroidism, and pheochromocytoma (120). Symptoms such as heart palpitations and chest pain occurring as part of panic disorder are not easily differentiated from manifestations of a primary cardiac disorder (120).

Many panic disorder patients seek treatment first in emergency rooms or other medical settings (54). Unfortunately, clinicians not familiar with panic disorder as a specific diagnostic entity may mistakenly attribute the symptoms to a physical condition. A Canadian study of patients presenting to emergency rooms with chest pain found that 98% of panic disorder goes unrecognized in this setting (78).

Individuals reporting a history of chest pain have four times the prevalence of panic disorder as other people (54). The presence of panic disorder, however, does not rule out cardiac disease: 21% of panic disorder patients admitted to a coronary care unit had medical findings, including myocardial infarction (120). Of acute coronary care inpatients with negative cardiac workups, more than half have panic disorder (120). Five variables have been identified in association with panic disorder among patients presenting to a hospital emergency department with chest pain: *(1)* absence of coronary artery disease, *(2)* atypical quality of chest pain, *(3)* female sex, *(4)* younger age, and *(5)* reporting high levels of anxiety (54).

Somatization disorder can be identified in as many as one-third or more of patients with irritable bowel syndrome and may account for the apparent association of psychiatric disorders such as panic disorder with irritable bowel syndrome (96, 132, 136). Because patients with somatization disorder complain of multiple medically unexplained symptoms, both physical and psychological, across multiple organ systems, co-occurring complaints of both panic and gastrointestinal symptoms may commonly occur in these patients.

How far to pursue a physical explanation for symptoms that may represent panic disorder depends on clinical judgment, but considerable resources are often invested in tests and consultations. A pharmacoeconomic review found the mean cost of medical treatment over the course of 1 year among panic disorder patients to be more than $1,100, approximately 5.5 times the health care cost of social phobia and 10 times the health care costs of controls over the same period (48). In one study (98), panic disorder patients received an average of five laboratory tests and two consultations with specialists. As the authors explained, "This is not unusual, since most patients did not consider their illness as psychiatric but saw themselves as persons suffering from undiagnosed physical conditions. This almost inevitably led to a search for an organic basis for the complaints. Sometimes the search was conducted against the physicians' better judgment in order that the patient might accept psychiatric referral. Even at that, the patients as a group were demanding and not easily satisfied. One patient's remark typified the attitude of many, 'I do not want to be told what I haven't got. I want the doctor to find something.' Another patient stated, 'I know I am nervous, I have always been nervous, but don't try to tell me that is what is wrong.'"

Panic attacks may be accompanied by hyperventilation, which in turn aggravates panic symptoms. Panic symptoms may occur with lowering of pCO_2 as well as other chemical alterations, including an elevation of lactic acid. Five deep breaths produced by yawning or sighing may be enough to alter pCO_2 and produce the characteristic symptoms (24): cerebral hypoxia, a slowing of the electroencephalogram, and respiratory alkalosis, which in turn can induce tetany. Apparently, some individuals are more susceptible than others to the effects of hyperventilation. The existence of a hyperventilation syndrome as a separate disorder has never been established, however. Psychiatric conditions such as somatization disorder or major depressive disorder can be the primary disorder, with hyperventilation or panic attacks occurring secondarily.

Panic attacks can occur as part of any psychiatric illness. Panic attacks commonly occur in major depressive disorder, obsessional illness, phobic disorder, somatization disorder, and alcoholism. Similarly, phobic symptoms are not confined to phobic disorders, and may accompany many other psychiatric disorders.

The mistake probably made most often in the evaluation of anxiety symptoms is that of overlooking major depressive disorder. Among other factors, a family history of mood disorder should alert one to the possibility that a patient with anxiety symptoms may have major depressive disorder with anxious features rather than an anxiety disorder. Also, anxiety that begins for the first time after the age of 40 is commonly part of a depressive syndrome rather than a manifestation of panic disorder. Among patients with well-documented histories of phobic disorder or panic disorder, the development of major depressive episodes with the full range of mood symptoms is common, and these episodes may be indistinguishable from major depressive disorder except for the prior history of significant phobic or panic symptoms. Such depressive episodes probably should be considered "secondary" (not implying etiological connotations with this nosologic distinction). Conversely, major depression not uncommonly presents with panic attacks or phobic qualities such as fearfulness of social situations or disease as part of the episode, potentially distracting the clinician from appreciating the major depressive disorder.

Most somatization disorder patients acknowledge significant problems with anxiety. Somatization disorder involves a broad range of medical complaints with frequent hospitalizations and operations not typical of panic and phobic disorders. Panic and phobic disorder patients do not undergo hospitalization and surgery more frequently than other individuals. The main differentiating feature is that panic and phobic disorders are not characterized by dramatic and medically unexplained complaints in nearly every area of the review of symptoms, as is the case in somatization disorder. Further, sexual and menstrual complaints and conversion symptoms (unexplained neurological complaints), common in somatization disorder, are not frequently encountered among patients with panic or phobic disorders.

Panic disorder, phobic disorder, and obsessive-compulsive disorder may be difficult to distinguish from one another. All three conditions begin early in life and have a chronic though sometimes fluctuating course. Phobias frequently accompany panic disorder. The distinction between phobic and panic disorder depends on whether phobias dominate the clinical picture. The most conspicuous feature of panic disorder is anxiety attacks unrelated to external situations in which the subjective experience of fear is accompanied by cardiorespiratory symptoms. Phobias and panic attacks also frequently occur in obsessive-compulsive disorder. Obsessive-compulsive disorder involves a panoply of obsessional symptoms and checking and compulsive rituals such as counting that are not a part of phobic or panic disorders. Although ruminations and compulsions may occur in mild or incomplete forms among patients with panic disorder, they are not characteristically severe.

Panic disorder can be mistaken for posttraumatic stress disorder. Panic disorder is not among the conditions most likely to be precipitated by exposure to a life-threatening event (97). In one series (91), patients who had experienced a life-threatening accident subsequently experienced a long period (6 months to 3 years) of free-floating anxiety, muscular tension, irritability, impaired concentration, repetitive nightmares of the accident, and social withdrawal. None of the patients, however, had cardiorespiratory or other autonomic symptoms, the hallmark of typical panic disorder.

Excessive worriers sometimes receive a diagnosis of generalized anxiety disorder. Despite the term, generalized anxiety disorder often involves anxiety about specific events such as work or school disturbance. The person is restless, easily tired, irritable, and may have trouble concentrating as well as sleep difficulty. Fears (which are usually chronic) in generalized anxiety disorder are distinguishable from phobia by their shifting focus and absence of avoidance behavior. Although generalized anxiety disorder has been said to afflict about 5% of the population at some time during their lives (139), the validity and reliability of the diagnosis remain questionable.

When phobic-like symptoms occur in schizophrenia, they are usually bizarre and unaccompanied by insight. Panic attacks occasionally occur in patients with schizophrenia, especially during exacerbations of psychosis.

Clinical Management

Psychiatric referral is rarely necessary for panic disorder if the patient's physician has diagnosed the disorder correctly, understands its natural history, and is willing to discuss the disorder with the patient. Telling the patient that there is nothing wrong physically is usually not enough. Some patients resent the implication that their symptoms might be "psychological." Others continue to believe that they have a serious illness. The physician should agree that something is wrong and should describe the syndrome in lay terms. Many patients are relieved by such an explanation and thereby become receptive to further reassurance.

As noted earlier, some patients with gastrointestinal or musculoskeletal complaints meet the criteria for panic disorder. In these cases, treatment should focus primarily on the basic underlying disorder—the panic disorder—so that the presenting physical complaints are viewed in this context and treated as conservatively as possible. In this process, however, clinicians should conduct a complete psychiatric evaluation to determine whether the patient has an anxiety disorder or whether the anxiety symptoms are a manifestation of another psychiatric disorder such as major depression or somatization disorder.

In the 1960s, Klein and colleagues in New York (66) and Marks and colleagues in England (82) found that antidepressants prevented panic attacks (99). The New York group focused on imipramine and the British group on monoamine oxidase inhibitors (MAOIs). Both types of drugs apparently had similar efficacy in preventing panic attacks, although there was some disagreement about the relief persisting after the drugs were discontinued and about the role of supportive or behavioral therapy in augmenting the effects of the drugs. The selective SSRI (e.g., fluoxetine, paroxetine) and serotonin-norepinephrine reuptake inhibitor (SNRI) (e.g., venlafaxine) antidepressants and other "newer generation" antidepressants (e.g., mirtazepine) are equally effective, better tolerated, and safer (8, 37, 104, 149). Their main side effects include gastrointestinal symptoms, headache, and sedation, particularly early in treatment, as well as sexual dysfunction and increased anxiety, but these can be managed by careful advancement of dosage and attention to the patient (11, 104). For these reasons, the SSRIs have become standard treatment for panic disorder and agoraphobia (18, 104). Despite this, benzodiazepine monotherapy remains the most widely used treatment for panic disorder in general practice (104, 129).

Benzodiazepines effectively prevent panic attacks, but large doses may be necessary (39, 129, 147). This type of medication generally does not work quickly enough to relieve panic attacks that are already underway (147). Benzodiazepines also reduce anticipatory anxiety between attacks. Adverse effects of benzodiazepines include drowsiness, ataxia, and cognitive and motor impairment (11). Additionally, potential for abuse and dependence limits selection of benzodiazepines as first-line agents and makes them a better short-term than long-term solution (11, 57, 147). In the treatment of comorbid major depression that is common in patients with panic disorder, antidepressants are preferable to benzodiazepines (57). Benzodiazepines are often administered concurrently with antidepressants for the treatment of panic disorder, especially initially in therapy. Although a benzodiazepine may accelerate the antidepressant response and reduce antidepressant-related stimulation (129), the advantage of benzodiazepine coadministration does not appear to last beyond about 3 months (104).

Recent research on the anticonvulsants valproic acid and gabapentin (but not carbamazepine) has some documented evidence of efficacy in panic disorder. Additionally, novel anticonvulsant medications pregabalin, tiagabine, and levatiracetam also show promise as potentially useful agents. Buspirone and beta blockers do not appear to be effective as monotherapy for panic disorder, but they may have potential for use as adjunctive agents (104).

Outside of the literature on agoraphobia, most available information from research on treatment of phobias has emerged from studies of social phobia. SSRIs are presently considered the first-line choice of treatment for social phobia, and the SNRI venlafaxine shows promise of similar efficacy (30, 125). The MAOIs such as phenelzine also appear to be quite effective, but their use is limited by the dietary and medication restrictions, side effects, and potential for hypertensive crises (31, 125). Although reversible inhibitors of monoamine oxidase type A (RIMAs) such as moclobemide and brofaramine appear to better tolerated and safer than MAOIs, these medications may not be as effective, and they lack availability and general acceptance as a treatment for social phobia at present (31, 125). Benzodiazepines are superior to placebo in treatment of social phobia, and they can be useful for individuals who fail to respond to or are not candidates for SSRI therapy, or as adjunctive to SSRI therapy (31, 125). Medications with selective action on the gamma-aminobutyric acid (GABA) system, for example, clonazepam, gabapentin, and pregabalin, have also been found helpful for social phobia (31). Because social phobia is a chronic disorder, relapse is common with discontinuation of medication, and long-term treatment is needed to maintain response (31, 125).

Tricyclic antidepressants, buspirone, and beta blockers have not been consistently shown to have efficacy for social phobia treatment (31, 121, 149). Despite anecdotal evidence and popular support for the use of beta blockers in performance anxiety (stage fright), placebo-controlled studies have provided no evidence of their effectiveness (13, 125).

Little research has focused on the pharmacotherapy of specific phobia. A review by Birk (13) concluded that anxiolytic medication for specific phobia and performance anxiety, unlike most other anxiety syndromes, not only lacks efficacy but is also contraindicated because it may reduce the effectiveness of exposure therapies and interfere with the extinction of fear responses. In a study of randomly assigned alprazolam pretreatment of 28 female flight attendants with phobias, Wilhelm and Roth (137) reported that the alprazolam was actually associated with increased physiological activation in the acute stress situation of flying, and it hindered therapeutic effects of exposure. Recent reports that D-cycloserine, an NMDA receptor agonist, has been found to increase extinction of conditioned fear in animal studies and that it may accelerate improvement of acrophobia in patients treated with virtual reality therapy (13, 32) suggest potential utility for this agent in the management of specific phobias, although further research is needed.

There has been much speculation about the action of antidepressant and benzodiazepine drugs in reducing anxiety and preventing panic attacks. Antidepressants appear to prevent panic attacks by decreasing norepinephrine turnover in the brain (6), and SSRIs may also reduce panic through activation of serotonin systems (15, 61, 126, 149). Benzodiazepines enhance inhibitory GABAergic transmission as well as acting on noradrenergic systems (129, 150).

Beta-adrenergic blocking agents such as propranolol, used for cardiac arrhythmias, were once considered a promising treatment for reducing the physiologic symptoms of panic disorder (107, 131). These medications have proven disappointing, however, as monotherapy for panic disorder in more recent placebo-controlled trials (113).

Before the emphasis on pharmacotherapy, the most popular approach to the treatment of specific and social phobias involved behavioral techniques based on learning theory, such as "systematic desensitization," introduced by Wolpe (140). This method consists of training patients to relax and then gradually exposing them to increasingly intensive versions of the phobic stimulus, which theoretically cancels the sensation of fear if the stimulus is not overwhelming. Exposure-based therapies used today have historic roots in desensitization therapy. Such therapies have historically invoked stimuli generated by the patient's imagination, but in recent applications, virtual reality technology provides real-seeming but imaginary scenes of phobic situations germane to patients' fears.

The main psychological treatments for panic and phobic disorders in current use involve cognitive-behavioral and cognitive therapy, exposure, and response-prevention therapies (14). The elements fundamental to cognitive-behavioral therapy are exposure, reduction of safety-seeking behaviors, attention focus modification, and cognitive restructuring (85). The main drawback to psychotherapies for panic and phobic disorders is the time commitment and effort required of the patient (11, 100). Prolonged and expensive forms of psychotherapy are rarely indicated.

A review of psychotherapeutic interventions for social phobia found cognitive and behavioral interventions superior to wait-list controls and supportive therapy (114). Comparison studies of cognitive-behavioral therapies and pharmacotherapy, however, have failed to demonstrate any consistent advantage of combining psychotherapy and pharmacotherapy over either intervention alone for phobic and panic disorders (14).

Regardless of the theoretical orientation of the treating clinician, it is generally agreed that at some point the patient must confront the feared situation. Most treatments—medications, psychotherapy, and behavior modification techniques—are designed to reduce panic and anxiety to the extent that the patient can tolerate exposure to his or her anxieties.

REFERENCES

1. Agras, W. S., Chapin, H. N., and Oliveau, D. C. The natural history of phobia. Course and prognosis. Arch. Gen. Psychiat., 26:315–317, 1972.

2. American Psychiatric Association. *Diagnostic and Statistical Manual of Mental Disorders*, 3rd edition. Washington, DC: Author, 1980.

3. American Psychiatric Association. *Diagnostic and Statistical Manual of Mental Disorders,* 3rd edition, revised. Washington, DC: Author, 1987.

4. American Psychiatric Association. *Diagnostic and Statistical Manual of Mental Disorders*, 4th edition. Washington, DC: Author, 1994.

5. American Psychiatric Association. *Diagnostic and Statistical Manual of Mental Disorders*, 4th edition, revised. Washington, DC: Author, 2000.

6. Bailey, J. E., Argyropoulos, S. V., Lightman, S. L., and Nutt, D. J. Does the brain noradrenaline network mediate the effects of the CO_2 challenge? J. Psychopharmacol., *17*:252–259, 2003.

7. Baillie, A. J., and Rapee, R. M. Panic attacks as risk markers for mental disorders. Soc. Psychiat. Psychiat. Epidemiol., *40*:240–244, 2005.

8. Bakker, A., van Balkom, A. J., and Spinhoven, P. SSRIs vs. TCAs in the treatment of panic disorder: a meta-analysis. Acta Psychiat. Scand., *106*:163–167, 2002.

9. Battaglia, M., Bertella, S., Bajo, S., Binaghi, F., and Bellodi, L. Anticipation of age at onset in panic disorder. Am. J. Psychiat., *155*:590–595, 1998.

10. Beard, G. M. Neurasthenia or nervous exhaustion. Boston Med. Surg. J., *3*:217, 1869.

11. Bennett, J. A., Moioffer, M., Stanton, S. P., Dwight, M., and Keck, P. E., Jr. A risk-benefit assessment of pharmacological treatments for panic disorder. Drug Safety, *18*:419–430, 1998.

12. Biederman, J., Petty, C., Faraone, S. V., Hirshfeld-Becker, D. R., Henin, A., Pollack, M. H., and Rosenbaum, J. F. Patterns of comorbidity in panic disorder and major depression: findings from a nonreferred sample. Depress. Anxiety, *21*:55–60, 2005.

13. Birk, L. Pharmacotherapy for performance anxiety disorders: occasionally useful but typically contraindicated. J. Clin. Psychol., *60*:867–879, 2004.

14. Black, D. W. Efficacy of combined pharmacotherapy and psychotherapy versus monotherapy in the treatment of anxiety disorders. CNS Spectr., *11*:29–33, 2006.

15. Bocola, V., Trecco, M. D., Fabbrini, G., Paladini, C., Sollecito, A., and Martucci, N. Antipanic effect of fluoxetine measured by CO_2 challenge test. Biol. Psychiat., *43*:612–615, 1998.

16. Bodinger, L., Hermesh, H., Aizenberg, D., Valevski, A., Marom, S., Shiloh, R., Gothelf, D., Zemishlany, Z., and Weizman, A. Sexual function and behavior in social phobia. J. Clin. Psychiat., *63*:874–879, 2002.

17. Boshuisen, M. L., Ter Horst, G. J., Paans, A. M., Reinders, A. A., and den Boer, J. A. rCBF differences between panic disorder patients and control subjects during anticipatory anxiety and rest. Biol. Psychiat., *52*:126–135, 2002.

18. Bruce, S. E., Vasile, R. G., Goisman, R. M., Salzman, C., Spencer, M., Machan, J. T., and Keller, M. B. Are benzodiazepines still the medication of choice for patients with panic disorder with or without agoraphobia? Am. J. Psychiat., *160*:1432–1438, 2003.

19. Bruce, S. E., Yonkers, K. A., Otto, M. W., Eisen, J. L., Weisberg, R. B., Pagano, M., Shea, M. T., and Keller, M. B. Influence of psychiatric comorbidity on recovery and recurrence in generalized anxiety disorder, social phobia, and panic disorder: a 12-year prospective study. Am. J. Psychiat., *162*:1179–1187, 2005.

20. Carpiniello, B., Baita, A., Carta, M. G., Sitzia, R., Macciardi, A. M., Murgia, S., and Altamura, A. C. Clinical and psychosocial outcome of patients affected by panic disorder with or without agoraphobia: results from a naturalistic follow-up study. Eur. Psychiat., *17*:394–398, 2002.

21. Carroll, B. J. The dexamethasone test for melancholia. Br. J. Psychiat., *140*:292–304, 1982.

22. Cassano, G. B., Petracca, A., Perugi, G., Toni, C., Tundo, A., and Roth, M. Derealization and panic attacks: a clinical evaluation on 150 patients with panic disorder/agoraphobia. Compr. Psychiat., *30*:5–12, 1989.

23. Chatel, J. C., and Peele, R. A centennial review of neurasthenia. J. Psychiat., *126*:1404–1413, 1970.

24. Christensen, B. Studies on hyperventilation. II: Electrocardiographic changes in normal man during voluntary hyperventilation. J. Clin. Invest., *24*:880, 1946.

25. Cohen, M., and White, P. Life situations, emotions, and neurocirculatory asthenia (anxiety neurosis, neurasthenia, effort syndrome). Ass. Res. Nerv. Dis. Proc., *29*:832–869, 1950.

26. Coryell, W. Panic disorder and mortality. Psychiat. Clin. N. Am., *11*:433–440, 1988.

27. Cosci, F., Schruers, K. R., Abrams, K., and Griez, E. J. Alcohol use disorders and panic disorder: a review of the evidence of a direct relationship. J. Clin. Psychiat., *68*:874–880, 2007.

28. Cowley, D. S., and Arana, G. W. The diagnostic utility of lactate sensitivity in panic disorder. Arch. Gen. Psychiat., *47*:277–284, 1990.

29. Dalessio, D. J. Hyperventilation: the vapors, effort syndrome, neurasthenia. JAMA, *239*:1401–1402, 1978.

30. Davidson, J. R. Social anxiety disorder under scrutiny. Depress. Anxiety, *11*:93–98, 2000.

31. Davidson, J. R. Pharmacotherapy of social phobia. Acta Psychiat. Scand. Suppl., *417*: 65–71, 2003.

32. Davis, M., Walker, D. L., and Myers, K. M. Role of the amygdala in fear extinction measured with potentiated startle. Ann. N. Y. Acad. Sci., *985*:218–232, 2003.

33. Diaconu, G., and Turecki, G. Panic disorder and suicidality: Is comorbidity with depression the key? J. Affect. Disord.,*66 Suppl.4*:2007.

34. Dindo, L., and Coryell, W. Comorbid major depression and panic disorder: significance of temporal sequencing to familial transmission. J. Affect. Disord., *82*:119–123, 2004.

35. Eaton, W. W., Dryman, A., and Weissman, M. M. Panic and phobia. In *Psychiatric Disorders in America: The Epidemiologic Catchment Area Study*, Robins, L. N., Regier, D. A. (eds.). New York: The Free Press, pp. 155–179, 1991.

36. Eaton, W. W., Kessler, R. C., Wittchen, H. U., and Magee, W. J. Panic and panic disorder in the United States. Am. J. Psychiat., *151*:413–420, 1994.

37. Feighner, J. P. Overview of antidepressants currently used to treat anxiety disorders. J. Clin. Psychiat., *60 Suppl 22*:18–22, 1999.

38. Finn, C. T., and Smoller, J. W. The genetics of panic disorder. Curr. Psychiat. Rep., *3*:131–137, 2001.

39. Fisekovic, S., and Loga-Zec, S. Sertraline and alprazolam in the treatment of panic desorder. Bosn. J. Basic Med. Sci., *5*:78–81, 2005.

40. Fleet, R. P., and Beitman, B. D. Cardiovascular death from panic disorder and panic-like anxiety: a critical review of the literature. J. Psychosom. Res., *44*:71–80, 1998.

41. Furmark, T. Social phobia: overview of community surveys. Acta Psychiat. Scand., 105:84–93, 2002.
42. Goldstein, R. B., Weissman, M. M., Adams, P. B., Horwath, E., Lish, J. D., Charney, D., Woods, S. W., Sobin, C., and Wickramaratne, P. J. Psychiatric disorders in relatives of probands with panic disorder and/or major depression. Arch. Gen. Psychiat., 51:383–394, 1994.
43. Goodwin, D. W. *Phobia: The Facts*. London: Oxford University Press, 1983.
44. Goodwin, R. D., Fergusson, D. M., and Horwood, L. J. Childhood abuse and familial violence and the risk of panic attacks and panic disorder in young adulthood. Psychol. Med., 35:881–890, 2005.
45. Gorman, J. M., Papp, L. A., Coplan, J. D., Martinez, J. M., Lennon, S., Goetz, R. R., Ross, D., and Klein, D. F. Anxiogenic effects of CO_2 and hyperventilation in patients with panic disorder. Am. J. Psychiat., 151:547–553, 1994.
46. Grasbeck, A., Rorsman, B., Hagnell, O., and Isberg, P. E. Mortality of anxiety syndromes in a normal population. The Lundby Study. Neuropsychobiol., 33:118–126, 1996.
47. Griez, E., and Schruers, K. Experimental pathophysiology of panic. J. Psychosom. Res., 45:493–503, 1998.
48. Grudzinski, A. N. Considerations in the treatment of anxiety disorders: a pharmacoeconomic review. Expert Opin. Pharmacother., 2:1557–1569, 2001.
49. Gruppo Italiano Disturbi d'Ansia. Familial analysis of panic disorder and agoraphobia. J. Affect. Dis., 17:1–8, 1989.
50. Guze, S. B., Woodruff, R. A., and Clayton, P. J. A study of conversion symptoms in psychiatric outpatients. Am. J. Psychiat., 128:643–646, 1971.
51. Hettema, J. M., Neale, M. C., and Kendler, K. S. A review and meta-analysis of the genetic epidemiology of anxiety disorders. Am. J. Psychiat., 158:1568–1578, 2001.
52. Hollifield, M., Katon, W., Skipper, B., Chapman, T., Ballenger, J. C., Mannuzza, S., and Fyer, A. J. Panic disorder and quality of life: variables predictive of functional impairment. Am. J. Psychiat., 154:766–772, 1997.
53. Hudson, J. I., Goldenberg, D. L., Pope, H. G., Jr., Keck, P. E., Jr., and Schlesinger, L. Comorbidity of fibromyalgia with medical and psychiatric problems. Am. J. Med., 92:363–367, 1992.
54. Huffman, J. C., and Pollack, M. H. Predicting panic disorder among patients with chest pain: an analysis of the literature. Psychosomat., 44:222–236, 2003.
55. Hybels, C. F., Blazer, D. G., and Kaplan, B. H. Social and personal resources and the prevalence of phobic disorder in a community population. Psychol. Med., 30:705–716, 2000.
56. Kaplan, D. S., Masand, P. S., and Gupta, S. The relationship of irritable bowel syndrome (IBS) and panic disorder. Ann. Clin. Psychiat., 8:81–88, 1996.
57. Kasper, S., and Resinger, E. Panic disorder: the place of benzodiazepines and selective serotonin reuptake inhibitors. Eur. Neuropsychopharmacol., 11:307–321, 2001.
58. Katschnig, H., and Amering, M. The long-term course of panic disorder and its predictors. J. Clin. Psychopharmacol., 18:6S–11S, 1998.

59. Kendler, K. S., Neale, M. C., Kessler, R. C., Heath, A. C., and Eaves, L. J. The genetic epidemiology of phobias in women. The interrelationship of agoraphobia, social phobia, situational phobia, and simple phobia. Arch. Gen. Psychiat., 49:273–281, 1992.

60. Kendler, K. S., Neale, M. C., Kessler, R. C., Heath, A. C., and Eaves, L. J. The clinical characteristics of major depression as indices of the familial risk to illness. Br. J. Psychiat., 165:66–72, 1994.

61. Kent, J. M., Coplan, J. D., and Gorman, J. M. Clinical utility of the selective serotonin reuptake inhibitors in the spectrum of anxiety. Biol. Psychiat., 44:812–824, 1998.

62. Kessler, R. C. The impairments caused by social phobia in the general population: implications for intervention. Acta Psychiat. Scand. Suppl., 417:19–27, 2003.

63. Kessler, R. C., Chiu, W. T., Demler, O., Merikangas, K. R., and Walters, E. E. Prevalence, severity, and comorbidity of 12-month DSM-IV disorders in the National Comorbidity Survey Replication. Arch. Gen. Psychiat., 62:617–627, 2005.

64. Kessler, R. C., McGonagle, K. A., Zhao, S., Nelson, C. B., Hughes, M., Eshleman, S., Wittchen, H. U., and Kendler, K. S. Lifetime and 12-month prevalence of DSM-III-R psychiatric disorders in the United States. Results from the National Comorbidity Survey. Arch. Gen. Psychiat., 51:8–19, 1994.

65. Khan, A., Leventhal, R. M., Khan, S., and Brown, W. A. Suicide risk in patients with anxiety disorders: a meta-analysis of the FDA database. J. Affect. Dis., 68:183–190, 2002.

66. Klein, D. F. Importance of psychiatric diagnosis in prediction of clinical drug effects. Arch. Gen. Psychiat., 16:118–126, 1967.

67. Klein, D. F. False suffocation alarms, spontaneous panics, and related conditions. An integrative hypothesis. Arch. Gen. Psychiat., 50:306–317, 1993.

68. Klein, D. F., Zitrin, C. M., Woerner, M. G., and Ross, D. C. Treatment of phobias. II. Behavior therapy and supportive psychotherapy: are there any specific ingredients? Arch. Gen. Psychiat., 40:139–145, 1983.

69. Koenigsberg, H. W., Pollak, C. P., Fine, J., and Kakuma, T. Cardiac and respiratory activity in panic disorder: effects of sleep and sleep lactate infusions. Am. J. Psychiat., 151:1148–1152, 1994.

70. Kouzis, A. C., and Eaton, W. W. Psychopathology and the initiation of disability payments. Psychiat. Serv., 51:908–913, 2000.

71. Kushner, M. G., Sher, K. J., and Beitman, B. D. The relation between alcohol problems and the anxiety disorders. Am. J. Psychiat., 147:685–695, 1990.

72. Lang, P. J. Fear reduction and fear behavior. "Problems in treating a construct." Chicago: 3rd Conference on Research in Psychotherapy, June, 1966.

73. Latas, M., Starcevic, V., and Vucinic, D. Predictors of work disabilities in patients with panic disorder with agoraphobia. Eur. Psychiat., 19:280–284, 2004.

74. Lavoie, K. L., Fleet, R. P., Laurin, C., Arsenault, A., Miller, S. B., and Bacon, S. L. Heart rate variability in coronary artery disease patients with and without panic disorder. Psychiat. Res., 128:289–299, 2004.

75. Lydiard, R. B. Social anxiety disorder: comorbidity and its implications. J. Clin. Psychiat., *62 Suppl* 1:17–23, 2001.

76. Lydiard, R. B. Increased prevalence of functional gastrointestinal disorders in panic disorder: clinical and theoretical implications. CNS Spectr., *10*:899–908, 2005.

77. Lydiard, R. B., Greenwald, S., Weissman, M. M., Johnson, J., Drossman, D. A., and Ballenger, J. C. Panic disorder and gastrointestinal symptoms: findings from the NIMH Epidemiologic Catchment Area project. Am. J. Psychiat., *151*:64–70, 1994.

78. Lynch, P., and Galbraith, K. M. Panic in the emergency room. Can. J. Psychiat., *48*:361–366, 2003.

79. Maddock, R. J. The lactic acid response to alkalosis in panic disorder: an integrative review. J. Neuropsychiat. Clin. Neurosci., *13*:22–34, 2001.

80. Maier, W., Lichtermann, D., Minges, J., Oehrlein, A., and Franke, P. A controlled family study in panic disorder. J. Psychiat. Res., *27 Suppl* 1:79–87, 1993.

81. Marcin, M. S., and Nemeroff, C. B. The neurobiology of social anxiety disorder: the relevance of fear and anxiety. Acta Psychiat. Scand. Suppl., *417*:51–64, 2003.

82. Marks, I., and Lader, M. Anxiety states (anxiety neurosis): a review. J. Nerv. Ment. Dis., *156*:3–18, 1973.

83. Marks, I. M. *Fears and Phobias.* New York: Academic Press, 1969.

84. Marks, I. M. The classification of phobic disorders. Br. J. Psychiat., *116*:377–386, 1970.

85. Marom, S., and Hermesh, H. Cognitive behavior therapy (CBT) in anxiety disorders. Isr. J. Psychiat. Relat. Sci., *40*:135–144, 2003.

86. Maron, E., Kuikka, J. T., Shlik, J., Vasar, V., Vanninen, E., and Tiihonen, J. Reduced brain serotonin transporter binding in patients with panic disorder. Psychiat. Res., *132*:173–181, 2004.

87. Massion, A. O., Dyck, I. R., Shea, M. T., Phillips, K. A., Warshaw, M. G., and Keller, M. B. Personality disorders and time to remission in generalized anxiety disorder, social phobia, and panic disorder. Arch. Gen. Psychiat., *59*:434–440, 2002.

88. McCraty, R., Atkinson, M., Tomasino, D., and Stuppy, W. P. Analysis of twenty-four hour heart rate variability in patients with panic disorder. Biol. Psychol., *56*:131–150, 2001.

89. McLellan, A. T., Luborsky, L., Woody, G. E., and O'Brien, C. P. An improved diagnostic evaluation instrument for substance abuse patients: the Addiction Severity Index. J. Nerv. Ment. Dis., *168*:26–33, 1980.

90. Miller, A., North, C. S., Clouse, R. E., Alpers, D. H., and Wetzel, R. D. Irritable bowel syndrome, psychiatric illness, personality, and abuse: is somatization disorder the missing link? Ann. Clin. Psychiat., *13*:25–30, 2001.

91. Modlin, H. C. Postaccident anxiety syndrome: psychosocial aspects. Am. J. Psychiat., *123*:1008–1012, 2003.

92. Morris, E. P., Stewart, S. H., and Ham, L. S. The relationship between social anxiety disorder and alcohol use disorders: a critical review. Clin. Psychol. Rev., *25*:734–760, 2005.

93. Myers, J. K., Weissman, M. M., Tischler, G. L., Holzer III, C. E., Leaf, P. J., Orvaschel, H., Anthony, J. C., Boyd, J. H., Burke Jr, J. D., Kramer, M., and Stoltzman, R. Six-month prevalence of psychiatric disorders in three communities. Arch. Gen. Psychiat., 41:959–967, 1984.

94. Nemiah, J. C. Phobic disorders (phobic neuroses). In *Comprehensive Textbook of Psychiatry*, 4th edition, Kaplan, H. I., Sadock, B. J. (eds.). Baltimore: Williams and Wilkins, 1985.

95. Ninan, P. T., and Dunlop, B. W. Neurobiology and etiology of panic disorder. J. Clin. Psychiat., *66 Suppl 4*:3–7, 2005.

96. North, C. S., Downs, D., Clouse, R. E., Alrakawi, A., Dokucu, M. E., Cox, J., Spitznagel, E. L., and Alpers, D. H. The presentation of irritable bowel syndrome in the context of somatization disorder. Clin. Gastroenterol. Hepatol., 2:787–795, 2004.

97. North, C. S., Nixon, S. J., Shariat, S., Mallonee, S., McMillen, J. C., Spitznagel, E. L., and Smith, E. M. Psychiatric disorders among survivors of the Oklahoma City bombing. JAMA, 282:755–762, 1999.

98. Noyes, R., Jr., and Clancy, J. Anxiety neurosis: a 5-year follow-up. J. Nerv. Ment. Dis., 162:200–205, 1976.

99. Noyes, R., Jr., and Perry, P. Maintenance treatment with antidepressants in panic disorder. J. Clin. Psychiat., *51 Suppl A*:24–30, 1990.

100. Otto, M. W., Pollack, M. H., and Maki, K. M. Empirically supported treatments for panic disorder: costs, benefits, and stepped care. J. Consult. Clin. Psychol., 68:556–563, 2000.

101. Papp, L. A., Martinez, J. M., Klein, D. F., Coplan, J. D., Norman, R. G., Cole, R., de Jesus, M. J., Ross, D., Goetz, R., and Gorman, J. M. Respiratory psychophysiology of panic disorder: three respiratory challenges in 98 subjects. Am. J. Psychiat., 154:1557–1565, 1997.

102. Perna, G., Caldirola, D., Arancio, C., and Bellodi, L. Panic attacks: a twin study. Psychiat. Res., 66:69–71, 1997.

103. Pitts, F. N., Jr., and McClure, J. N., Jr. Lactate metabolism in anxiety neurosis. N. Engl. J. Med., 277:1329–1336, 1967.

104. Pollack, M. H. The pharmacotherapy of panic disorder. J. Clin. Psychiat., *66 Suppl 4*:23–27, 2005.

105. Ponto, L. L., Kathol, R. G., Kettelkamp, R., Watkins, G. L., Richmond, J. C., Clark, J., and Hichwa, R. D. Global cerebral blood flow after CO_2 inhalation in normal subjects and patients with panic disorder determined with [15o]water and PET. J. Anxiety Dis., 16:247–258, 2002.

106. Pope, A. R., Conrad, K. J., Baxter, W., Elbaum, P., Lisiecki, M. A., Daghestani, A., Hultman, C., and Lyons, J. Case managed residential care for homeless addicted veterans: Evanston/VA. Alc. Treat. Q., 10:155–169, 1993.

107. Ravaris, C. L., Friedman, M. J., Hauri, P. J., and McHugo, G. J. A controlled study of alprazolam and propranolol in panic-disordered and agoraphobic outpatients. J. Clin. Psychopharmacol., 11:344–350, 1991.

108. Regier, D. A., Farmer, M. E., Rae, D. S., Locke, B. Z., Keith, S. J., Judd, L. L., and Goodwin, F. K. Comorbidity of mental-disorders with alcohol and other drug

abuse. Results from the Epidemiologic Catchment Area (ECA) study. JAMA, 264:2511–2518, 1990.

109. Reiman, E. M. The study of panic disorder using positron emission tomography. Psychiat. Dev., 5:63–78, 1987.

110. Reiman, E. M., Raichle, M. E., Butler, F. K., Herscovitch, P., and Robins, E. A focal brain abnormality in panic disorder, a severe form of anxiety. Nature, 310:683–685, 1984.

111. Robins, L. N., Helzer, J. E., Weissman, M. M., Orvaschel, H., Gruenberg, E., Burke, J. D., and Regier, D. A. Lifetime prevalence of specific psychiatric disorders in three sites. Arch. Gen. Psychiat., 41:949–958, 1984.

112. Robins, L. N., Locke, B. Z., and Regier, D. A. An overview of psychiatric disorders in America. In *Psychiatric Disorders in America: The Epidemiologic Catchment Area Study*, Robins, L. N., Regier, D. A. (eds.). New York: The Free Press, pp. 328–386, 1991.

113. Rosenbaum, J. F., Pollack, M. H., and Fredman, S. J. The pharmacotherapy of panic disorder. In *Panic Disorder and Its Treatment*, Rosenbaum, J. F., Pollack, M. H. (eds.). New York: Marcel Dekker, pp. 153–180, 1998.

114. Rowa, K., and Antony, M. M. Psychological treatments for social phobia. Can. J. Psychiat., 50:308–316, 2005.

115. Rubin, H. C., Rapaport, M. H., Levine, B., Gladsjo, J. K., Rabin, A., Auerbach, M., Judd, L. L., and Kaplan, R. Quality of well being in panic disorder: the assessment of psychiatric and general disability. J. Affect. Disord., 57:217–221, 2000.

116. Sakai, Y., Kumano, H., Nishikawa, M., Sakano, Y., Kaiya, H., Imabayashi, E., Ohnishi, T., Matsuda, H., Yasuda, A., Sato, A., Diksic, M., and Kuboki, T. Cerebral glucose metabolism associated with a fear network in panic disorder. NeuroReport, 16:927–931, 2005.

117. Sanderson, W. C., Wetzler, S., and Asnis, G. M. Alprazolam blockade of CO_2-provoked panic in patients with panic disorders. Am. J. Psychiat., 151:1220–1222, 1994.

118. Shih, R. A., Belmonte, P. L., and Zandi, P. P. A review of the evidence from family, twin and adoption studies for a genetic contribution to adult psychiatric disorders. Int. Rev. Psychiat., 16:260–283, 2004.

119. Simon, G. E., and VonKorff, M. Somatization and psychiatric disorder in the NIMH Epidemiologic Catchment Area study. Am. J. Psychiat., 148:1494–1500, 1991.

120. Simon, N. M., and Fischmann, D. The implications of medical and psychiatric comorbidity with panic disorder. J. Clin. Psychiat., 66 Suppl 4:8–15, 2005.

121. Simpson, H. B., Schneier, F. R., Campeas, R. B., Marshall, R. D., Fallon, B. A., Davies, S., Klein, D. F., and Liebowitz, M. R. Imipramine in the treatment of social phobia. J. Clin. Psychopharmacol., 18 A:132–135, 1998.

122. Smoller, J. W., and Tsuang, M. T. Panic and phobic anxiety: defining phenotypes for genetic studies. Am. J. Psychiat., 155:1152–1162, 1998.

123. Snaith, R. P. A clinical investigation of phobias. Br. J. Psychiat., 114:673–697, 1968.

124. Sperber, A. D., Atzmon, Y., Neumann, L., Weisber, I., Shalit, Y., Abu-Shkrah, M., Fich, A., and Buskila, D. Fibromyalgia in the irritable bowel syndrome: studies of prevalence and clinical implications. Am. J. Gastroenterol., 94:3541–3546, 1999.

125. Stein, D. J., Ipser, J. C., and Balkom, A. J. Pharmacotherapy for social phobia. Cochrane Database Syst. Rev. CD001206, 2004.

126. Stein, D. J., and Stahl, S. Serotonin and anxiety: current models. Int. Clin. Psychopharmacol., 15 *Suppl* 2:S1–S6, 2000.

127. Stinson, F. S., Dawson, D. A., Patricia, C. S., Smith, S., Goldstein, R. B., June, R. W., and Grant, B. F. The epidemiology of DSM-IV specific phobia in the USA: results from the National Epidemiologic Survey on Alcohol and Related Conditions. Psychol. Med., 37:1047–1059, 2007.

128. Sullivan, P. F., Smith, W., and Buchwald, D. Latent class analysis of symptoms associated with chronic fatigue syndrome and fibromyalgia. Psychol. Med., 32:881–888, 2002.

129. Susman, J., and Klee, B. The role of high-potency benzodiazepines in the treatment of panic disorder. Prim. Care Comp. J. Clin. Psychiat., 7:5–11, 2005.

130. Swoboda, H., Amering, M., Windhaber, J., and Katschnig, H. The long-term course of panic disorder: an 11 year follow-up. J. Anxiety Dis., 17:223–232, 2003.

131. Tyrer, P. Current status of beta-blocking drugs in the treatment of anxiety disorders. Drugs, 36:773–783, 1988.

132. Walker, E. A., Gelfand, A. N., Gelfand, M. D., and Katon, W. J. Psychiatric diagnoses, sexual and physical victimization, and disability in patients with irritable bowel syndrome or inflammatory bowel disease. Psychol. Med., 25:1259–1267, 1995.

133. Weissman, M. M., Myers, J. K., and Harding, P. S. Psychiatric disorders in a U.S. urban community: 1975–1976. Am. J. Psychiat., 135:459–462, 1978.

134. Weissman, M. M., Wickramaratne, P., Adams, P. B., Lish, J. D., Horwath, E., Charney, D., Woods, S. W., Leeman, E., and Frosch, E. The relationship between panic disorder and major depression. A new family study. Arch. Gen. Psychiat., 50:767–780, 1993.

135. Westphal, C. Agoraphobie: eine neuropathische Erscheinuung. Arch. Psychiat. Nervenk., 3:138–221, 1871.

136. Whitehead, W. E., and Crowell, M. D. Psychologic considerations in the irritable bowel syndrome. Gastroenterol. Clin. N. Am., 20:249–267, 1991.

137. Wilhelm, F. H., and Roth, W. T. Acute and delayed effects of alprazolam on flight phobics during exposure. Behav. Res. Ther., 35:831–841, 1997.

138. Wittchen, H. U., and Fehm, L. Epidemiology and natural course of social fears and social phobia. Acta Psychiat. Scand. Suppl., 417:4–18, 2003.

139. Wittchen, H. U., Zhao, S., Kessler, R. C., and Eaton, W. W. DSM-III-R generalized anxiety disorder in the National Comorbidity Survey. Arch. Gen. Psychiat., 51:355–364, 1994.

140. Wolpe, J. *Psychotherapy by Reciprocal Inhibition*. Stanford, CA: Stanford University Press, 1958.

141. Woodruff, R. A., Jr., Guze, S. B., and Clayton, P. J. Anxiety neurosis among psychiatric outpatients. Compr. Psychiat., 13:165–170, 1972.

142. Yamada, K., Tsutsumi, T., and Fujii, I. Serum cholesterol levels in patients with panic disorders: a comparison with major depression and schizophrenia. Psychiat. Clin. Neurosci., 51:31–34, 1997.

143. Yeragani, V. K., Pohl, R., Balon, R., Jampala, V. C., and Jayaraman, A. Twenty-four-hour QT interval variability: increased QT variability during sleep in patients with panic disorder. Neuropsychobiol., 46:1–6, 2002.

144. Yeragani, V. K., Tancer, M., and Uhde, T. Heart rate and QT interval variability: abnormal alpha-2 adrenergic function in patients with panic disorder. Psychiat. Res., 121:185–196, 2003.

145. Yonkers, K. A., Bruce, S. E., Dyck, I. R., and Keller, M. B. Chronicity, relapse, and illness—course of panic disorder, social phobia, and generalized anxiety disorder: findings in men and women from 8 years of follow-up. Depress. Anxiety, 17:173–179, 2003.

146. Yonkers, K. A., Dyck, I. R., and Keller, M. B. An eight-year longitudinal comparison of clinical course and characteristics of social phobia among men and women. Psychiat. Serv., 52:637–643, 2001.

147. Zamorski, M. A., and Albucher, R. C. What to do when SSRIs fail: eight strategies for optimizing treatment of panic disorder. Am. Fam. Physician, 66:1477–1484, 2002.

148. Zimmerman, M., and Mattia, J. I. Axis I diagnostic comorbidity and borderline personality disorder. Compr. Psychiat., 40:245–252, 1999.

149. Zohar, J., and Westenberg, H. G. Anxiety disorders: a review of tricyclic antidepressants and selective serotonin reuptake inhibitors. Acta Psychiat. Scand. Suppl., 403:39–49, 2000.

150. Zwanzger, P., and Rupprecht, R. Selective GABAergic treatment for panic? Investigations in experimental panic induction and panic disorder. J. Psychiat. Neurosci., 30:167–175, 2005.

151. American Psychiatric Association. *Diagnostic and Statistical Manual of Mental Disorders*, 4th edition, text revision. Washington, DC: Author, 2000.

·

5

Posttraumatic Stress Disorder

Posttraumatic stress disorder (PTSD) is currently defined an anxiety disorder emerging after exposure to an extreme traumatic stressor involving actual or threatened death or serious injury. In the first two editions of the American Psychiatric Association's *Diagnostic and Statistical Manual of Mental Disorders* (*DSM-I* and *DSM-II*), in 1952 and 1968, stress-related disorders were classified as transient situational personality disorders under the names "gross stress reaction" and "transient situational disturbance," respectively (5, 6). It was not until *DSM-III*, the third edition of the diagnostic manual, in 1980, that PTSD was introduced as a specific disorder in its own right (7). The posttraumatic symptoms were organized into categories of intrusion and avoidance/denial proposed by Horowitz (101), and a third category representing hyperarousal. Definition of the diagnosis continued to evolve thereafter. Specification of the originating traumatic event was revised from the 1980 *DSM-III* definition evoking "significant symptoms of distress in almost everyone" to a traumatic experience that is "outside the range of usual human experience" in the 1987 revision (*DSM-III-R*). *DSM-III-R* further allowed that the traumatic event could be experienced either personally or by witnessing a traumatic event, if the individual reacted to the event "with intense fear, helplessness, or horror." The fourth edition of the diagnostic criteria, *DSM-IV*, in 1994, clarified that the stressor event must comprise a physical threat of death or serious injury (8).

The current diagnostic criteria for PTSD are listed in Table 5.1. By definition, PTSD cannot occur without exposure to a traumatic event. One of few other diagnostic categories including an environmental precipitant in its definition is the very broad category of adjustment disorders in which symptoms are associated with psychosocial stressors not characterized as "traumatic." Thus, these diagnostic labels attempt to describe pathological response(s) to a traumatic event. What kind of stressor, one might ask, would rise to the level of traumatic stress, and does traumatic stress differ from other types of stress? To

TABLE 5.1 Criteria for Posttraumatic Stress Disorder (*DSM-IV-TR*)

A. The person has been exposed to a traumatic event in which both of the following were present:

    (1) The person experienced, witnessed, or was confronted with an event or events that involved actual or threatened death or serious injury or a threat to the physical integrity of self or others.

    (2) The person's response involved intense fear, helplessness, or horror. Note: In children, this may be expressed instead by disorganized or agitated behavior.

B. The traumatic event is persistently re-experienced in one (or more) of the following ways:

    (1) Recurrent and intrusive distressing recollections of the event, including images, thoughts, or perceptions Note: In young children, repetitive play may occur in which themes or aspects of the trauma are expressed.

    (2) Recurrent distressing dreams of the event Note: In children, there may be frightening dreams without recognizable content.

    (3) Acting or feeling as if the traumatic event were recurring (includes a sense of reliving the experience, illusions, hallucinations, and dissociative flashback episodes, including those that occur on awakening or when intoxicated) Note: In young children, trauma-specific reenactment may occur.

    (4) Intense psychological distress at exposure to internal or external cues that symbolize or resemble an aspect of the traumatic event

    (5) Physiological reactivity on exposure to internal or external cues that symbolize or resemble an aspect of the traumatic event

C. Persistent avoidance of stimuli associated with the trauma and numbing of general responsiveness (not present before the trauma), as indicated by three (or more) of the following:

    (1) Efforts to avoid thoughts, feelings, or conversations associated with the trauma

    (2) Efforts to avoid activities, places, or people that arouse recollections of the trauma

    (3) Inability to recall an important aspect of the trauma

    (4) Markedly diminished interest or participation in significant activities

    (5) Feeling of detachment or estrangement from others

    (6) Restricted range of affect (e.g., unable to have loving feelings)

    (7) Sense of a foreshortened future (e.g., does not expect to have a career, marriage, children, or a normal life span)

continued

TABLE 5.1 (Continued)

D. Persistent symptoms of increased arousal (not present before the trauma), as indicated by two (or more) of the following:

(1) Difficulty falling or staying asleep
(2) Irritability or outbursts of anger
(3) Difficulty concentrating
(4) Hypervigilance
(5) Exaggerated startle response

E. Duration of the disturbance (symptoms in Criteria B, C, and D) is more than 1 month.
F. The disturbance causes clinically significant distress or impairment in social, occupational, or other important areas of functioning.

Specify if:

Acute: if duration of symptoms is less than 3 months
Chronic: if duration of symptoms is 3 months or more

Specify if:

With Delayed Onset: if onset of symptoms is at least 6 months after the stressor

---

Adapted from diagnostic criteria in the *Diagnostic and Statistical Manual of Mental Disorders,* fourth edition text revision. Washington, DC: American Psychiatric Association, 2000.

qualify as "traumatic," the stressful event must pose a threat to life or limb. Purely emotional events such as being fired or being confronted with divorce would not qualify unless tangible physical danger was involved. Two individuals exposed to the same life-threatening event may not find it equally traumatic; one may be horrified, the other fearless. Only the former would be a potential candidate for a diagnosis of PTSD.

According to *DSM-IV-TR*, the traumatic event may be experienced directly, personally witnessed, or experienced vicariously through the exposure of a loved one to a traumatic event. Examples of directly experienced traumatic events are exposure to the physical dangers of military combat, being physically attacked or sexually assaulted, suffering a bad traffic accident, or experiencing a disaster such as a tornado or a plane crash. Examples of witnessed events are seeing people injured or killed in a bad traffic accident, seeing someone murdered, or unexpectedly discovering a dead body. Indirect exposure to events vicariously through the direct experience of loved ones could occur with learning of the sudden unexpected death or life-threatening experience of a close family member involving a severe heart attack, suicide, homicide, or an automobile accident.

Criterion A (the "stressor criterion") is the entry point for diagnostic candidacy. This criterion has been applied inappropriately in claims of PTSD in litigation and applications for disability compensation (202, 203). For example, one woman complained in a lawsuit against her employer that she had developed PTSD because she was not promoted on her job in as timely a manner as she desired. Another woman filed a lawsuit against her beauty shop claiming PTSD on the basis of damage to her hair. It could be argued that these experiences do not rank with amputation of one's hand in a chain saw accident or witnessing a co-worker being crushed to death by heavy equipment. Although it has been observed that related symptoms commonly occur outside the context of traumatic events as defined here, it is the origination of the symptoms in association with a traumatic event that differentiates PTSD from other kinds of stress-related complaints, symptoms, or syndromes (31).

Diagnosis of PTSD further requires the development of new trauma-related symptoms after the traumatic event, that continue for more than 1 month, in three categories: intrusive re-experience, avoidance and numbing, and hyper-arousal. Intrusive re-experience consists of symptoms such as flashbacks, night-mares, and recurrent vivid images related to the event. Avoidance and numbing symptoms signify overwhelming inability to cope with the event. Reminders may be actively avoided and the individual may feel emotionally numb or distant from others. Hyperarousal symptoms are exaggerated startle response, sleep disturbance, loss of concentration, and excessive vigilance for danger.

It should be noted that PTSD has been a topic of great interest for researchers and clinicians particularly in the last 30 years. However, PTSD remains a diagnosis in evolution because of the relative newness of the diag-nosis, the complexity of the concept (emotional response to a particular type of stressor), changing conceptualization of entry point, difficulties with delimita-tion from "normal response," and other reasons (see later in this chapter). The data-based references in this chapter are cited for what they contribute to the developing knowledge base. The reader should not conclude that the amount of research or findings, or even the inclusion of this diagnosis in this text, signifies validity of the current definition of the disorder.

Historical Background

Emotional responses to catastrophic events were recorded as long as 4,000 years ago in cuneiform records of the destruction of the city of Ur (2000 B.C.) (114):

> In its places, where the festivities of the land took place, the people lay
>   in heaps.
> At night a bitter lament having been raised unto me,

I, although, for that night tremble,
Fled not before that night's violence.
The storm's cyclone like destruction—verily its terror has filled me full.
Because of its [affliction] in my nightly sleeping place,
In my nightly sleeping place verily there is no peace for me. (Verses
   95–99 and 217)

Homer's *Iliad* described military soldiers' reactions to the horrors of war. These reactions were grief, guilt over fallen comrades, feeling dead, and berserk rage attacks (187), not unlike the descriptions of posttraumatic reactions among combat soldiers, especially among Vietnam veterans commonly depicted in feature films.

A witness to the 1666 Great Fire of London described recurrent sleep disturbances and intrusive images associated with the experience (53):

How strange that to this very day I cannot sleep at night without great
fear of being overcome by fire. And last night I lay awake until almost
2 o'clock in the morning because I could not stop thinking about the fire.

Medical literature on psychiatric trauma syndromes can be traced to 1867 when John Erichsen described railroad spine syndrome in connection with collisions occurring with use of the newfangled steam-powered train in England (70, 214). Symptoms of railroad spine syndrome were sleep disturbance, distressing dreams, anxiety, irritability, memory and concentration problems, and multiple somatic symptoms. Erichsen considered the syndrome organically based, involving physical damage to the spinal cord (p. 77) (68):

[I] direct your attention to a class of cases in which the injury inflicted
upon the back is either very slight in degree, or in which the blow, if
more severe, has fallen upon some other part of the body than the
spine, and in which, consequently, its influence upon the cord has
been of a less direct and often of a less instantaneous character.
Nothing is more common than that the symptoms of spinal mischief
do not develop for several days after heavy falls on the back.

Page (158), however, disagreed, arguing in favor of extreme fear as the cause. Around the same time, however, Putnam (166) considered railroad spine syndrome to represent a form of hysterical neurosis. Railway spine evolved into a pejorative term that included "obscure affections of the brain and spinal cord" (191) and "real or imaginary affections of the spine" (91). It may be no accident that personal insurance was introduced around the same time as railway transportation. Railway accidents were among the first tragedies for which people could sue for damages (117).

American Civil War soldiers emerging from battlefields developed a syndrome consisting of exertional chest pain, rapid feeble pulse, shortness of breath, sleep disturbance with unpleasant dreams and jerking during sleep, headaches, dizziness, and gastrointestinal symptoms, chiefly diarrhea (93). Da Costa (52) formally named this constellation of complaints irritable heart syndrome, reflecting his belief that overreaction and excessive excitement caused irritability of the heart. The syndrome has also been referred to as Da Costa syndrome, soldier's heart, and effort syndrome. The possibility of emotional origins to these combat-related symptoms was not entertained, perhaps in part because conditions considered "hysterical" had not been observed to occur regularly in men (210). In the late nineteenth century, however, Briquet and Charcot (137) described several male cases of hysteria. Charcot proposed that neurological damage precipitated by traumatic events led to hysteria (64). Babinski and Froment (13) disagreed, however, invoking the process of suggestion as producing the symptoms rather than neurological damage from traumatic events.

Observing alleged sexual trauma in early childhood as a recurring feature of hysteria, Freud elaborated a traumatic theory of hysterical neurosis (75). Just 2 years later, however, he abandoned this position (74) in favor of a view that the reported traumatic events represented fantasies (109). Contemporaneously, Janet concluded that the shocking events alleged as etiologic in hysteria might actually be imaginary (104). He proposed instead that dissociative processes are central to the psychopathology of hysteria and traumatic neurosis (219). (Dissociation is a theoretical process involving postulated disruption in the integrative functions of consciousness, memory, identity, or perception of the environment. Classical dissociative presentations include dissociative amnesia; fugue; depersonalization, which is a sensation of change or unreality of oneself; and derealization, which is a perception of change or unreality of one's environment or world.) Although it has been hypothesized that dissociative disorders are caused by the experience of unbearable trauma (204), empirical support is lacking, and dissociative disorders are not among those typically observed in studies of disaster survivors and combat veterans.

World War I saw the emergence of "soldier's heart," a posttraumatic syndrome with many associated nervous symptoms, leading to 80,000 discharges from the U.S. Army (50). Finding no cardiac abnormalities in these cases, MacKenzie concluded that they were psychiatrically based (124). Myers applied the term "shell shock" to combat-related psychological syndromes (143).

As described by Mott, shell shock constituted a variety of hysterical symptoms (paralysis, contractions, and disordered gait), neurasthenia symptoms (lassitude, fatigue, headaches, and terrifying dreams), exaggerated startle reflex, chronic jerking mannerisms, and spasms of the head and neck stimulated by noise (140).

At the end of World War I, skepticism was growing over the concept of shell shock, and suspicions of malingering arose (18, 103). By the beginning of World War II, the syndrome of shell shock had given way to the concept of war neurosis, implying psychogenic origins (109, 128).

Although reference to "trauma" had previously been reserved for physical, as opposed to psychological, experiences, in World War II and the Korean War, extreme psychological stress first came under the broad umbrella of emotional "trauma" (109). Studies of World War II prisoners of war and survivors of the horrors of Nazi concentration camps revealed ensuing problems of irritability and anger, restlessness and tension, chronic fears, depression, paranoia, decreased interest, poor concentration, social isolation, and changes in personality (17, 25, 221). The Vietnam War galvanized attention to posttraumatic psychiatric syndromes, which further increased in the 1980s and 1990s (117).

Posttraumatic syndromes have long been described in civilian victims of disasters and in industrial and occupational medicine. Following the 1871 passage of damage claims laws in Germany and in the midst of subsequent economic crisis in Germany, concerns arose about illness faked for compensation (98). In this context, a new term, "compensation neurosis," was introduced (70). American compensation laws passed in 1911 heralded a sharp increase in cases of industrial neurosis (61). Significant economic repercussions soon followed, fostering vigilance for "unscrupulous malingerers" faking injuries to obtain compensation (138). Persistent concerns about motivation for compensation complicated the evaluation of claims of Holocaust survivors and Vietnam veterans (79, 202).

The first community-based study of disasters is attributed to Stierlin (209), who in 1911 found sleep disturbance and nightmares in 25% of survivors of the Messina earthquake. Stierlin described two associated psychological syndromes. The first, considered to represent a psychotic or hysterical state, termed "fright psychosis," involved features of clouded consciousness, amnesia, disorientation, fearful affect, and hallucinations persisting 3 days. A second, longer lasting, "traumatic neurosis" consisted of sleep disturbance and autonomic changes, including rapid or labile pulse, hyperactive patellar reflexes, tremor, and fatigue.

A landmark study of the Coconut Grove fire in Boston in 1943 established the feasibility of systematic investigation into the psychological effects of major disasters (3). The following two decades saw the publication of a number of studies in the wake of major disasters, including a tornado in Mississippi in 1952 (23), the 1962 Alaska earthquake (118), the sinking of the Andrea Doria (78), and the Bristol floods (16).

In 1950, publication of an article on extreme stress in studies of animals (186) heralded new approaches to research into neuroendocrine mechanisms of stress. This study also first introduced the word *stress* into everyday speech in reference to psychological experiences (117). More recently, the word *trauma* has been used loosely in common parlance to represent anything emotionally upsetting. Having to give a speech in class, being embarrassed by a colleague's comment, and sitting for a difficult examination are examples of emotionally stressful events popularly labeled "traumatic." Unfortunately, the use of the word *trauma* to describe purely emotionally stressful events has blurred the distinction between emotional stress and trauma in general usage.

Recent studies have linked PTSD with childhood molestation, depression, anxiety disorders, borderline personality disorder, somatization disorder, multiple personality disorder, smoking, alcohol and drug abuse, irritable bowel syndrome, and just about any label/problem/disorder imaginable. The literature describing the interrelationships of these problems has assumed a causal role of childhood trauma in the pathogenesis of borderline personality and PTSD (96), although causal relationships have not been sufficiently documented in these groups.

Epidemiology

Posttraumatic stress disorder does not represent the unified construct that has been established for other validated psychiatric disorders identified in this text. Validation (and reliability) of PTSD as a psychiatric diagnosis, in a process outlined several years ago by Robins and Guze (174), awaits more definitive research, especially determination that the symptoms correlate more with each other than with other disorders, demonstration that the disorder is distinguishable from other disorders (which may not be possible given the degree of symptom overlap with anxiety and depressive disorders), and documentation that the disorder runs in families (145, 155, 178, 206).

The epidemiology of PTSD varies with characteristics of the associated traumatic event and the population affected. Thus, estimation of the disorder's prevalence is dependent on how many people were sufficiently exposed to a specific type of qualifying event.

Historically, most knowledge about human response to traumatic experiences has emerged from research on combat veterans (40, 117) and, more recently, disaster victims (30). In a study of more than 10,000 Vietnam veterans by the Centers for Disease Control (213), 15% were diagnosed with combat-related PTSD. The National Vietnam Veterans Readjustment Study (NVVRS) (116) identified post-combat PTSD in 31% of male and 26% of female military veterans, and current PTSD in 15% of male and 9% of female veterans (115) interviewed between 1986 and 1988 (116). A recent study of soldiers returning from deployment to military combat in Iraq estimated PTSD in 12%–20% (99). This study used a symptom checklist survey providing a "broad screening definition" of disorders rather than a diagnostic instrument, however, reducing confidence in the accuracy of the prevalence rates provided.

Nearly 15 years after the Vietnam War, 715 military veterans who served in Southeast Asia were studied along with their military veteran twins who did not serve in Southeast Asia. Current (6-month) prevalence of PTSD was 17% among the Southeast Asia veterans compared to 5% of their non-Vietnam veteran twins (84).

Combat-related PTSD has been predicted by pre-service variables (such as pre-existing psychiatric diagnosis and lower educational achievement), military variables (including exposure to grotesque death and life threat), and post-military variables (such as lack of social support and negative life events) (86, 198, 208). Schnurr and colleagues (184) examined 131 military veterans who had completed the MMPI as college students prior to combat exposure. No MMPI scale predicted combat exposure. MMPI Depression, Hypomania, and Social Introversion scale scores predicted post-deployment PTSD.

Studies of prisoners of war (POWs) demonstrate markedly higher rates of PTSD than in other war veterans. Among veterans of the Korean conflict, 78% of 36 former POWs compared to 18% of 29 non-captured veterans (212) were diagnosed with PTSD.

Posttraumatic stress disorder may present differently in populations affected by community-wide disasters. Also, from one disaster to another, PTSD incidence varies considerably. Low rates were identified in association with a volcano eruption (2%) (189), after torrential rain and mudslides (4%) (45), and following combined flooding and dioxin contamination (8% or less) (194). Higher rates of PTSD were described among survivors of the Oklahoma City bombing (34%) (151), a dam break and flood (44%) (88), and an airplane crash landing (54%) (192). Even after major catastrophic events, however, the majority of people usually do not develop PTSD (80, 151, 183).

Some disaster experts consider disasters of willful human causation more likely than technological accidents or natural disasters to precipitate PTSD (14, 15, 73, 83, 148). Agreement on this point is not universal, however (179). Intensity of exposure to a disaster and severity of the disaster incident (reflected, for example, in number of casualties and amount of property destruction) are associated with PTSD and have not been teased apart from the type of disaster in research to date (151, 179).

Violent trauma is an endemic part of community life. In a study of 1,007 young adults in an urban health maintenance organization, Breslau's group studied found that 39% had been exposed to violent trauma at some time during their lives (35). Studying a community sample of 1,000 adults, Norris (147) encountered a 69% lifetime rate of exposure to at least one traumatic event, 21% in the last year alone. The National Women's Study telephone survey of a national probability household sample of 4,008 adult women found that 69% had been exposed to a traumatic event in their lives (172). The National Comorbidity Study of 5,877 noninstitutionalized U.S. civilians ages 15 to 54 reported that 56% had experienced at least one traumatic event in their lives, and most of these described other traumatic experiences as well (108). The most commonly reported types of traumatic events were witnessing a serious or fatal injury (25%), being in a life-threatening accident (19%), and experiencing a natural disaster (17%).

Posttraumatic stress disorder following traumatic events is not nearly as prevalent as the traumatic events leading to the disorder. Among people exposed to traumatic events, PTSD was diagnosed in 24% in the Breslau et al. study (35), 18% in the National Women's Study (172), and 14% in the National Comorbidity Study (108).

The likelihood of PTSD following traumatic events appears to vary according to the type of event. In the Breslau et al. study (35), the type of event most associated with PTSD was rape, with a PTSD rate of 49%. Other events were associated with somewhat lower rates of PTSD: being badly beaten up (32%), other sexual assault (24%), and serious accident or injury (17%). In the National Comorbidity Study, incidents most likely to lead to PTSD were rape (49%) and combat (39%); far less likely to result in PTSD were witnessing serious or fatal injury (6%) and experiencing a natural disaster (5%).

The first general population prevalence data on PTSD in the community were gathered in St. Louis and North Carolina as part of the Epidemiologic Catchment Area study, using the Diagnostic Interview Schedule, a structured interview providing estimates of psychiatric diagnosis conforming to accepted diagnostic criteria. The lifetime rates of PTSD in this study were 1%–2% (57, 94). More recent general population studies have described lifetime PTSD population prevalence around 8%–9% (35, 108). Rates of PTSD in women are twice those in men (94, 108).

Exposure to traumatic events is not a random occurrence. The risk factors for exposure to traumatic events are not the same as risk factors for PTSD following such events (28, 34, 36). Exposure to a traumatic event is associated with lack of education, early conduct problems, pre-existing psychiatric illness, substance abuse, and personality traits of novelty seeking and risk taking.

Two characteristics of individuals have repeatedly emerged as robust predictors of PTSD: female gender (106, 123, 139, 179, 207, 220) and pre-existing psychopathology (41, 132, 151, 152, 168, 193, 220). Specifically, pre-existing personality characteristics predict PTSD (47, 122, 125, 132, 201). Early life history of adversity and chaotic family background, which may occur in association with pre-existing psychopathology, also predict PTSD (35, 236). These powerful individual predictors of psychopathology may account at least in part for effects previously attributed to exposure to the traumatic event (33, 69, 97, 218), because of the confounding of pre-existing characteristics that convey risk for trauma as well as for psychopathology following that trauma. Other negative life events occurring after disasters also predict PTSD (67, 125, 151).

Posttraumatic stress disorder may be especially prevalent in certain populations. A study of 900 homeless people randomly sampled from St. Louis shelters and street locations by North and colleagues (153) found that more than 40% had a history of past violent trauma. The trauma had usually preceded the onset of homelessness. Posttraumatic stress disorder was identified in 34% of homeless women and 18% of homeless men.

In summary, the disparity in reported prevalence rates from epidemiologic studies of PTSD may be a reflection of the uncertain validity of the current state of development of diagnostic criteria for the disorder. Regardless, acknowledgement of diagnostic criteria is prevalent in many special populations. Because trauma is not a random occurrence in populations, confounding of risk for trauma with risk for psychiatric disorder following a traumatic event creates difficulties in understanding relationships among pre-existing personal characteristics and psychiatric sequelae of trauma. Clinicians and researchers are cautioned to avoid premature assumptions about causalities within these relationships in their evaluation of individual patients and specific populations.

Clinical Picture

Most people directly exposed to major disasters describe symptoms of intrusive re-experience and hyperarousal. Among directly exposed survivors of the Oklahoma City bombing, 96% reported having at least one posttraumatic symptom (151). The most frequently reported symptoms are nightmares, sleep disturbance, difficulties concentrating, and jumpiness (151, 209, 212). People indirectly exposed (e.g., members of an affected community) or only remotely affected (such as those hearing about a disaster in news broadcasts) may also describe such symptoms. In a Pew poll of the American public conducted shortly after the September 11 terrorist attacks, 7 out of 10 people acknowledged feeling depressed, nearly one-half described poor concentration, and 1 in 3 reported sleep difficulties (1).

Posttraumatic symptoms not so commonly encountered after disasters pertain to avoidance and numbing, and psychogenic amnesia and restricted range of affect are especially infrequent (151, 176, 212). These infrequent avoidance and numbing symptoms, however, constitute the essence of PTSD as currently defined (37, 151). In the Oklahoma City bombing study, 94% of directly exposed survivors with three or more avoidance and numbing symptoms met full criteria for the diagnosis of PTSD (151). These avoidance and numbing symptoms were also associated with other indicators of illness: pre-existing psychopathology, postdisaster disorders, interference with functioning, seeking treatment, taking medication, and consuming alcohol or drugs to cope. Several other studies have also demonstrated avoidance and numbing symptoms to be pivotal to the diagnosis of PTSD in other populations (37, 63, 71, 135, 222).

Symptoms of intrusive re-experience and hyperarousal are so commonly reported that they may be considered the norm, or *normative* (i.e., described by most people). These common re-experience and hyperarousal symptoms would not be assumed to be evidence of illness in the absence of prominent avoidance and numbing responses, but rather emotional distress of nonpathologic proportion. Analysis by Breslau and colleagues confirmed that posttraumatic symptoms below the level required to qualify for a diagnosis of PTSD do not represent the same pathological process experienced by patients meeting PTSD criteria (37).

Posttraumatic stress disorder may vary in its symptomatic expression, depending on the setting and the population involved. For example, intrusive re-experience was found particularly in association with combat exposure, but denial was more often reported after witnessing abusive violence (215). In other studies, hyperarousal was prominent in descriptions of symptoms by former prisoners, and avoidance was foremost among rape victims (95). Although sleep complaints, including insomnia and nightmares, are prevalent in populations exposed to traumatic events (151), sleep laboratory studies fail to document the frequency and severity of subjective complaints, which were found to be out of proportion to objective findings (119).

A recurring theme in descriptions of PTSD in various settings is psychiatric comorbidity. In all populations PTSD more often presents in the company of other co-existing psychiatric disorders than emerging solo. High rates of psychiatric comorbidity are well documented in association with PTSD, 80% or more observed among combat veterans with PTSD (59, 107, 116, 156, 190), 60%–80% in disaster survivors with PTSD (134, 135, 151), and 70%–90% of individuals with PTSD in community samples (29, 30, 108, 112, 159). The comorbid disorders most often described are major depression (28%–79%), other anxiety disorders (25%–94%), and substance abuse/dependence (43%–50%) (66, 112, 212). Bipolar disorder and psychotic disorders such as schizophrenia are not among those observed to arise in the immediate aftermath of trauma exposure.

Comorbidity of personality and somatoform disorders with PTSD is less well studied (136). While borderline personality, antisocial, and somatoform comorbidities have been described in association with PTSD in populations selected from treatment settings, these problems have often been found to predate the traumatic exposure (72, 149–152, 167). A study of 34 Vietnam combat veteran inpatients and outpatients with PTSD found the most prevalent comorbid personality disorders to be Cluster B personality disorders, especially borderline personality disorder (76%) (201). Other prevalent personality disorders identified were obsessive-compulsive (44%), avoidant (41%), paranoid (38%), and passive-aggressive (35%) personality disorders (43, 87, 212). Gunderson and Sabo emphasized the overlap of features of PTSD and borderline personality in psychiatric patients (89). A study of 50 selected patients from the Boston PTSD center found that 26% met criteria for a personality disorder, almost all of which was represented by either antisocial personality disorder or mixed personality disorder with antisocial features. The average number of personality disorder diagnoses was 3.8 (107). Southwick and colleagues (201) considered the possibility that the associated character pathology represents enduring posttrauma changes, as well as possibly representing pre-existing characteristics that render individuals more susceptible to traumatic events and posttraumatic difficulties.

Posttraumatic stress disorder has been linked with dissociation, a condition considered by its specialists to have origins in early psychologically traumatic experiences. In clinical settings, many patients with comorbid personality disorders of the "Cluster B" ("acting-out") group, in which childhood abuse is prevalent, present with dissociative symptoms. Dissociative disorders, however, are infrequently observed in populations affected by disasters (223, 234). The clinical significance and validity of "dissociative" symptoms in the disaster setting have not been adequately determined. A diagnosis of acute stress disorder was developed to provide a diagnostic category for distressed trauma survivors in the first month, before a diagnosis of PTSD can be applied, and this diagnosis encompasses dissociative symptoms alongside the characteristic symptoms of PTSD. Although the occurrence of acute stress disorder predicts subsequent development of PTSD (42), research to establish diagnostic validity of this entity presently falls far short of progress in the incomplete body of work on diagnostic validity of PTSD.

It is unclear whether the comorbidity of other psychiatric disorders with PTSD is merely a consequence of overlap of criteria for other psychiatric disorders (87, 174, 201), most notably major depression, generalized anxiety and phobic disorders (107), and dissociation (33) as opposed to true co-occurring pathology (39, 87, 201, 205). The extensive comorbidity of PTSD with other psychiatric disorders, as previously noted, represents a challenge to the validity and reliability of the diagnosis of PTSD (32, 33, 39, 84, 87, 107, 174, 196).

In clinical practice, the remarkable comorbidity of other psychiatric disorders with PTSD (151) points to the utility of continuing the search for psychiatric disorders after PTSD is assessed. Diagnostic comorbidity with PTSD represents a marker for severity of illness and disability, and identifies cases that merit special attention (151). The comorbid disorders may be at least as important as PTSD itself to the treatment, course, and outcome of PTSD.

Biological Findings

Numerous biological investigations have attempted to understand the physiological underpinnings of pathological responses to traumatic events. These investigations have yielded a number of theories, which are reviewed in the following text.

Many recent investigations into PTSD have pursued the role of sympathetic dysregulation in the fear response circuitry. In patients with PTSD, exposure to traumatic reminders elicits physiologic hyperreactivity (e.g., precipitous elevations in heart rate and blood pressure) associated with exaggerated increases in catecholamine excretion (60, 77, 113, 120, 130, 195, 232). Such catecholamine responses, however, are not consistently observed in PTSD patients at rest or in response to nontraumatic stressors (131, 142, 163, 165). The glutaminergic system is thought to be involved in modulation of the HPA axis through increasing corticotropin-releasing factor (CRF) that acts to release norepinephrine from the locus ceruleus, suggesting a role for antiglutamatergic agents for reducing posttraumatic anxiety and hyperarousal (144).

Posttraumatic stress disorder has also been found to be associated with reduced platelet alpha-2 adrenergic receptor binding (26, 160) that may reflect receptor down-regulation in response to chronic sympathetic stimulation (77).

Further demonstrating the role of the sympathetic nervous system in PTSD, pharmacologic probes can alter adrenergic function in PTSD. Administration of the alpha-2 adrenergic receptor blocker yohimbine has been shown to provoke physiologic reactivity (199) and antiadrenergic agents clonidine, guanfacine, prazosin, and propranolol to suppress noradrenergic hyperreactivity (24, 102, 110, 164, 169, 211) in response to traumatic reminders in individuals with PTSD.

Research has not fully differentiated the degree to which sympathetic arousal in relation to disaster is a function of disaster exposure per se (as part of the "fight or flight" reaction mediated by release of norepinephrine from the locus ceruleus) or a part of the PTSD that follows. A study of survivors of the Oklahoma City bomb blast (15% of whom had PTSD) found that physiologic reactivity did not correlate with PTSD symptoms; blast survivors did, however, demonstrate greater physiologic reactivity to reminders of the event compared to an unexposed group (217). A study of mental health treatment–seeking patients who survived the September 11 attacks on the World Trade Center found that norepinephrine excretion was not associated with a diagnosis of PTSD. The level of norepinephrine secretion did, however, appear to diminish with time elapsed since the event (19).

Other research into biologic mechanisms of PTSD implicates changes in the hypothalamic-pituitary-adrenal (HPA) axis and abnormalities in cortisol regulation in association with traumatic stress. Trauma exposure stimulates a rapid surge in cortisol production. Cortisol appears to enable the organism to meet the challenge of extreme stress by directing physiologic responses to heighten vigilance and arousal and prepare for action. An inability to mount a brisk cortisol surge in the immediate face of trauma may be involved in PTSD. A study of motor accident victims admitted to a hospital for treatment of injuries found that cortisol levels measured in the first 15 hours after the accident were lower among those who would develop PTSD by 1 month (60). Chronically subnormal cortisol levels are also observed in PTSD (77, 127, 133, 224, 233), suggesting a down-regulation of the HPA axis in PTSD (60). Published findings on these variables have not been consistent, however, and a longstanding controversy surrounding the short- and long-term cortisol response in association with PTSD persists today (60, 120, 162, 173, 227).

Further evidence of dysregulation of the HPA axis in PTSD is drawn from studies demonstrating increased lymphocyte glucocorticoid receptors in PTSD and excessive suppression of cortisol in PTSD patients administered dexamethasone (a synthetic glucocorticoid) (90, 228–231). In PTSD, low cortisol levels are paradoxically coupled with high levels of corticotropin-releasing factor (CRF). Administration of dexamethasone results in excessive suppression of adrenocorticotropic hormone (ACTH) in PTSD patients (230). These findings implicate reduced ACTH production in the pituitary rather than sluggish adrenal output as the potential mechanism for the enhanced HPA axis cortisol feedback inhibition postulated to be fundamental to the neurobiology of PTSD (225, 230). Interestingly, among intensive care unit patients suffering septic shock or recovering from cardiac surgery who were suspected to have critical illness-related corticosteroid insufficiency, those administered stress doses of glucocorticoids in controlled trials had a significant reduction of PTSD symptoms (181).

The degree to which the state of HPA axis dysregulation in PTSD is a product of acquired down-regulation of the endocrine stress system stemming from the traumatic experience or is a reflection of antecedent constitutional predisposition to PTSD vulnerability is not entirely clear at present (48, 226). Regardless, the pattern of these findings in PTSD is in distinct contrast with findings in patients with major depression, in whom elevated cortisol levels and reduced cortisol response to dexamethasone are observed (195).

The medial prefrontal cortex in the human brain normally functions to inhibit the amygdala, where fear responses are generated (27, 48). In the face of danger, the norepinephrine surge inhibits the prefrontal cortex, allowing activation of the rapid "default" subcortical response, promoting survival of the organism (11, 20, 195). In PTSD, chronic hypoactivity of the medial prefrontal cortex may contribute to disinhibition of the amygdala, resulting in sympathetic overdrive and producing PTSD symptoms. Provocation studies have determined that confrontation with traumatic reminders among PTSD patients is followed by reduced blood flow to the medial prefrontal cortex and increased blood flow to the amygdala (27, 27, 171, 188).

Neuroimaging studies of individuals with PTSD have demonstrated reduced hippocampal volume, which is further associated with subnormal 24-hour urinary cortisol secretion (170). The hippocampus is an especially plastic and vulnerable part of the brain, and it is postulated that it may sustain damage with exposure to severely traumatic stress. Glucocorticoid stress hormones have been implicated in processes involved in hippocampal atrophy in PTSD. Animal models point to excitatory amino acids such as glutamate, acting on the N-methyl-D-aspartate (NMDA) receptor, in hippocampal atrophy and neuronal death (2, 46, 129). The causal pathways characterizing the association of reduced hippocampal volume in PTSD remain undetermined. It may be that reduced hippocampal volume reflects pre-existing characteristics that render the brain vulnerable to psychopathological responses or neurotoxic effects of psychological trauma (82).

Significant hippocampal volume loss in any condition would ordinarily be expected to be accompanied by demonstrable deficits in declarative, episodic, spatial, and contextual memory performance. Hippocampal atrophy is non-specific in PTSD, and it is also found in association with diverse conditions, including Cushing syndrome, recurrent depressive illness, normal aging preceding dementia, and Alzheimer disease (129). Additionally, comorbid disorders, such as major depression and alcohol abuse, and pre-existing brain characteristics may represent serious confounders in determining proposed relationships with other conditions, including PTSD. Despite these findings and associated theories of causation, no replicable neurological finding has been definitely linked with PTSD.

Natural History

The concepts of onset and recovery in PTSD have not been sufficiently defined. Inadequate attention to definitions of onset and recovery, however, are apparent across general definitions of psychiatric disorders. Onset of PTSD refers to "onset of symptoms" (p. 429) (9). In *DSM-IV-TR*, definition of remission from psychiatric disorders is subdivided into categories of full remission, which refers to the absence of any symptoms of the disorder, and partial remission, defined as continuing symptoms that have fallen below the diagnostic threshold.

Authors of a recent article noted that prevailing applications of PTSD onset are ambiguous as to whether they require onset of *any* posttraumatic symptoms or fulfillment of the full diagnostic criteria for PTSD. The authors of this article represented the timing of onset of PTSD as the point at which full criteria are met (10). A long history of epidemiologic research (175) and current *DSM-IV* definition, however, identify the onset of a psychiatric disorder as the point at which any symptoms of the disorder begin. This difference in definition is a likely source of discrepancy in claims surrounding PTSD onset (10). Close inspection reveals that reports of delayed-onset PTSD largely represent individuals with PTSD symptoms beginning within 6 months of the event but not meeting full criteria until later. Most of these cases are actually subthreshold, usually demonstrating many symptoms but short of diagnostic threshold by one or two avoidance/numbing symptoms and later meeting full criteria with the subsequent appearance of these additional symptoms (154).

Disaster studies permit the study of circumscribed populations with a well-defined traumatic event that may not be subject to selection biases inherent with exposure to other kinds of trauma in general community settings. Disaster research has revealed important aspects of the course of PTSD in exposed populations. Posttraumatic stress disorder tends to commence quickly in disaster survivors. Among 182 directly exposed survivors of the Oklahoma City bombing, 76% of those with PTSD retrospectively reported onset of symptoms the day of the bombing, 94% within the first week, and 98% within the first month. Delayed-onset PTSD (symptoms beginning more than 6 months after the incident) is generally not observed after disasters, as demonstrated in studies of the Oklahoma City bombing (151) and a mass murder episode in Killeen, Texas (152, 154). Delayed-onset PTSD has more often been described in other populations, such as adult survivors of childhood sexual abuse and combat veterans (65, 85, 180, 185).

Posttraumatic stress disorder tends to follow a chronic course, lasting on average a year or longer. Chronic PTSD is defined in *DSM-IV-TR* as lasting for at least 3 months. One-third of people with PTSD in the general population describe their symptom(s) as having persisted for at least a decade (33, 108). All PTSD identified in Oklahoma City bombing survivors was, by definition, chronic (symptoms lasting at least 3 months) (151). Following a mass murder episode in Killeen, Texas, about one-half of the PTSD cases identified among survivors within 2 months of the event were still symptomatic a year later (154).

The definition of remission requires further elaboration, as it may seem counterintuitive that an individual might have a continuing reaction to a stressor a decade later, and because patients do not commonly see psychiatrists for 10 years in relation to a stressful event, even after horrible accidents. According to *DSM-IV-TR*, a person must be free of *any* symptoms or signs of PTSD to have full remission from the disorder after having once met full criteria. Thus, an individual who, for example, still avoids discussion of the event but has no other symptoms would technically be considered still symptomatic and only in partial remission, even if that individual is no longer experiencing any functional impairment from the symptom. Because DSM definitions of remission from psychiatric illness have not been uniformly applied to PTSD, studies including partially remitted cases in the remitted category have described more optimistic rates of recovery from PTSD (10, 81).

Predictors of PTSD chronicity in the general population are greater severity of PTSD, psychiatric comorbidity, interpersonal numbing, emotional reactivity, female gender, and family history of antisocial behavior. Few predictors of PTSD recovery have been identified.

Complications

The diagnosis of PTSD predicts impaired functioning and quality of life, specifically problems in family and other interpersonal relationships, sexual functioning, employment, legal problems, violence, suicide, and substance abuse (49, 100, 197). Relationships identified between PTSD and social maladjustment, however, could reflect either negative effects of the disorder on ability to function, or pre-existing psychiatric characteristics that predisposed to both PTSD and functional difficulties.

Posttraumatic stress disorder may surpass major depression and other anxiety disorders in its frequency of association with physical health and functioning problems (235). Specifically, excessive health complaints, medical disorders, and health care utilization have been reported in association with PTSD (44, 62).

Family Studies

Two family history studies by Davidson and colleagues described elevated rates of anxiety disorders and alcoholism among relatives of PTSD patients and depression in relatives of depressed patients (54, 55). These studies suggest a specific genetic link between PTSD and anxiety but not major depression.

Other studies have described a broad array of psychiatric findings in families. A family history study of 6,744 male twins from the Vietnam Era Twin Registry found risk of exposure to traumatic events to be associated with family history of mood disorders as well as with pre-existing conduct disorder and substance dependence. Risk for PTSD following traumatic exposure was not associated with family history but with lack of education and history of conduct disorder, generalized anxiety disorder, and major depression. The association of familial psychopathology with PTSD may be mediated, at least in part, by shared risk of traumatic exposure and pre-existing psychopathology (111). A review of 2,647 studies of PTSD and meta-analysis of 68 studies concluded that family history of psychopathology was a significant, but small, predictor of PTSD (157). Most of the above studies obtained information about family members by asking the probands, rather than studying the family members directly. Studies that interview family members directly are needed.

A study of 4,042 Vietnam-era veteran male twin pairs found approximately twice the concordance (i.e., agreement between paired cases) for combat exposure in monozygotic compared to dizygotic pairs (215). Controlling for concordance of combat exposure between the monozygotic and dizygotic twin pairs, genetic factors accounted for nearly one-third of the concordance in PTSD symptoms. Combat exposure accounted for concordance in few symptoms, including symptoms of the re-experiencing symptom cluster and avoidance of reminders. Shared family life experiences contributed little to concordance in susceptibility to posttraumatic symptoms, predicting only painful memories.

Another study of Vietnam-era twins concluded that the association of comorbid major depression and substance use disorders with PTSD within individuals was not due to the combat exposure itself, but that genetic and environmental contributors tended to increase risk for both PTSD and these other disorders (182).

Differential Diagnosis

As described earlier in this chapter, posttraumatic symptoms appear to overlap with manifestations of other anxiety disorders, major depression, dissociative disorders, and certain personality disorders (76). The physiologic reactivity to reminders of the traumatic event and exaggerated startle response of PTSD resemble features of panic attacks in panic disorder, including tachycardia and palpitations, sweating, and tremor. Symptoms of PTSD overlapping with generalized anxiety disorder include feeling "keyed up" or "on edge" and sleep disturbance. Symptoms of PTSD overlapping with major depression are loss of interest, sleep disturbance, psychomotor agitation, and difficulty concentrating. Some PTSD symptoms such as flashbacks and emotional numbing appear similar to dissociative syndromes, but these symptoms are considered conceptually distinct from the emotional analgesia and dissociated perceptual states of dissociation (38).

Because patients with somatization disorder and borderline personality disorder habitually endorse multiple symptoms of many psychiatric disorders without meeting criteria for those disorders (121), they may also endorse many posttraumatic symptoms. Given the characteristic chaotic and dysfunctional family backgrounds, exaggerated reporting styles, and suggestibility associated with these disorders, reports of childhood abuse are common and, especially if true, provide fertile soil for elaboration of posttraumatic symptom complaints. Posttraumatic stress disorder must also be distinguished from malingering in settings of potential financial compensation such as in civil litigation and disability benefits (12, 105).

The most fundamental differentiating posttraumatic symptoms from symptoms of these other disorders is the defining occurrence of posttraumatic symptoms in association with a sudden, unexpected event that threatens life or limb. If the symptoms arise anew following traumatic exposure and/or are thematically associated with the event, they may be counted toward a diagnosis of PTSD; otherwise, they may represent symptoms of another disorder. PTSD-like symptoms in the absence of a qualifying traumatic event are common presenting complaints in patients with personality disorders or somatization disorder (223). Symptoms insufficient to meet PTSD criteria following sufficient exposure to a qualifying event may represent normal experiences, emotional distress of nondiagnostic proportion, or response to other life stressors.

Clinical Management

An important principle in psychiatric assessment and management of PTSD is that the disorder more often than not presents with comorbid disorders that may be at least as important as the PTSD in determining clinical outcome and choice of treatment. Therefore, clinicians should continue the search for other disorders even after considering the diagnosis of PTSD. Cases of PTSD with psychiatric comorbidity can be expected to have more severe symptoms and greater functional disability than PTSD-only cases (151). Comorbid disorders can be treated in conjunction with treatment of PTSD, and many of the medications used in the treatment of PTSD are also effective for other anxiety disorders and major depression that may accompany PTSD.

In the treatment of psychologically traumatized patients with a history of childhood abuse, it is recommended that psychiatric disorders be diagnosed and treated in the usual manner as described in other chapters of this text. Although childhood abuse is a potentially important problem for a patient, its recognition should not circumvent a complete assessment and treatment of psychiatric disorders and should not overshadow recognition of the multiple early background and family problems of many patients with this history. Psychotherapists are cautioned to avoid assumptions of causality from childhood abuse to current problems or psychiatric disorders and to base psychotherapy on practical management of current psychosocial issues in the patient's life (141).

A comprehensive review of treatment research in anxiety disorders found no published studies meeting rigorous criteria for evaluation of psychotherapeutic or pharmacologic approaches to PTSD (22). A recent report by the Institute of Medicine concluded that there is insufficient evidence to determine the efficacy of any medication for treatment of PTSD (with one dissenting opinion regarding SSRI and novel antipsychotic agents), and the only form of psychotherapy with sufficient evidence of efficacy was exposure therapy (146). Despite a general shortage of evidence-based literature, several studies have provided indications of potential utility of various other treatment methods such as cognitive-behavioral therapy for PTSD and pharmacologic agents such as prazosin for traumatic nightmares.

Antidepressant medications have been considered a mainstay of pharmacotherapy for PTSD. Two medications, sertraline and paroxetine, have received FDA indications for pharmacotherapy of PTSD. All three PTSD symptom clusters (re-experiencing, avoidance/numbing, hyperarousal) have been found to respond (56). Promising research evidence indicates that other serotonin-selective reuptake inhibitor (SSRI) medications and other classes of antidepressant agents may also have therapeutic potential. The therapeutic effects of the approved agents for PTSD appear to be independent of their antidepressant effects (58, 126, 216). Although research on older psychopharmacologic agents—tricyclic antidepressants and monoamine oxidase inhibitors—has suggested efficacy for PTSD, the SSRIs are generally preferred for their more tolerable side effect profiles and lower potential for toxicities (4, 56). Other agents investigated with potential to augment pharmacotherapy for PTSD are antipsychotics, β-blockers, α-2 agonists, α-1 antagonists, anticonvulsants, and lithium.

Benzodiazepines, sedative-hypnotics, antipsychotics, and mood stabilizers are not first-line agents of pharmacotherapy for PTSD (51, 76). There is little empirical support for the efficacy of benzodiazepines in the treatment of PTSD, and benzodiazepine withdrawal may exacerbate PTSD symptoms (4). Members of these other medication classes, however, are sometimes used to augment standard pharmacotherapy in treatment-resistant PTSD, especially for short-term, adjunctive use (4). When needed, potentially abusable medications should be carefully monitored in PTSD patients, particularly in the context of comorbid substance abuse and the presence of Cluster B personality disorders that confer risk for problems with substance misuse and behavioral disinhibition.

Psychotherapy has been found useful in the treatment of PTSD, and it is also an available adjunct to medication in the treatment of PTSD (21, 200). Exposure therapy, which helps patients with their traumatic experience by confronting it directly, has proven efficacy (92, 146), but this method is intensive and requires considerable training and skill to administer effectively and safely. People with PTSD, who by definition have prominent avoidance and numbing, may have difficulties with therapies focusing on memories of the experience of the event (76, 161). Once the avoidance and numbing have declined to more tolerable levels (such as with pharmacotherapeutic intervention), psychotherapy may proceed more readily. Supportive and cognitive therapies are also modalities that may be utilized adjunctively.

Psychological debriefing is a widely used approach designed to assist with the processing of traumatic experiences and emotions. This typically single-session group intervention is provided for people who have experienced a traumatic event collectively, such as firefighter responders to a particularly gruesome incident with many casualties, or employees exposed to a violent workplace attack. Psychological debriefing became a popular tool for post-trauma intervention around the globe with little evidence supporting its efficacy. Because the procedure is typically applied in methodologically diverse ways by those utilizing it, evaluation of this technique has been difficult. Several recent studies addressing single-session debriefing, reviewed by Rose and colleagues (177), have established little, if any, psychiatric benefit from debriefing in terms of preventing or resolving PTSD.

Preventing or treating PTSD, however, is not a reasonable benchmark for evaluating the success of debriefing. Many debriefing participants have reported that it provided them helpful opportunities for emotional processing, education, reassurance, and social support. Of concern, however, is an identified potential for psychological harm resulting from this procedure, and those with prominent avoidance and numbing responses may be unable to tolerate the unpleasant memories of the traumatic event provoked by debriefing. Importantly, people already developing PTSD (especially those with prominent avoidance symptoms) may be re-traumatized by debriefing that involves confrontation with material that they may not be able to process. Therefore, highly traumatized individuals such as those with PTSD or prominent avoidance and numbing should instead be referred for psychiatric evaluation, and it is recommended that participation in psychological debriefing should not be made mandatory for all members of groups exposed to traumatic events.

REFERENCES

1. Poll: Americans depressed, sleepless. Washington, DC: Associated Press. Available at: http://www.chron.com/cs/CDA/story.hts/special/terror/impact/1055126. Accessed on 1/21/2006.
2. Adamec, R. E., Burton, P., Shallow, T., and Budgell, J. NMDA receptors mediate lasting increases in anxiety-like behavior produced by the stress of predator exposure—implications for anxiety associated with posttraumatic stress disorder. Physiol. Behav., 65:723–737, 1999.
3. Adler, A. Neuropsychiatric complications in victims of Boston's Coconut Grove disaster. JAMA., 123:1098–1101, 1943.
4. Albucher, R. C., and Liberzon, I. Psychopharmacological treatment in PTSD: a critical review. J. Psychiat. Res., 36:355–367, 2002.

5. American Psychiatric Association. *Diagnostic and Statistical Manual: Mental Disorders*, 1st edition. Washington, DC: Author, 1952.

6. American Psychiatric Association. *Diagnostic and Statistical Manual of Mental Disorders*, 2nd edition. Washington, DC: Author, 1968.

7. American Psychiatric Association. *Diagnostic and Statistical Manual of Mental Disorders*, 3rd edition. Washington, DC: Author, 1980.

8. American Psychiatric Association. *Diagnostic and Statistical Manual of Mental Disorders*, 4th edition. Washington, DC: Author, 1994.

9. American Psychiatric Association. *Diagnostic and Statistical Manual of Mental Disorders*, 4th edition, text revision. Washington, DC: Author, 2000.

10. Andrews, B., Brewin, C. R., Philpott, R., and Stewart, L. Delayed-onset posttraumatic stress disorder: a systematic review of the evidence. Am. J. Psychiat., *164*: 1319–1326, 2007.

11. Arnsten, A. F., and Goldman-Rakic, P. S. Noise stress impairs prefrontal cortical cognitive function in monkeys: evidence for a hyperdopaminergic mechanism. Arch. Gen. Psychiat., *55*:362–368, 1998.

12. Atkinson, R. M., Henderson, R. G., Sparr, L. F., and Deale, S. Assessment of Viet Nam veterans for posttraumatic stress disorder in Veterans Administration disability claims. Am. J. Psychiat., *139*:1118–1121, 1982.

13. Babinski, J., and Froment, J. *Hysteria or Pithiatism and Reflect Nervous Disorders in the Neurology of War*. London: University of London Press, 1918.

14. Baum, A., Fleming, R., and Davidson, L. M. Natural disaster and technological catastrophe. Env. Behav., *15*:333–354, 1983.

15. Beigel, A., and Berren, M. Human-induced disasters. Psychiat. Ann., *15*:143–150, 1985.

16. Bennett, G. Bristol floods 1968: controlled survey of effects on health of local community disaster. Br. J. Med., *3*:454–458, 1970.

17. Bensheim, H. Die K.Z. Neurose rassisch Verfolgter: Ein Beitrag zur Psychopathologie der Neurosen [The concentration camp neurosis of the racially persecuted: a contribution on the psychopathology of neuroses]. Der Nervenarzt, *31*:462–469, 1960.

18. Benton, G. H. "War" neurosis and allied conditions in ex-service men: as observed in the United States Public Health Service Hospitals for Psychoneurotics. JAMA, *17*:360–365, 1931.

19. Bierer, L. M., Tischler, L., Labinsky, E., Cahill, S., Foa, E., and Yehuda, R. Clinical correlates of 24-h cortisol and norepinephrine excretion among subjects seeking treatment following the world trade center attacks on 9/11. Ann. N. Y. Acad. Sci., *1071*:514–520, 2006.

20. Birnbaum, S., Gobeske, K. T., Auerbach, J., Taylor, J. R., and Arnsten, A. F. A role for norepinephrine in stress-induced cognitive deficits: alpha-1-adrenoceptor mediation in the prefrontal cortex. Biol. Psychiat., *46*:1266–1274, 1999.

21. Bisson, J. I., Ehlers, A., Matthews, R., Pilling, S., Richards, D., and Turner, S. Psychological treatments for chronic post-traumatic stress disorder. Systematic review and meta-analysis. Br. J. Psychiat., *190*:97–104, 2007.

22. Black, D. W. Efficacy of combined pharmacotherapy and psychotherapy versus monotherapy in the treatment of anxiety disorders. CNS Spectr., 11:29–33, 2006.

23. Block, D. A., Silber, E., and Perry, S. E. Some factors in the emotional reaction of children to disaster. Am. J. Psychiat., 412:416–422, 1956.

24. Boehnlein, J. K., and Kinzie, J. D. Pharmacologic reduction of CNS noradrenergic activity in PTSD: the case for clonidine and prazosin. J. Psychiat. Pract., 13:72–78, 2007.

25. Bradford, J. M., and Bradford, E. J. Neurosis in escaped prisoners of war. Br. J. Med. Psychol., 20:422–435, 1947.

26. Bremner, J. D., Krystal, J. H., Southwick, S. M., and Charney, D. S. Noradrenergic mechanisms in stress and anxiety: II. Clinical studies. Synapse, 23:39–51, 1996.

27. Bremner, J. D., Staib, L. H., Kaloupek, D., Southwick, S. M., Soufer, R., and Charney, D. S. Neural correlates of exposure to traumatic pictures and sound in Vietnam combat veterans with and without posttraumatic stress disorder: a positron emission tomography study. Biol. Psychiat., 45:806–816, 1999.

28. Breslau, N. Epidemiology of trauma and posttraumatic stress disorder. In *Psychological Trauma*, Yehuda, R. (ed.). Washington, DC: American Psychiatric Press, pp. 1–29, 1998.

29. Breslau, N. Outcomes of posttraumatic stress disorder. J. Clin. Psychiat., *62 Suppl 17*:55–59, 2001.

30. Breslau, N. The epidemiology of posttraumatic stress disorder: what is the extent of the problem? J. Clin. Psychiat., 62:16–22, 2001.

31. Breslau, N., Chase, G. A., and Anthony, J. C. The uniqueness of the DSM definition of post-traumatic stress disorder: implications for research. Psychol. Med., 32:573–576, 2002.

32. Breslau, N., and Davis, G. C. Posttraumatic stress disorder: the etiologic specificity of wartime stressors. Am. J. Psychiat., 144:578–583, 1987.

33. Breslau, N., and Davis, G. C. Posttraumatic stress disorder in an urban population of young adults: risk factors for chronicity. Am. J. Psychiat., 149:671–675, 1992.

34. Breslau, N., Davis, G. C., and Andreski, A. Risk factors for PTSD-related traumatic events: a prospective analysis. Am. J. Psychiat., 152:529–535, 1995.

35. Breslau, N., Davis, G. C., Andreski, P., and Peterson, E. Traumatic events and posttraumatic stress disorder in an urban population of young adults. Arch. Gen. Psychiat., 48:216–222, 1991.

36. Breslau, N., Kessler, R. C., Chilcoat, H. D., Schultz, L. R., Davis, G. C., and Andreski, P. Trauma and posttraumatic stress disorder in the community: the 1996 Detroit area survey of trauma. Arch. Gen. Psychiat., 55:626–632, 1998.

37. Breslau, N., Lucia, V. C., and Davis, G. C. Partial PTSD versus full PTSD: an empirical examination of associated impairment. Psychol. Med., 34:1205–1214, 2004.

38. Brett, E. A. Classifications of posttraumatic stress disorder in DSM-IV: anxiety disorder, dissociative disorder, or stress disorder? In *Posttraumatic Stress Disorder: DSM-IV and Beyond*, Davidson, J. R. T., Foa, E. B. (eds.). Washington, DC: American Psychiatric Press, pp. 191–204, 1993.

39. Brett, E. A., Spitzer, R. L., and Williams, J. B. W. DSM-III-R criteria for post-traumatic stress disorder. Am. J. Psychiat., *145(10)*:1232–1236, 1988.

40. Brewin, C. R., Andrews, B., and Valentine, J. D. Meta-analysis of risk factors for posttraumatic stress disorder in trauma-exposed adults. J. Consult. Clin. Psychol., *68*:748–766, 2000.

41. Bromet, E. J., Parkinson, D. K., and Schulberg, H. C. Mental health of residents near the Three Mile Island reactor: a comparative study of selected groups. J. Prevent. Psychiat., *1*:225–276, 1982.

42. Bryant, R. A., Moulds, M. L., and Guthrie, R. M. Acute Stress Disorder Scale: a self-report measure of acute stress disorder. Psychol. Assess., *12*:61–68, 2000.

43. Buydens-Branchey, L., Noumair, D., and Branchey, M. Duration and intensity of combat exposure and posttraumatic stress disorder in Vietnam veterans. J. Nerv. Ment. Dis., *178(9)*:582–587, 1990.

44. Calhoun, P. S., Bosworth, H. B., Grambow, S. C., Dudley, T. K., and Beckham, J. C. Medical service utilization by veterans seeking help for posttraumatic stress disorder. Am. J. Psychiat., *159*:2081–2086, 2002.

45. Canino, G., Bravo, M., Rubio-Stipec, M., and Woodbury, M. The impact of disaster on mental health: prospective and retrospective analyses. Int. J. Ment. Health, *19*:51–69, 1990.

46. Chambers, R. A., Bremner, J. D., Moghaddam, B., Southwick, S. M., Charney, D. S., and Krystal, J. H. Glutamate and post-traumatic stress disorder: toward a psycho-biology of dissociation. Semin. Clin. Neuropsychiat., *4*:274–281, 1999.

47. Chen, C. C., Yeh, T. L., Yang, Y. K., Chen, S. J., Lee, I. H., Fu, L. S., Yeh, C. Y., Hsu, H. C., Tsai, W. L., Cheng, S. H., Chen, L. Y., and Si, Y. C. Psychiatric morbidity and post-traumatic symptoms among survivors in the early stage following the 1999 earthquake in Taiwan. Psychiat. Res., *105*:13–22, 2001.

48. Cohen, H., Kaplan, Z., Kotler, M., Kouperman, I., Moisa, R., and Grisaru, N. Repetitive transcranial magnetic stimulation of the right dorsolateral prefrontal cortex in posttraumatic stress disorder: a double-blind, placebo-controlled study. Am. J. Psychiat., *161*:515–524, 2004.

49. Connor, K. M., and Davidson, J. R. T. The role of serotonin in posttraumatic stress disorder: neurobiology and pharmacotherapy. CNS Spectr., *3*:43–51, 1998.

50. Culpin, M. The need for psychopathology. Lancet, *2*:725–726, 1930.

51. Cyr, M., and Farr, M. K. Treatment for posttraumatic stress disorder. Ann. Pharmacother., *34*:366–376, 2000.

52. Da Costa, J. M. On irritable heart: a clinical study of a form of functional cardiac disorder and its consequence. Am. J. Med. Sci., *16*:17–52, 2003.

53. Daly, R. J. Samuel Pepys and post-traumatic stress disorder. Br. J. Psychiat., *143*:64–68, 1983.

54. Davidson, J., Smith, R., and Kudler, H. Familial psychiatric illness in chronic posttraumatic stress disorder. Compr. Psychiat., *30*:339–345, 1989.

55. Davidson, J., Swartz, M., Storck, M., Krishnan, R. R., and Hammett, E. A diagnostic and family study of posttraumatic stress disorder. Am. J. Psychiat., *142*:90–93, 1985.

56. Davidson, J. R. Pharmacotherapy of posttraumatic stress disorder: treatment options, long-term follow-up, and predictors of outcome. J. Clin. Psychiat., 61Suppl: 52–59, 2000.

57. Davidson, J. R. T., Hughes, D., Blazer, D. G., and George, L. K. Post-traumatic stress disorder in the community: an epidemiological study. Psychol. Med., 21:713–721, 1991.

58. Davidson, J. R. T., Rothbaum, B. O., van der Kolk, B. A., Sikes, C. R., and Farfel, G. M. Multicenter, double-blind comparison of sertraline and placebo in the treatment of posttraumatic stress disorder. Arch. Gen. Psychiat., 58:485–492, 2001.

59. Deering, G. G., Glover, S. G., Ready, D., Eddlelman, H. C., and Alarcon, D. Unique patterns of comorbidity in posttraumatic stress disorder from different sources of trauma. Compr. Psychiat., 37:336–346, 1996.

60. Delahanty, D. L., Raimonde, A. J., and Spoonster, E. Initial posttraumatic urinary cortisol levels predict subsequent PTSD symptoms in motor vehicle accident victims. Biol. Psychiat., 48:940–947, 2000.

61. Denham, R. H., and Currier, F. P. The traumatic neurosis and the relation to the surgeon. J. Mich. State Med. Soc., 23:299–303, 1924.

62. Deykin, E. Y., Keane, T. M., Kaloupek, D., Fincke, G., Rothendler, J., Siegfried, M., and Creamer, K. Posttraumatic stress disorder and the use of health services. Psychosom. Med., 63:835–841, 2001.

63. Difede, J., and Barocas, D. Acute intrusive and avoidant PTSD symptoms as predictors of chronic PTSD following burn injury. J. Trauma. Stress, 12:363–369, 1999.

64. Ellenberger, H. F. *The Discovery of the Unconscious.* New York: Basic Books, 1970.

65. Elliott, D. M., and Briere, J. Posttraumatic stress associated with delayed recall of sexual abuse: a general population study. J. Trauma. Stress, 8:629–647, 1995.

66. Engdahl, B. E., Speed, N., Eberly, R. E., and Schwartz, J. Comorbidity of psychiatric disorders and personality profiles of American World War II prisoners of war. J. Nerv. Ment. Dis., 179:181–187, 1991.

67. Epstein, R., Fullerton, C., and Ursano, R. Posttraumatic stress disorder following an air disaster: a prospective study. Am. J. Psychiat., 155:934–938, 1998.

68. Erichsen, J. *On Concussion of the Spine: Nervous Shock and Other Obscure Injuries of the Nervous System. [Reprinted in New York: William Wood; 1886, pp. 36–37].* London: Longmans, Green, 1875.

69. Feinstein, A., and Dolan, R. Predictors of post-traumatic stress disorder following physical trauma: an examination of the stressor criterion. Psychol. Med., 21:85–91, 1991.

70. Fischer-Homberger, E. Railway Spine and traumatische neurose: seele and rückenmark [Railway Spine and traumatic neurosis: soul and spine]. Gesnerus, 27:96–111, 1970.

71. Foa, E. B., Riggs, D. S., and Gershuny, B. S. Arousal, numbing, and intrusion; symptoms structure of PTSD following assault. Am. J. Psychiat., 152:116–120, 1995.

72. Fontana, A., and Rosenheck, R. The role of war-zone trauma and PTSD in the etiology of antisocial behavior. J. Nerv. Ment. Dis., *193*:203–209, 2005.

73. Frederick, C. J. Effects of natural vs. human-induced violence upon victims. Eval. Change, *Special Issue*:71–75, 1980.

74. Freud, S. My views on the part played by sexuality in the aetiology of the neuroses. In *A Case of Hysteria, Three Essays on Sexuality and Other Works [The Standard Edition of the Complete Psychological Works of Sigmund Freud, Volume VII (1901–1905)]*, Strachey, J. (ed. and trans.). London: The Hogarth Press and the Institute of Psychoanalysis, pp. 269–279, 1906.

75. Freud, S. The etiology of hysteria. In *The Standard Edition of the Complete Psychological Works of Sigmund Freud Vol. 3*, J. Strachey (ed.). London: The Hogarth Press, 1962, pp. 186–221, 1896.

76. Friedman, M. J. Toward rational pharmacotherapy for posttraumatic stress disorder: an interim report. Am. J. Psychiat., *145*:281–285, 1988.

77. Friedman, M. J. Biological approaches to the diagnosis and treatment of post-traumatic stress disorder. J. Trauma. Stress, *4*:67–91, 1991.

78. Friedman, P., and Linn, L. Some psychiatric notes on the Andrea Doria disaster. Am. J. Psychiat., *114*:426–432, 1957.

79. Frueh, B. C., Smith, D. W., and Barker, S. E. Compensation seeking status and psychometric assessment of combat veterans seeking treatment for PTSD. J. Trauma. Stress, *9*:427–439, 1996.

80. Galea, S., Ahern, J., Resnick, H., Kilpatrick, D., Bucuvalis, M., Gold, J., and Vlahov, D. Psychological sequelae of the September 11 terrorist attacks in New York City. N. Engl. J. Med., *346*:982–987, 2002.

81. Galea, S., Vlahov, D., Resnick, H., Ahern, J., Susser, E., Gold, J., Bucuvalas, M., and Kilpatrick, D. Trends of probable post-traumatic stress disorder in New York City after the September 11 terrorist attacks. Am. J. Epidemiol., *158*:514–524, 2003.

82. Gilbertson, M. W., Shenton, M. E., Ciszewski, A., Kasai, K., Lasko, N. B., Orr, S. P., and Pitman, R. K. Smaller hippocampal volume predicts pathologic vulnerability to psychological trauma. Nat. Neurosci., *5A*:1242–1247, 2002.

83. Gleser, G. C., Green, B. L., and Winget, C. N. *Prolonged Psychosocial Effects of Disaster: A Study of Buffalo Creek*. New York: Academic Press, 1981.

84. Goldberg, J., True, W. R., Eisen, S. A., and Henderson, W. G. A twin study of the effects of the Vietnam War on posttraumatic stress disorder. JAMA, *263*:1227–1232, 1990.

85. Green, A. H. Comparing child victims and adult survivors: clues to the pathogenesis of child sexual abuse. J. Am. Acad. Psychoanal., *23*:655–670, 1995.

86. Green, B. L., Grace, M. C., Lindy, J. D., Gleser, G. C., and Leonard, A. Risk factors for PTSD and other diagnoses in a general sample of Vietnam veterans. Am. J. Psychiat., *147(6)*:729–733, 1990.

87. Green, B. L., Lindy, J. D., and Grace, M. C. Posttraumatic stress disorder: toward DSM-IV. J. Nerv. Ment. Dis., *173*:406–411, 1985.

88. Green, B. L., Lindy, J. D., Grace, M. C., Gleser, G. C., Leonard, A. C., Korol, M., and Winget, C. Buffalo Creek survivors in the second decade: stability of stress symptoms. Am. J. Orthopsychiat., 60:43–54, 1990.

89. Gunderson, J. G., and Sabo, A. N. The phenomenological and conceptual interface between borderline personality disorder and PTSD. Am. J. Psychiat., 150:19–27, 1993.

90. Halbreich, U., Olympia, J., Carson, S., Glogowski, J., Yeh, C. M., Axelrod, S., and Desu, M. M. Hypothalamo-pituitary-adrenal activity in endogenously depressed post-traumatic stress disorder patients. Psychoneuroendocrinology, 14:365–370, 1989.

91. Hall, J. C. Medical evidence in railway accidents. Br. Med. J., i:216–217, 272–274, 325–327, 1868.

92. Hamner, M. B., Robert, S., and Frueh, B. C. Treatment-resistant posttraumatic stress disorder: strategies for intervention. CNS Spectr., 9:740–752, 2004.

93. Hawthorne, H. On heart disease in the army. Am. J. Med. Sci., 48:89–92, 1863.

94. Helzer, J. E., Robins, L. N., and McEvoy, L. Post-traumatic stress disorder in the general population. Findings of the epidemiologic catchment area survey. N. Engl. J. Med., 317:1630–1634, 1987.

95. Henigsberg, N., Folnegovic-Smalc, V., and Moro, L. Stressor characteristics and post-traumatic stress disorder symptom dimensions in war victims. Croat. Med. J., 42:543–550, 2001.

96. Herman, J., and van der Kolk, B. A. Traumatic antecedents of borderline personality disorder. In *Psychological Trauma*, van der Kolk, B. A. (ed.). Washington, DC: American Psychiatric Press, 1987.

97. Hocking, F. Psychiatric aspects of extreme environmental stress. Dis. Nerv. Syst., 31:542–545, 1970.

98. Hoffman, J. Erfahrungen über die Traumatische Neurose [Experiences with traumatic neurosis]. Berliner Klinische Wochenschrift, 27:655–660, 1890.

99. Hoge, C. W., Castro, C. A., Messer, S. C., McGurk, D., Cotting, D. I., and Koffman, R. L. Combat duty in Iraq and Afghanistan, mental health problems, and barriers to care. N. Engl. J. Med., 351:13–22, 2004.

100. Holbrook, T. L., Hoyt, D. B., Stein, M. B., and Sieber, W. J. Perceived threat to life predicts posttraumatic stress disorder after major trauma: risk factors and functional outcome. J. Trauma. Stress, 51:287–292, 2001.

101. Horowitz, M. J. *Stress Response Syndromes*. New York: Jason Aronson, 1976.

102. Horrigan, J. P. Guanfacine for PTSD nightmares. J. Am. Acad. Child Adolesc. Psychiat., 35:975–976, 1996.

103. Inman, T. G. Some comparisons between war neuroses and those of civilian life. J. Calif. State Med. Soc., 18:184–186, 1920.

104. Janet, P. *The Major Symptoms of Hysteria: 15 Lectures Given in the Medical School of Harvard University*. New York: Macmillan, 1907.

105. Johnson, R. K. Psychologic assessment of patients with industrial hand injuries. Hand Clin., 9:221–229, 1993.

106. Kasl, S. V., Chisholm, R. E., and Eskenazi, B. The impact of the accident at Three Mile Island on the behavior and well-being of nuclear workers. Am. J. Publ. Health, 71:472–495, 1981.

107. Keane, T. M., and Wolfe, J. Comorbidity in post-traumatic stress disorder: an analysis of community and clinical studies. J. Appl. Soc. Psychol., 20:1776–1778, 1990.

108. Kessler, R. C., Sonnega, A., Bromet, E., Hughes, M., and Nelson, C. B. Posttraumatic stress disorder in the National Comorbidity Survey. Arch. Gen. Psychiat., 52:1048–1060, 1995.

109. Kinzie, J. D., and Goetz, R. R. A century of controversy surrounding posttraumatic stress-spectrum syndromes: the impact on DSM-III and DSM-IV. J. Trauma. Stress, 9:159–179, 1996.

110. Kinzie, J. D., and Leung, P. Clonidine in Cambodian patients with posttraumatic stress disorder. J. Nerv. Ment. Dis., 177:546–550, 1989.

111. Koenen, K. C., Harley, R., Lyons, M. J., Wolfe, J., Simpson, J. C., Goldberg, J., Eisen, S. A., and Tsuang, M. A twin registry study of familial and individual risk factors for trauma exposure and posttraumatic stress disorder. J. Nerv. Ment. Dis., 190:209–218, 2002.

112. Koenen, K. C., Moffitt, T. E., Caspi, A., Gregory, A., Harrington, H., and Poulton, R. The developmental mental-disorder histories of adults with posttraumatic stress disorder: a prospective longitudinal birth cohort study. J. Abnorm. Psychol., 117:460–466, 2008.

113. Kosten, T. R., Mason, J. W., Giller, E. L., Ostroff, R. B., and Harkness, L. Sustained urinary norepinephrine and epinephrine elevation in post-traumatic stress disorder. Psychoneuroendocrinology, 12:13–20, 1987.

114. Kramer, S. N. A Sumerian Lamentation. In *Ancient Near Eastern Texts Relating to the Old Testament*, Pritchard, J. B. (ed.). Trenton, NJ: Princeton University Press, pp. 455–463, 1969.

115. Kulka, R. A., Schlenger, W. E., Fairbank, J. A., Hough, R. L., Jordan, B. K., and Marmar, C. R. National Vietnam V (ed.). *National Vietnam Veterans Readjustment Study (NVVRS): Description, Current Status, and Initial PTSD Prevalence Rates.* Research Triangle Park, N.C.: Research Triangle Institute, 1988.

116. Kulka, R. A., Schlenger, W. E., Fairbank, J. A., Hough, R. L., Jordan, B. K., Marmar, C. R., and Weiss, D. S. *Trauma and the Vietnam War Generation: Report of the Findings From the National Vietnam Veterans Readjustment Study.* New York: Bruner/Mazel, 1990.

117. Lamprecht, F., and Sack, M. Posttraumatic stress disorder revisited. Psychosom. Med., 64:222–237, 2002.

118. Langdon, J. R., and Parker, A. H. Psychiatric aspects of the March 7, 1954 earthquake. Alaska Med., 6:33–35, 1954.

119. Lavie, P. Sleep disturbances in the wake of traumatic events. N. Engl. J. Med., 345:1825–1832, 2001.

120. Lemieux, A. M., and Coe, C. L. Abuse-related posttraumatic stress disorder: evidence for chronic neuroendocrine activation in women. Psychosom. Med., 57:105–115, 1995.

121. Lenze, E. L., Miller, A., Munir, Z., Pornoppadol, C., and North, C. S. Psychiatric symptoms endorsed by somatization disorder patients in a psychiatric clinic. Ann. Clin. Psychiat., 11:73–79, 1999.

122. Liao, W. C., Lee, M. B., Lee, Y. J., Wang, T., Shih, F. Y., and Ma, M. H. Association of psychological distress with psychological factors in rescue workers within two months after a major earthquake. J. Formos. Med. Assoc., 101:169–176, 2002.

123. Lopez-Ibor, J. J., Jr., Canas, S. F., and Rodriguez-Gamazo, M. Psychological aspects of the toxic oil syndrome catastrophe. Br. J. Psychiat., 147:352–365, 1985.

124. MacKenzie, J. The soldier's heart and war neurosis: a study in symptomatology. Br. Med. J., Part II:530–534, 1920.

125. Maes, M., Mylle, J., Delmeire, L., and Janca, A. Pre- and post-disaster negative life events in relation to the incidence and severity of post-traumatic stress disorder. Psychiat. Res., 105:1–12, 2001.

126. Marshall, R. D., Beebe, K. L., Oldham, M., and Zaninelli, R. Efficacy and safety of paroxetine treatment for chronic PTSD: a fixed-dose, placebo-controlled study. Am. J. Psychiat., 158:1982–1988, 2001.

127. Mason, J. W., Giller, E. L., Kosten, T. R., Ostroff, R. B., and Podd, L. Urinary free-cortisol levels in posttraumatic stress disorder patients. J. Nerv. Ment. Dis., 174:145–149, 1986.

128. Mathers, A. T. The psychoneuroses in wartime. Can. Med. Ass. J., 47:103–111, 1942.

129. McEwen, B. S. Possible mechanisms for atrophy of the human hippocampus. Mol. Psychiat., 2:255–262, 1997.

130. McFall, M. E., Murburg, M. M., Ko, G. N., and Veith, R. C. Autonomic responses to stress in Vietnam combat veterans with posttraumatic stress disorder. Biol. Psychiat., 27:1165–1175, 1990.

131. McFall, M. E., Veith, R. C., and Murburg, M. M. Basal sympathoadrenal function in posttraumatic distress disorder. Biol. Psychiat., 31:1050–1056, 1992.

132. McFarlane, A. C. The aetiology of post-traumatic morbidity: predisposing, precipitating and perpetuating factors. Br. J. Psychiat., 154:221–228, 1989.

133. McFarlane, A. C., Atchison, M., and Yehuda, R. The acute stress response following motor vehicle accidents and its relation to PTSD. Ann. N. Y. Acad. Sci., 821:437–441, 1997.

134. McFarlane, A. C., and Papay, P. Multiple diagnoses in posttraumatic stress disorder in the victims of a natural disaster. J. Nerv. Ment. Dis., 180:498–504, 1992.

135. McMillen, J. C., North, C. S., and Smith, E. M. What parts of PTSD are normal: intrusion, avoidance, or arousal? Data from the Northridge, California earthquake. J. Trauma. Stress, 13:57–75, 2000.

136. Mellman, T. A., Randolph, C. A., Brawman-Mintzer, O., Flores, L. P., and Milanes, F. J. Phenomenology and course of psychiatric disorders associated with combat-related posttraumatic stress disorder. Am. J. Psychiat., 149:1568–1574, 1992.

137. Micale, M. Charcot and the idea of hysteria in the male: gender, mental science, and medical diagnosis of the late nineteenth century in France. Med. Hist., 34:363–411, 1990.

138. Moleen, G. A. Nervous disturbances as a result of injury, with special reference to the true and false traumatic neurasthenia. Colorado Med., 21:87–91, 1924.

139. Moore, H. E., and Friedsam, H. J. Reported emotional stress following a disaster. Soc. Forces, 38:135–138, 1959.

140. Mott, F. W. *War Neurosis and Shell Shock*. London: Oxford University Press, 1919.

141. Mullen, P. E., Martin, J. L., Anderson, J. C., Romans, S. E., and Herbison, G. P. Childhood sexual abuse and mental health in adult life. Br. J. Psychiat., 163:721–732, 1993.

142. Murburg, M. M., McFall, M. E., Lewis, N., and Veith, R. C. Plasma norepinephrine kinetics in patients with posttraumatic stress disorder. Biol. Psychiat., 38:819–825, 1995.

143. Myers, C. S. A contribution to the study of shell shock. Lancet, i:316–320, 1915.

144. Nair, J., and Singh, A. S. The role of the glutamatergic system in posttraumatic stress disorder. CNS Spectr., 13:585–591, 2008.

145. National Academy of Sciences Institute of Medicine. *Posttraumatic Stress Disorder: Diagnosis and Assessment*. Washington, DC: National Academy Press, 2006.

146. National Academy of Sciences Institute of Medicine. *Treatment of Posttraumatic Stress Disorder: An Assessment of the Evidence*. Washington, DC: The National Academies Press, 2007.

147. Norris, F. H. Epidemiology of trauma: frequency and impact of different potentially traumatic events on different demographic groups. J. Consult. Clin. Psychol., 60:409–418, 1992.

148. Norris, F. H., Friedman, M. J., Watson, P. J., Byrne, C. M., Diaz, E., and Kaniasty, K. 60,000 disaster victims speak: Part I. An empirical review of the empirical literature, 1981–2001. Psychiat., 65:207–239, 2002.

149. North, C. S. Somatization in survivors of catastrophic trauma: a methodological review. Environ. Health Perspect., 110:637–640, 2002.

150. North, C. S., Kawasaki, A., Spitznagel, E. L., and Hong, B. A. The course of PTSD, major depression, substance abuse, and somatization after a natural disaster. J. Nerv. Ment. Dis., 192:823–829, 2004.

151. North, C. S., Nixon, S. J., Shariat, S., Mallonee, S., McMillen, J. C., Spitznagel, E. L., and Smith, E. M. Psychiatric disorders among survivors of the Oklahoma City bombing. JAMA, 282:755–762, 1999.

152. North, C. S., Smith, E. M., and Spitznagel, E. L. Posttraumatic stress disorder in survivors of a mass shooting. Am. J. Psychiat., 151:82–88, 1994.

153. North, C. S., Smith, E. M., and Spitznagel, E. L. Violence and the homeless: an epidemiologic study of victimization and aggression. J. Trauma. Stress, 7:95–110, 1994.

154. North, C. S., Smith, E. M., and Spitznagel, E. L. One-year follow-up of survivors of a mass shooting. Am. J. Psychiat., 154:1696–1702, 1997.

155. North, C. S., Suris, A. M., Davis, M., and Smith, R. P. Toward validation of the diagnosis of posttraumatic stress disorder. Am. J. Psychiat., 166:1–8, 2009.

156. Orsillo, S. M., Weathers, F. W., Litz, B. T., Steinberg, H. R., Huska, J. A., and Keane, T. M. Current and lifetime psychiatric disorders among veterans with war zone-related posttraumatic stress disorder. J. Nerv. Ment. Dis., 184:307–313, 1996.

157. Ozer, E. J., Best, S. R., Lipsey, T. L., and Weiss, D. S. Predictors of posttraumatic stress disorder and symptoms in adults: a meta-analysis. Psychol. Bull., 129:52–73, 2003.

158. Page, H. W. *Injuries of the Spine and Spinal Cord without Apparent Mechanical Lesions and Nervous Shock in Their Surgical and Medical Legal Aspects.* London: J.A. Churchill, 1885.

159. Perkonigg, A., Kessler, R. C., Storz, S., and Wittchen, H. U. Traumatic events and post-traumatic stress disorder in the community: prevalence, risk factors and comorbidity. Acta Psychiat. Scand., 101:46–59, 2000.

160. Perry, B. D., Giller, E. L., Jr., and Southwick, S. M. Altered platelet alpha 2-adrenergic binding sites in posttraumatic stress disorder. Am. J. Psychiat., 144:1511–1512, 1987.

161. Pitman, R. K., Altman, B., Greenwald, E., Longpre, R. E., Macklin, M. L., Poire, R. E., and Steketee, G. S. Psychiatric complications during flooding therapy for posttraumatic stress disorder. J. Clin. Psychiat., 52:17–20, 1991.

162. Pitman, R. K., and Orr, S. P. Twenty-four hour urinary cortisol and catecholamine excretion in combat-related posttraumatic stress disorder. Biol. Psychiat., 27:245–247, 1990.

163. Pitman, R. K., Orr, S. P., Forgue, D. F., Altman, B., de Jong, J. B., and Herz, L. R. Psychophysiologic responses to combat imagery of Vietnam veterans with post-traumatic stress disorder versus other anxiety disorders. J. Abnorm. Psychol., 99:49–54, 1990.

164. Pitman, R. K., Sanders, K. M., Zusman, R. M., Healy, A. R., Cheema, F., Lasko, N. B., Cahill, L., and Orr, S. P. Pilot study of secondary prevention of posttraumatic stress disorder with propranolol. Biol. Psychiat., 51:189–192, 2002.

165. Prins, A., Kaloupek, D. G., and Keane, T. M. Psychophysiological evidence for autonomic arousal and startle in traumatized adult populations. In *Neurobiological and Clinical Consequences of Stress: From Normal Adaptation to Post-traumatic Stress Disorder*, Friedman, M. J., Charney, D. S., Deutch, A. Y. (eds.). Philadelphia: Lippincott-Raven, pp. 291–314, 1995.

166. Putnam, J. J. Recent investigation into the so-called concussion of the spine. Med. Surg. J., 109:217–220, 1883.

167. Raja, M., Onofri, A., Azzoni, A., Borzellino, B., and Melchiorre, N. Post-traumatic stress disorder among people exposed to the Ventotene street disaster in Rome. Clin. Pract. Epidemol. Ment. Health, 4:5, 2008.

168. Ramsay, R. Post-traumatic stress disorder: a new clinical entity? J. Psychosomat. Res., 34:355–365, 1990.

169. Raskind, M. A., Peskind, E. R., Kanter, E. D., Petrie, E. C., Radant, A., Thompson, C. E., Dobie, D. J., Hoff, D., Rein, R. J., Straits-Troster, K., Thomas, R. G., and McFall, M. M. Reduction of nightmares and other PTSD symptoms in combat veterans by prazosin: a placebo-controlled study. Am. J. Psychiat., 160:371–373, 2003.

170. Rauch, S. L., Shin, L. M., Whalen, P. J., and Pitman, R. K. Neuroimaging and the neuroanatomy of posttraumatic stress disorder. CNS Spectr., 3:31–41, 1998.

171. Rauch, S. L., van der Kolk, B. A., Fisler, R. E., Alpert, N. M., Orr, S. P., Savage, C. R., Fischman, A. J., Jenike, M. A., and Pitman, R. K. A symptom provocation study of posttraumatic stress disorder using positron emission tomography and script-driven imagery. Arch. Gen. Psychiat., 53:380–387, 1996.

172. Resnick, H. S., Kilpatrick, D. G., Dansky, B. S., Saunders, B. E., and Best, C. L. Prevalence of civilian trauma and posttraumatic stress disorder in a representative national sample of women. J. Consult. Clin. Psychol., 61:984–991, 1993.

173. Resnick, H. S., Yehuda, R., Pitman, R. K., and Foy, D. W. Effect of previous trauma on acute plasma cortisol level following rape. Am. J. Psychiat., 152:1675–1677, 1995.

174. Robins, L. N. Steps toward evaluating post-traumatic stress reaction as a psychiatric disorder. J. Appl. Soc. Psychol., 20:1674–1677, 1990.

175. Robins, L. N., and Regier, D. A. *Psychiatric Disorders in America: The Epidemiologic Catchment Area Study.* New York: The Free Press, 1991.

176. Roca, R. P., Spence, R. J., and Munster, A. M. Posttraumatic adaptation and distress among adult burn survivors. Am. J. Psychiat., 149:1234–1238, 1992.

177. Rose, S., Bisson, J., and Wessely, S. A systematic review of single-session psychological interventions ("debriefing") following trauma. Psychother. Psychosom., 72:176–184, 2003.

178. Rosen, G. M., and Lilienfeld, S. O. Posttraumatic stress disorder: an empirical evaluation of core assumptions. Clin. Psychol. Rev., 28:837–868, 2008.

179. Rubonis, A. V., and Bickman, L. Psychological impairment in the wake of disaster: the disaster-psychopathology relationship. Psychol. Bull., 109:384–399, 1991.

180. Ruzich, M. J., Looi, J. C., and Robertson, M. D. Delayed onset of posttraumatic stress disorder among male combat veterans: a case series. Am. J. Geriatr. Psychiat., 13:424–427, 2005.

181. Schelling, G., Roozendaal, B., Krauseneck, T., Schmoelz, M., DE Quervain, D., and Briegel, J. Efficacy of hydrocortisone in preventing posttraumatic stress disorder following critical illness and major surgery. Ann. N. Y. Acad. Sci., 1071:46–53, 2006.

182. Scherrer, J. F., Xian, H., Lyons, M. J., Goldberg, J., Eisen, S. A., True, W. R., Tsuang, M., Bucholz, K. K., and Koenen, K. C. Posttraumatic stress disorder; combat exposure; and nicotine dependence, alcohol dependence, and major depression in male twins. Compr. Psychiat., 49:297–304, 2008.

183. Schlenger, W. E., Caddell, J. M., Ebert, L., Jordan, B. K., Rourke, K. M., Wilson, D., Thalji, L., Dennis, J. M., Fairbank, J. A., and Kulka, R. A. Psychological reactions to terrorist attacks: findings from the National Study of Americans' Reactions to September 11. JAMA, *288*:581–588, 2002.

184. Schnurr, P. P., Friedman, M. J., and Rosenberg, S. D. Premilitary MMPI scores as predictors of combat-related PTSD symptoms. Am. J. Psychiat., *150*:479–483, 1993.

185. Schnurr, P. P., Lunney, C. A., Sengupta, A., and Waelde, L. C. A descriptive analysis of PTSD chronicity in Vietnam veterans. J. Trauma Stress, *16*:545–553, 2003.

186. Selye, H., and Fortier, C. Adaptive reaction to stress. Psychosomat. Med., *12*:149–157, 1950.

187. Shay, J. Learning about combat stress through Homer's *Iliad*. J. Trauma. Stress, *4*:561–579, 1991.

188. Shin, L. M., Kosslyn, S. M., McNally, R. J., Alpert, N. M., Thompson, W. L., Rauch, S. L., Macklin, M. L., and Pitman, R. K. Visual imagery and perception in posttraumatic stress disorder. A positron emission tomographic investigation. Arch. Gen. Psychiat., *54*:233–241, 1997.

189. Shore, J. H., Tatum, E. L., and Vollmer, W. M. The Mount St. Helens stress response syndrome. In *Disaster Stress Studies: New Methods and Findings*, Shore, J. H. (ed.). Washington, DC: American Psychiatric Press, pp. 77–97, 1986.

190. Sierles, F. S., Chen, J.-J., Messing, M. L., Besyner, J. K., and Taylor, M. A. Concurrent psychiatric illness in non-Hispanic outpatients diagnosed as having posttraumatic stress disorder. J. Nerv. Ment. Dis., *174*:171–173, 1986.

191. Skey, F. C. Compensation for railway injuries. Lancet, *ii*:161–163, 1865.

192. Sloan, P. Posttraumatic stress in survivors of an airplane crash-landing: a clinical and exploratory research intervention. J. Trauma. Stress, *1*:211–229, 1988.

193. Smith, E. M., North, C. S., McCool, R. E., and Shea, J. M. Acute postdisaster psychiatric disorders: identification of persons at risk. Am. J. Psychiat., *147*:202–206, 1990.

194. Smith, E. M., Robins, L. N., Przybeck, T. R., Goldring, E., and Solomon, S. D. Psychosocial consequences of a disaster. In *Disaster Stress Studies: New Methods and Findings*, Shore, J. H. (ed.). Washington, DC: American Psychiatric Association, pp. 49–76, 1986.

195. Smith, R. P., Katz, C. L., Charney, D. S., and Southwick, S. M. Neurobiology of disaster exposure: fear, anxiety, trauma, and resilience. In *Textbook of Disaster Psychiatry*, Ursano, R. J., Fullerton, C. S., Weisaeth, L., Raphael, B. (eds.). Cambridge, England: Cambridge University Press, pp. 97–117, 2007.

196. Solomon, S. D., and Canino, G. J. Appropriateness of DSM-III-R criteria for post-traumatic stress disorder. Compr. Psychiat., *31*:227–237, 1990.

197. Solomon, Z. PTSD and social functioning. A three year prospective study. Soc. Psychiat. Psychiat. Epidemiol., *24*:127–133, 1989.

198. Solomon, Z., Mikulincer, M., and Hobfoll, S. Objective versus subjective measurement of stress and social support: combat-related reactions. J. Consult. Clin. Psychol., *55*:577–583, 1987.

199. Southwick, S. M., Krystal, J. H., Morgan, C. A., Johnson, D., Nagy, L. M., Nicolaou, A., Heninger, G. R., and Charney, D. S. Abnormal noradrenergic function in posttraumatic stress disorder. Arch. Gen. Psychiat., 50:266–274, 1993.

200. Southwick, S. M., and Yehuda, R. The interaction between pharmacotherapy and psychotherapy in the treatment of posttraumatic stress disorder. Am. J. Psychother., 47:404–410, 1993.

201. Southwick, S. M., Yehuda, R., and Giller, E. L. Personality disorders in treatment-seeking combat veterans with posttraumatic stress disorder. Am. J. Psychiat., 150:1020–1023, 1993.

202. Sparr, L. F. Legal aspects of posttraumatic stress disorder, uses and abuses. In *Posttraumatic Stress Disorder: Etiology, Phenomenology, and Treatment*, Wolfe, M. E., Mosniam, A. D. (eds.). Washington, DC: American Psychiatric Press, 1990.

203. Sparr, L. F. Post-traumatic stress disorder: does it exist? Neurol. Clin., 13:413–429, 1995.

204. Spiegel, D. Multiple personality as a post-traumatic stress disorder. Psychiat. Clin. N. Am., 7:101–110, 1984.

205. Spiegel, D., Hunt, T., and Dondershine, H. E. Dissociation and hypnotizability in posttraumatic stress disorder. Am. J. Psychiat., 145:301–305, 1988.

206. Spitzer, R. L., First, M. B., and Wakefield, J. C. Saving PTSD from itself in DSM-V. J. Anxiety Disord., 21:233–241, 2007.

207. Steinglass, P., and Gerrity, E. Natural disasters and posttraumatic stress disorder: short-term vs. long-term recovery in two disaster-affected communities. J. Appl. Soc. Psychol., 20:1746–1765, 1990.

208. Steinglass, P., Weisstub, E., and De-Nour, A. K. Perceived personal networks as mediators of stress reactions. Am. J. Psychiat., 145:1259–1264, 1988.

209. Stierlin, E. Nervöse and psychische Störungen nach Katastrophen [Nervous and psychological disturbances following catastrophes]. Deutsche Medizinische Wochenschrift, 37:2028–2035, 1911.

210. Stinson, B. Battle fatigue and how it was treated in the Civil War. Civil War Times Illustrated, 4:40–44, 1965.

211. Strawn, J. R., and Geracioti, T. D., Jr. Noradrenergic dysfunction and the psychopharmacology of posttraumatic stress disorder. Depress. Anxiety, 2007.

212. Sutker, P. B., Allain, A. N., and Winstead, D. K. Psychopathology and psychiatric diagnoses of World War II Pacific theater prisoner of war survivors and combat veterans. Am. J. Psychiat., 150:240–245, 1993.

213. The Centers for Disease Control Vietnam Experience Study. Health status of Vietnam veterans. I. Psychosocial characteristics. JAMA, 259:2701–2708, 1988.

214. Trimble, M. R. *Post-Traumatic Neurosis from Railway Spine to Whiplash*. Chichester, England: Wiley and Sons, 1981.

215. True, W. R., Rice, J., Eisen, S. A., Heath, A. C., Goldberg, J., Lyons, M. J., and Nowak, J. A twin study of genetic and environmental contributions to liability for posttraumatic stress symptoms. Arch. Gen. Psychiat., 50:257–260, 1993.

216. Tucker, P., Zaninelli, R., Yehuda, R., Ruggiero, L., Dillingham, K., and Pitts, C. D. Paroxetine in the treatment of chronic posttraumatic stress disorder: results of a placebo-controlled, flexible-dosage trial. J. Clin. Psychiat., 62:860–868, 2001.

217. Tucker, P. M., Pfefferbaum, B., North, C. S., Kent, A., Burgin, C. E., Parker, D. E., Hossain, A., Jeon-Slaughter, H., and Trautman, R. P. Physiologic reactivity despite emotional resilience several years after direct exposure to terrorism. Am. J. Psychiat., 164:230–235, 2007.

218. Ursano, R. J., Boystun, J. A., and Wheatley, R. D. Psychiatric illness in U.S. Air Force Vietnam prisoners of war: a five-year follow up. Am. J. Psychiat., 138:310–314, 1981.

219. van der Kolk, B., and van der Hart, O. Pierre Janet and the breakdown of adaptation in psychological trauma. Am. J. Psychiat., 146:1530–1540, 1989.

220. Weisæth, L. Post-traumatic stress disorder after an industrial disaster. In *Psychiatry—The State of the Art*, Pichot, P., Berner, P., Wolf, R., Thau, K. (eds.). New York: Plenum Press, pp. 299–307, 1985.

221. Whiles, H. A study of neurosis among repatriated prisoners of war. Br. Med. J., 2:697–698, 1945.

222. Wolfe, J., Brown, P. J., and Bucsela, M. L. Symptom responses of female Vietnam veterans to Operation Desert Storm. Am. J. Psychiat., 149:676–679, 1992.

223. Yargic, L. I., Sar, V., Tutkun, H., and Alyanak, B. Comparison of dissociative identity disorder with other diagnostic groups using a structured interview in Turkey. Compr. Psychiat., 39:345–351, 1998.

224. Yehuda, R. Recent developments in the neuroendocrinology of posttraumatic stress disorder. CNS Spectr., 3:23–29, 1998.

225. Yehuda, R. Biology of posttraumatic stress disorder. J. Clin. Psychiat., 62 Suppl 17:41–46, 2001.

226. Yehuda, R. Current status of cortisol findings in post-traumatic stress disorder. Psychiat. Clin. North Am., 25:341–68, vii, 2002.

227. Yehuda, R. Advances in understanding neuroendocrine alterations in PTSD and their therapeutic implications. Ann. N. Y. Acad. Sci., 1071:137–166, 2006.

228. Yehuda, R., Boisoneau, D., Lowy, M. T., and Giller, E. L., Jr. Dose-response changes in plasma cortisol and lymphocyte glucocorticoid receptors following dexamethasone administration in combat veterans with and without posttraumatic stress disorder. Arch. Gen. Psychiat., 52:583–593, 1995.

229. Yehuda, R., Boisoneau, D., Mason, J. W., and Giller, E. L. Glucocorticoid receptor number and cortisol excretion in mood, anxiety, and psychotic disorders. Biol. Psychiat., 34:18–25, 1993.

230. Yehuda, R., Golier, J. A., Halligan, S. L., Meaney, M., and Bierer, L. M. The ACTH response to dexamethasone in PTSD. Am. J. Psychiat., 161:1397–1403, 2004.

231. Yehuda, R., Lowy, M. T., Southwick, S. M., Shaffer, D., and Giller, E. L. Lymphocyte glucocorticoid receptor number in posttraumatic stress disorder. Am. J. Psychiat., 148:499–504, 1991.

232. Yehuda, R., Southwick, S., Giller, E. L., Ma, X., and Mason, J. W. Urinary catecholamine excretion and severity of PTSD symptoms in Vietnam combat veterans. J. Nerv. Ment. Dis., 180:321–325, 1992.

233. Yehuda, R., Southwick, S. M., Nussbaum, G., Wahby, V., Giller, E. L., Jr., and Mason, J. W. Low urinary cortisol excretion in patients with posttraumatic stress disorder. J. Nerv. Ment. Dis., 178:366–369, 1990.

234. Zanarini, M. C., Ruser, T., Frankenburg, F. R., and Hennen, J. The dissociative experiences of borderline patients. Compr. Psychiat., 41:223–227, 2000.

235. Zayfert, C., Dums, A. R., Ferguson, R. J., and Hegel, M. T. Health functioning impairments associated with posttraumatic stress disorder, anxiety disorders, and depression. J. Nerv. Ment. Dis., 190:233–240, 2002.

236. Zohar, J., Sasson, Y., Amital, D., Iancu, I., and Zinger, Y. Current diagnostic issues and epidemiological insights in PTSD. CNS Spectr., 3:12–14, 1998.

6

Obsessive-Compulsive Disorder

Obsessions are persistent distressing thoughts, images, or impulses experienced as unwanted and senseless but irresistible. *Compulsions* are repetitive behaviors aimed to prevent or reduce anxiety or distress but not to provide pleasure or gratification. Obsessive-compulsive disorder (OCD) is a chronic illness dominated by obsessions and compulsions occurring in the absence of another psychiatric disorder. Obsessional neurosis was a synonym in vogue before *DSM-III* was published in 1980.

Historical Background

The term *obsessional neurosis* apparently originated with Karl Westphal (1833–1890), a German neurologist who wrote about obsessional conditions and phobias. Kraepelin described obsessional neurosis (*Zwangsneurose*) in his textbooks in the early part of the twentieth century, and the same term was adopted by Freud, whose classical description of the clinical picture, published in 1917, follows (30):

> The obsessional neurosis takes this form: the patient's mind is occupied with thoughts that do not really interest him, he feels impulses which seem alien to him, and he is impelled to perform actions which not only afford him no

pleasure but from which he is powerless to desist. The thoughts (obsessions) may be meaningless in themselves or only of no interest to the patient; they are often only absolutely silly.

Recognition of obsessional traits, however, substantially antedated psychiatrists' description of the syndrome. In the early seventeenth century Richard Flecknoe, in discussing "enigmaticall characters," described one such character as an "irresolute Person" (42):

> He hovers in his choice, like an empty Ballance with no waight of Judgement to incline him to either scale . . . everything he thinks on, is matter of deliberation . . . and he does nothing readily, but what he thinks not on . . . when he begins to deliberate, never makes an end . . . . Has some dull demon cryes, do not, do not still, when hee's on point of doing anything . . . . He plays at shall I, shall I? so long, till opportunity be past . . . and then repents at leisure.

In the seventeenth century, obsessions were often referred to as "scruples," defined by Jermey A. Taylor (96) as

> a great trouble of mind preceding from a little motive, and a great indisposition, by which the conscience though sufficiently determined by proper arguments, dares not proceed to action, or if it do, it cannot rest . . . some persons dare not eat for fear of gluttony, they fear that they shall sleep too much, and that keeps them waking, and troubles their heads more and then their scruples increase. When they are married they are afraid to do their duty, for fear it be secretly an indulgence to the flesh, and to be suspected of carnality, and yet they dare not omit it, for fear they should be unjust, and yet their fear that the very fearing it to be unclean should be a sin, and suspect that if they do not fear so it is too great a sign they adhere to Nature more than to the Spirit . . . . Scruple is a little stone in the foot, if you set it upon the ground it hurts you; if you hold it up you cannot go forward; it is a trouble where the trouble is over, a doubt when doubts are resolved . . . very often it hath no reason at all for its inducement.

The content of obsessions, today as in years past, is often religious. In his monograph *Of Religious Melancholy* (68), published in 1692, John Moore described "naughty and sometimes blasphemous thoughts which start in the mind while they are exercised in the worship of God despite all their endeavors to stiffle and suppress them." In fact, he wrote, "the more they struggle with them, the more they increase." Bishop Moore had difficulty understanding this state as the sufferers were "mostly good People," whereas "bad men . . . rarely know anything of these kinds of Thoughts." Like others, he argued that this was good reason "to judge them to be Distempers of the body rather than Faults of the Mind." He was particularly concerned about the phobic avoidances that could result from such obsessions and wrote, "I exhort you not to quit your Employment . . . for no business at all is as bad for you as too much: and there is always more Melancholy to be found in a Cloyster than in the Marketplace."

The obsessional fear of suffering from syphilis was also well recognized as a manifestation of mental illness by the clergy and later by psychiatrists. In the past, the word *superstition* was often used to describe obsessive behaviors by today's conventions. Samuel Johnson apparently had this in mind when he wrote that "the superstitious are often melancholic, and the melancholic almost always superstitious." As will be noted later, obsessions are common in depressive states and vice versa.

Epidemiology

Obsessive-compulsive disorder was once considered rare, but studies in the mid-1980s suggested that the disorder may affect 2% of the general population, making it one of the more common forms of serious psychopathology (55, 82, 87). Comparison of prevalence rates of OCD in seven countries found the rates to be remarkably consistent, falling in the 1%–2% range (80). Only a small proportion of OCD patients visit psychiatrists. Less than 5% of psychiatric inpatients and outpatients receive the diagnosis. According to some studies, OCD occurs more frequently in women than in men (11, 80). When compared with all other psychiatric patients, those with OCD reportedly differ in the following ways: (1) they belong to higher social classes, (2) they make higher scores on intelligence tests, and (3) they have a higher educational level (44, 61, 82, 89).

Clinical Picture

When medical attention is finally sought for OCD (often years after the illness began), it may be because of depression, acute anxiety, exacerbation of obsessions, or social incapacity resulting from any of these conditions (14, 60, 78) (Table 6.1). The onset of symptoms often seems associated with a life

TABLE 6.1 Diagnostic Criteria for Obsessive-Compulsive Disorder

A. Either obsessions or compulsions:

Obsessions as defined by:

    (1) Recurrent and persistent thoughts, impulses, or images that are experienced, at some time during the disturbance, as intrusive and inappropriate and that cause marked anxiety or distress

    (2) The thoughts, impulses, or images are not simply excessive worries about real-life problems.

    (3) The person attempts to ignore or suppress such thoughts, impulses, or images, or to neutralize them with some other thought or action.

    (4) The person recognizes that the obsessional thoughts, impulses, or images are a product of his or her own mind (not imposed from without as in thought insertion).

Compulsions as defined by:

    (1) Repetitive behaviors (e.g., hand washing, ordering, checking) or mental acts (e.g., praying, counting, repeating words silently) that the person feels driven to perform in response to an obsession, or according to rules that must be applied rigidly

    (2) The behaviors or mental acts are aimed at preventing or reducing distress or preventing some dreaded event or situation; however, these behaviors or mental acts either are not connected in a realistic way with what they are designed to neutralize or prevent or are clearly excessive.

B. At some point during the course of the disorder, the person has recognized that the obsessions or compulsions are excessive or unreasonable.
Note: This does not apply to children.

C. The obsessions or compulsions cause marked distress, are time consuming (take more than 1 hour a day), or significantly interfere with the person's normal routine, occupational (or academic) functioning, or usual social activities or relationships.

D. If another psychiatric disorder is present, the content of the obsessions or compulsions is not restricted to it (e.g., preoccupation with food in the presence of an eating disorder; hair pulling in the presence of trichotillomania; concern with appearance in the presence of body dysmorphic disorder; preoccupation with drugs in the presence of a substance use disorder; preoccupation with having a serious illness in the presence of hypochondriasis; preoccupation with sexual urges or fantasies in the presence of a paraphilia; or guilty ruminations in the presence of major depressive disorder).

E. The disturbance is not due to the direct physiological effects of a substance (e.g., a drug of abuse, a medication) or a general medical condition.

Adapted from diagnostic criteria in the *DSM-IV-TR* (104).

event: the death of a relative, a sexual conflict, overwork, or pregnancy (44, 61). Just as often, however, no precipitating factors can be identified.

Common presenting complaints are the obsessional fears of contamination or injuring oneself or another person, often a child or close relative. Fearful of losing control, these patients may develop avoidances or rituals that lead in turn to social incapacity. They may refuse to leave the house and may avoid sharp objects or wash repeatedly.

On reflection, they may identify the obsessional idea as illogical, but not always. Sometimes the ideas are not, strictly speaking, illogical (e.g., germs do produce disease) and sometimes, even when obviously absurd, the ideas are not viewed as such. What distinguishes an obsession from a delusion is not so much insight (recognizing the idea's absurdity) as the person's struggle against the obsessional experience itself. Individuals with the disorder strive to free themselves from the obsession but cannot and feel increasingly uncomfortable until the idea temporarily runs its course or the compulsive act has been completed (60).

The frequency of obsessional symptoms in patients with OCD has been studied systematically by three groups, and their results indicate that the illness may assume one or more of the following forms (2, 26, 56):

Obsessional ideas: Thoughts that repetitively intrude into consciousness (words, phrases, rhymes) and interfere with the normal train of thought, causing distress to the person. Often the thoughts are obscene, blasphemous, or nonsensical.

Obsessional images: Vividly imagined scenes, often of a violent, sexual, or disgusting nature (images of a child being killed, cars colliding, excrement, parents having sexual intercourse) that repeatedly come to mind.

Obsessional convictions: Notions that are often based on the magical formula of thought equals act: "Thinking ill of my son will cause him to die." Unlike delusions, obsessional beliefs are characterized by ambivalence: The person believes and simultaneously does not believe. As Jaspers expressed it, there is a "constant going on between a consciousness of validity and non-validity. Both push this way and that, but neither can gain the upper hand" (51).

Obsessional rumination: Prolonged, inconclusive thinking about a subject to the exclusion of other interests. The subject is often religion or metaphysics—why and wherefore questions that are as unanswerable, as they are endlessly ponderable. Indecisiveness in ordinary matters is very common: "Which necktie should I wear?" Doubt may lead to extremes in caution, both irksome and irresistible. "Did I turn off the gas?" "Lock the door?" "Write the correct address?" The individual checks and rechecks, stopping only when exhausted or on checking a predetermined "magical" number of times. Several studies suggest that obsessional doubts—*manie du doute*—may well be the most prominent feature in obsessive-compulsive illness (2, 26, 90). As with other obsessions, ruminations are resisted. The person tries to turn his or her attention elsewhere, but cannot; often the more he or she tries, the more intrusive and distressing the thoughts become.

Obsessional impulses: Typically relates to self-injury (leaping from a window); injury to others (smothering an infant); or embarrassing behavior (shouting obscenities in church).

Obsessional fears: Often of dirt, disease, contamination; of potential weapons (razors, scissors); of being in specific situations or performing particular acts.

Obsessional rituals (compulsions): Repetitive, stereotyped acts of counting, touching, arranging objects, moving, washing, tasting, looking in specific ways. Compulsions may be inseparable from obsessions. About one-quarter of patients display no compulsions (2).

Counting rituals are especially common. The person feels compelled to count letters or words or the squares in a tile floor or to perform arithmetical operations. Certain numbers, or their multiples, may have special significance (the person "must" lay down her pencil three times or step on every fifth sidewalk crack). Other rituals concern the performance of excretory functions and such everyday acts as preparing to go to bed. Also common are rituals involving extremes of cleanliness (handwashing compulsions, relentless emptying of wastebaskets) and complicated routines assuring orderliness and punctuality. Women apparently have a higher prevalence of contamination phobia and of compulsive cleaning behavior than do men (26).

According to a study of patients with OCD (14), four kinds of rituals occur most frequently: counting, checking, cleaning, and avoidance rituals. Each occurred in half of the patients. Avoidance rituals were similar to those seen in phobic disorders (see section "Differential Diagnosis"). An example can be seen in a patient who avoided anything colored brown. Her inability to approach brown objects greatly limited her activities.

Other less common rituals include slowing, striving for completeness, and extreme meticulousness. With slowing, such simple tasks as buttoning a shirt or tying a shoelace might take up to 15 minutes. Striving for completeness may be seen in dressing also. Asked why he spends so much time with a single button, the patient might reply that he was trying to prove to himself that he had "buttoned the button properly."

A common form of pathological meticulousness is a concern that objects be arranged in a special way. Pencils, for example, may have to be arranged so that the points are directed away from the person. Students may spend so much time arranging pencils, pens, erasers, and so on that they cannot do their work.

Rituals, ridiculous as they may seem to the person, are accompanied by a profound dread and apprehension that assures their performance because they alone give relief. "I'll explode if I don't do it," a patient may say. Occasionally patients believe that failure to perform a given ritual will result in harm to themselves or others; often the ritual is as inexplicable to patients as it is to observers.

Obsessional symptoms often are accompanied by a dysphoric mood. The patient may be irritable, tense, or depressed. This may lead to an erroneous diagnosis of a mood disorder because the mood element at the time of examination may overshadow the obsessional content.

Obsessional symptoms rarely occur singly (57). As with most psychiatric illnesses, obsessional disorder presents a cluster of symptoms that, individually, are variable and inconstant over time but as a group maintain characteristics unique to the illness. Thus, a patient may now have one set of obsessional impulses, fears, and rituals and later another set, but the symptoms remain predominantly obsessional.

R. J. obsessed so much about eating contaminated food that he was 30 pounds underweight. He worried so much that he might gun the accelerator and run people over at an intersection that he always put the car in park. He was so compulsive that he copied serial numbers off dollar bills and dressed and undressed so many times in the morning that it was noon before he was ready to go to work as a school custodian.

Occasionally, however, a single obsession dominates the clinical picture:

A thirty-five-year-old banker, P. T. had an obsession concerning the length of his trousers. He would buy a pair of trousers but fail to convince himself that they were the correct length. He would then go back to the tailor repeatedly to have them adjusted—returning as many as a dozen times and stopping only when his embarrassment became acute as the tailor became more frustrated. Then he would adjust the length himself. He would stand endlessly before mirrors, trying to decide whether the length was correct. Whenever he crossed his leg and the pant was hiked up, showing a part of his sock, he worried that there was too much sock showing or too little. Again he would alter the pants.

The obsession made him miserable. He could not concentrate on his work. He repeatedly asked fellow employees whether they thought his pants were too long or too short and was convinced that they thought he was crazy (which perhaps they did). He had legitimate fears of losing his position at the bank. He started staying home more and more, hating himself for succumbing to what he recognized was a foolish fear. But he could not stop the fear. It came to occupy most of his waking hours as he altered between studying the pant leg to see if it should be a millimeter shorter or longer and castigating himself for being a weak and feckless fellow in worrying about such matters.

Although P. T. had mild-to-moderate symptoms of depression, the obsession dominated his clinical picture. It had begun in his early twenties and had persisted more or less intensely since then. He had no other obsessions. In previous times the symptom would have been called a monomania.

Biological Findings

While neuroimaging studies, including positron emission tomography (PET) and magnetic resonance imaging (MRI), have been undertaken, they have not demonstrated convergence of findings to allow early causal inference.

Natural History

The onset of obsessive-compulsive illness is usually before age 25 (13). The median age of onset in one study (82) was 23, and clear-cut obsessional symptoms often develop by age 15. The illness may begin as early as age 6. Fewer than 15% of cases begin after age 35 (29, 44, 57, 71).

Though the mean age of onset of symptoms is roughly 20 in both sexes, the first psychiatric contact is made on the average about 7 years later. If hospitalized, most patients are in their 30s by the time they enter a hospital, and hospitalization for the first time after age 40 is rare (33).

The mode of onset may be acute or insidious (57). The course of the disorder may be unremitting (with or without social incapacity), episodic, or characterized by incomplete remissions that permit normal social functioning.

In one outpatient study, the majority of patients had episodic courses with exacerbations that usually lasted less than a year (78). Most investigators who study patients requiring hospitalization, however, have found the course to be steady, with exacerbations often attributed to fatigue or medical illness and with a tendency for the severity of the illness to wane gradually over many years (44, 61).

Patients with mild obsessional symptoms requiring only outpatient therapy appear to have a rather good prognosis; as many as 60%–80% are asymptomatic or improved 1–5 years after diagnosis (51, 78). The prognosis is not as good for hospitalized patients, who comprise a more severely ill group. One-third or fewer are improved symptomatically on reexamination several years after discharge; two-thirds or more, however, are functioning as well socially as before hospitalization (44, 57). Between 5%–10% of clear-cut cases of OCD do have a course marked by progressive social incapacity (88). Favorable prognosis is reported to be associated with three factors: *(1)* mild or atypical symptoms, including predominance of phobic-ruminative ideas and absence of compulsions (44, 57); *(2)* short duration of symptoms before treatment is begun (78); and *(3)* good premorbid personality without childhood symptoms or abnormal personality traits (57, 58). The specific content of obsessions is not believed to have prognostic significance (Table 6.2).

TABLE 6.2 Follow-up Studies of Obsessive-Compulsive Disorder

Sample Characteristics				Length of Follow-up (to Nearest Year)	Condition on Follow-up (%)		
Author	Place	Pt. Source	N*		Asymp- tomatic	Improved	Unimproved
Balslev- Olesen and Geert-Jorgensen (9)	Denmark	I, O	52	0–8	6	58	37
Coryell (20)	U.S.	I	36	1–32	22	57	22
Grimshaw (36)	England	O	97	1–14	40	24	35
Hastings (39)	U.S.	I	23	6–12	13	40	47
Ingram (44)	England	I	46	1–11	9	30	61
Kringlen (57)	Norway	I	85	13–20	4	45	45
Langfeldt (58)	Norway	I	27	1–11	26	41	33
Lewis (60)	England	I, O	50	>5	32	34	34
Lo (61)	Hong Kong	I, O	87	1–14	20	36	44
Luff and Garrod (62)	England	O	49	3	39	27	34
Pollitt (78)	England	I, O	66	0–15	24	48	28
Rennie (86)	U.S.	I	47	20	36	38	26
Rüdin (89)	Germany	I, O	130	1–16	12	26	61

*Excluded are lobotomized cases and patients dead on follow-up. The sex ratio differs from study to study but approaches unity when all studies are combined.

I, inpatient; O, outpatient.

Adapted from Goodwin et al. (33).

Complications

Depression—often indistinguishable symptomatically from major depression—is probably the most common complication of obsessional disorder. Failure to marry also may be a complication of OCD. Additionally, those who marry appear to be more likely than married people in the general population to experience substantial marital maladjustment (18, 66). Further, fertility rates appear to be reduced among people with OCD (72). Despite the frequency with which suicide may figure in obsessional thinking (36, 44), completed suicide is rare in these patients, less than 1%.

Patients with OCD sometimes fear they will injure someone by an impulsive act. They fear they will lose control in some manner and embarrass themselves. They worry about becoming addicted to drugs prescribed by their physician. These fears are generally unwarranted (20). There is little evidence that OCD predisposes to homicide, criminal behavior, alcoholism, or drug addiction (44, 57).

Finally, people with OCD may fear they will "lose" their minds, become totally disabled, or need chronic hospitalization. None of these events is a common complication of OCD. If schizophrenia is clearly ruled out at the beginning, schizophrenia probably develops in these individuals no more often than in anyone else. Patients with OCD infrequently become totally disabled, and they usually do not require long-term hospitalization (36, 44, 78).

Family History

Initial family studies of OCD were limited by substantial methodological difficulties, but they suggested a greater frequency of obsessional illness in families of OCD patients than in families of other patients or the general population (13, 46). More recent studies (70, 75) have strongly supported the familial nature of OCD. There is also substantial evidence of a link to Tourette syndrome (53, 59, 76). About half of people with Tourette syndrome also have obsessive-compulsive symptoms. In one study, relatives of patients with Tourette syndrome had an increased rate of OCD, regardless of whether the Tourette probands had OCD symptoms. Surprisingly, no increase in other anxiety disorders was found among the family members of Tourette patients (76). The association between OCD and Tourette syndrome is firmly established, but family studies of the disorders yield conflicting results.

Studies of twins with obsessional illness indicate that monozygotic twins are more concordant for OCD than dizygotic twins (45, 82). About 80%–90% of monozygotic twins are concordant for OCD versus a concordance rate in dizygotic twins of no more than 50% and probably much lower. This does not prove the existence of genetic factors in obsessional illness; all of the twin pairs were raised together and identical twins may emulate each other more than fraternal twins. However, in instances where twins have little contact, environmental explanations seem implausible, as illustrated by the following case histories adapted from a published report (67).

The "W" twins. Jean, a housewife, developed her symptoms at age 24 when she acquired a fear of contamination by dirt with severe washing and cleansing rituals. At the time of her referral for hospitalization 3 years later she was washing her hands between 60 and 80 times per day, spending 12 hours a day cleaning and disinfecting her house, and using up to 20 quarts of liquid disinfectant a week. Her daughter, aged 2.5 years, was not toilet trained and was restricted to one room of the house in order to avoid spread of contamination, and her husband had been obliged to give up sports for fear that his soiled sports clothes would introduce dirt to their home. When she was admitted to the hospital, the skin on her hands was roughened, red, cracked, and bleeding.

Jill, the co-twin, a social worker, developed her symptoms at age 22 when she and Jean were leading separate lives and had little contact with each other. Her traits of neatness and cleanliness became more pronounced, and she developed rituals concerned with washing up the dishes and utensils, which had to be started immediately when a meal was finished; any delay resulted in severe anxiety. The washing of the dishes and utensils had to proceed in a specific order and failure to comply with the routine, or an attempt by others to relieve her of her task, provoked great discomfort. She attempted to resist carrying out her rituals, which she considered silly and unnecessary, but the time spent on them increased and interfered with her social life.

Their father, a retired clerk, was fastidiously neat and orderly in his habits, but neither he nor other family members had received psychiatric treatment. Their early development and childhood were unremarkable, and at school both did well academically. They attended separate universities. Both were normally outgoing and sociable and both had personality traits of orderliness, determination, and conscientiousness. Neither had suffered any previous illness and they only learned of their similar obsessional problems after Jean began treatment.

The "K" twins. Linda, a secretary, began having obsessional thoughts at age 25 when she felt envious of a roommate who had formed a close relationship with a man. Aware of her envy and associated guilt, she began to think of imaginary pleasant scenes of herself with her friend, but within a few weeks these thoughts became recurrent, intrusive, difficult to resist, and were no longer associated with relief of unpleasant feelings. Obsessional thoughts troubled her to a varying degree for several years, with exacerbations during times of stress or unhappiness. Often she would have to repeat a conversation in her mind and, if interrupted before it was completed, she felt bound to repeat the whole conversation again. Sometimes she was compelled to touch an object to signify completion of an obsessional thought and this sometimes had a magical aspect; for example, if the object was a clock, the numbers indicating the time became her "lucky numbers" for the rest of the day.

Ann, the co-twin, an actress, also developed obsessional thoughts in her mid-20s. She was not in regular contact with Linda at this time and only years later learned of her similar difficulties. Ann also used "good thoughts" to counter anxiety, which was usually caused by parental disapproval of her career. The thoughts soon developed an obsessional quality and were associated with compulsive behavior. For example, if a "bad thought" occurred to her while speaking on the telephone, after the call ended she felt compelled to repeat the conversation and create "good thoughts." If she passed a shop window and could not recall its contents, she would have to go back and check them. She also spent hours arranging clothing in her wardrobe according to the color or type of garment. Although she considered her obsessions to be irrational, any attempts to resist them gave rise to the fears of impending disaster.

The father was an accountant described as being "compulsively neat." Their mother had older twin sisters who both had a lifelong phobia of birds.

Twin and family studies implicate a genetic etiology for OCD (3, 69, 91). Few details of the genetic nature of this disorder have been elucidated (73), and no specific genes for OCD have been identified (91). Multiple new molecular genetic methodologies, including segregation analysis, linkage analyses, and association studies, are currently being applied in attempts to map the heritability of OCD (3, 15, 25, 34, 38, 91, 103).

Differential Diagnosis

Obsessions occur in children, in healthy adults, and in patients with a variety of psychiatric and medical illnesses. The rituals and superstitions of children—avoidance of sidewalk cracks, insistence on a given routine, carrying of amulets and charms—may resemble the compulsive acts of OCD, but with a difference:

Children usually do not complain about these acts, which seem natural to them and produce little distress. Further, obsessional children do not view the behavior as unreasonable.

Only a small proportion of children manifesting obsessional behavior can be classified by usual standards as having obsessional disorder. It is not known whether children who are exceptionally ritualistic and superstitious have a greater risk of developing OCD than their less-obsessional peers.

Many adults with OCD give a history of obsessional symptoms in childhood (33, 61, 89), but the commonness of such symptoms and the influence of retrospective distortion make such data hard to interpret. Adults with OCD commonly cite phobias and rituals as childhood symptoms (44, 57, 61). They rarely give a history of stealing, truancy, or tantrums in childhood (57, 61).

Obsessional personality (currently termed "obsessive-compulsive personality disorder" in DSM-IV-TR) is more a description than a diagnosis. No investigator has followed a group with clearly defined obsessional personalities over time to determine their fate; hence, this characteristic has no predictive value and is not in this sense a diagnosis. The individual with an obsessional personality is punctual, orderly, scrupulous, meticulous, and dependable. He is also rigid, stubborn, pedantic, and something of a bore. He has trouble making up his mind, but once made up, is single-minded and obstinate (67).

Many individuals with obsessional disorder have obsessional personalities antedating the illness (57, 78, 89), although one study (13) found no relationship between OCD and obsessional personality. The proportion of obsessional personalities who develop OCD, depression, or other psychiatric illness is not known.

Phobias are commonly associated with OCD, and patients with OCD often have anxiety symptoms. Obsessional phobias have a compulsive quality and are almost always accompanied by rituals as well as other obsessional phenomena (57). The phobias of phobic disorders, on the other hand, are characterized primarily by simple avoidance of the anxiety-provoking object or situation.

Obsessions and depression occur together so commonly that discriminating symptom from illness may be difficult. The difficulty is compounded by the fact that people with OCD may develop depressive symptoms as florid as those seen in major depression or bipolar illness. During the depression the obsessional symptoms may remain unchanged, worsen, or disappear. Similarly, after the depression lifts, the obsessions may be worse, better, or unchanged (the last being the most common outcome) (31).

Episodes of depression, in a substantial number of cases, are accompanied by obsessions (31). These are usually ruminative in nature, characterized by guilt and self-deprecation, and mild by comparison with the depressed mood.

In more atypical depressions, however, obsessions may dominate the picture. According to one study, one-third of patients with major depression have obsessional personality traits premorbidly and during remissions (60). Obsessional traits apparently precede depression as often as they precede OCD (60).

Obsessive-compulsive disorder in some instances may be as cyclical as bipolar disorder, with alternating remissions and exacerbations having no apparent relation to life events (44, 61, 78). The episodicity may suggest a mood disorder. Some clinicians treat patients with cyclical obsessions as if they had depressive illness, that is, with antidepressant drugs or electrotherapy.

In distinguishing between OCD and major depression, the following points may be helpful: Compared with patients with major depression and bipolar disorder who have obsessional symptoms, OCD patients who develop a depression do so at an earlier age, have more depressive episodes in their history, exhibit obsessional symptoms episodically during each depression, have a lower rate of attempted suicide, and lack a history of mania (31).

Family history is of diagnostic value when it includes clear-cut depressive episodes, mania, suicide, or alcoholism, which are found more regularly in the families of patients with major depression than in the families of patients with any other illness (102).

Mistaking OCD for schizophrenia is not unusual, especially in the early stages of the illness. Error may arise from difficulty in distinguishing obsessions from delusions and from equating bizarreness or disablement with schizophrenia. Early onset and insidious development are common in both illnesses.

Schizophrenia is characterized by delusions, hallucinations, and *formal* thought disorder (form referring to the flow and connections of thought). Obsessive-compulsive disorder is primarily a disorder of thought *content*. The speech of OCD patients is understandable; only their ideas are weird. The fact that people with OCD recognize their ideas are weird is one of the chief distinctions between OCD and schizophrenia. According to one study, obsessions occur in schizophrenia in about 3% of cases, usually early in the course and almost always in the paranoid type (94). When obsessions and schizophrenia symptoms occur together, schizophrenia is usually the appropriate diagnosis.

Obsessions have been observed in the following medical conditions: encephalitis lethargia, especially during oculogyric crises; early stages of arteriosclerotic dementia; post-encephalitic states; hearing loss with tinnitus; and hypothyroidism (33). Each of these conditions may be accompanied by the sense that one's mind is working independently, that it is not an integrated part of oneself (60), and by repetitive behavior resembling compulsions.

However, the "forced thinking" and "organic orderliness" (32) occasionally observed in brain-damaged patients are said to be less well organized than those that occur in OCD, and they also lack the sense of internal compulsion that distinguishes OCD.

The hallmarks of brain syndromes—confusion, disorientation, memory loss—are not seen in OCD. Their presence makes the diagnosis comparatively simple. Past history; neurological examination; blood, urine, and spinal fluid studies; plus special imaging techniques help establish the specific cause.

Clinical Management

The data on OCD justify a certain measure of optimism about its natural course. Spontaneous improvement often occurs, and the patient can be informed of this. She can be reassured that her impulses to commit injury or socially embarrassing acts almost certainly will not be carried out and that she will not—as she often fears—lose her mind. If she needs to be hospitalized, she can be assured that the hospitalization is unlikely to be a long one.

Obsessive-compulsive disorder is rarely helped by psychotherapy alone. "Insight" therapy may even be contraindicated. "A searching, interpretive, in-depth approach," wrote one therapist, "in many instances facilitates an introspective obsessive stance" (64). Pessimism about psychotherapy for OCD is reflected by the scarcity of quality research testing its efficacy. A recent literature review conducted by Black (12) found only four methodologically adequate studies comparing monotherapy involving only psychotherapy or pharmacotherapy alone with combined treatment involving both psychotherapy and pharmacotherapy. Two studies comparing combined fluoxetine and exposure therapy to be superior to exposure therapy alone found combined fluoxetine and psychotherapy was superior to psychotherapy alone, but only in the short term (22, 41). A third study, however, showed no benefit to adding fluoxetine to exposure therapy or cognitive therapy for OCD (101). A fourth study found that both exposure therapy and clomipramine were effective for OCD; however, there was no added benefit of combining clomipramine with exposure therapy compared to exposure therapy alone, and adding exposure therapy to clomipramine was superior to clomipramine alone (28). Black concluded from his review that available evidence is limited for the use of combined treatments for OCD.

Behavior therapy derives from learning theory. According to learning theory, obsessional thoughts are conditioned responses to anxiety-provoking stimuli. Compulsions are established when the individual discovers that the compulsive act reduces the anxiety attendant on obsessional thought. The reduction in anxiety reinforces the compulsive act.

The techniques of behavior therapy are manifold, but their application to OCD usually involves a single principle: The patient must be exposed to the fear-inducing stimulus. After repeated exposure and refraining from the compulsion it presents, the fear disappears because, at bottom, it is unfounded. As fear subsides, so do the obsessions and compulsions. The various techniques for achieving this goal bear such names as desensitization, implosion, paradoxical intention, operant shaping, and cognitive rehearsal (7, 16, 19, 27, 29, 54).

Many studies indicate that behavior therapy produces relief from compulsive rituals in many patients; the relief is maintained for at least 2–3 years following treatment (65, 93). Behavior therapy may take up to 30 sessions in the therapist's office plus self-exposure homework, sometimes with relatives cooperating as exposure co-therapists. Some patients are too apprehensive to submit to such an ordeal. Others are too depressed. Frequently a cognitive component is added to challenge the false beliefs, thereby reducing relapse by supporting the patient.

Many medications have been used in the treatment of obsessional disorder. They include phenothiazines, monoamine oxidase inhibitors (MAOIs), lysergic acid diethylamide (LSD), L-tryptophan, and tricyclic antidepressants (48). With the exception of clomipramine, a tricyclic antidepressant, the only evidence for efficacy of the above agents has come from single case reports or open trials. Double-blind, placebo-controlled studies (5, 6, 47, 64, 97) of clomipramine have repeatedly demonstrated the antiobsessional effects from this drug.

Until the late 1980s, clomipramine was clearly the drug that showed the most promise as a specific antiobsessional agent. There has been much speculation about its mode of action. Clomipramine inhibits serotonin reuptake and thus potentiates serotonergic activity, the latter believed to have a mood-altering effect (24, 37, 48, 50, 95). Tryptophan, the amino acid precursor of serotonin, is reported to relieve obsessional symptoms (4), supporting the idea that serotonin in some way is related to obsessional thinking. (Tryptophan has been withdrawn from the market.)

Following the introduction of selective serotonin-reuptake inhibitors (SSRIs), the role of serotonin and OCD has received considerable attention. Multiple selective SSRIs, fluoxetine (Prozac), fluvoxamine (Luvox), sertraline (Zoloft), paroxetine (Paxil), and citalopram (Celexa), have been studied for treatment of OCD. Review of the SSRI treatment studies reveals that 40%–70% of OCD patients have a significant response to their first SSRI treatment (1, 77, 81). Noteworthy also are the limited side effect profiles and general acceptance of the selective SSRIs compared with the anticholinergic, antihistaminic, and anti-alpha-1-adrenergic effects of clomipramine. The mechanism of action for these medications is unclear. Studies of blood serotonin concentration in OCD patients have produced mixed results, one (37) showing that OCD patients had *higher* pretreatment blood levels of serotonin than controls. This contradicts the idea that the mechanism of action of SSRIs is to *increase* serotonin levels. Imaging studies suggest that SSRIs may normalize cerebral metabolism, said to be subnormal in OCD (10, 95). Although OCD patients respond to SSRIs, the improvement usually does not include complete remission (17, 81). Response includes reduction in the frequency of symptoms and an increase in the quality of their lives. Discontinuation of the medication can result in relapse (17, 71, 74, 85).

Monoamine oxidase inhibitors (MAOIs) are available in the United States, and one study (100), as well as single case reports with phenelzine sulfate (49) and tranylcypromine sulfate, (52) described marked improvement in obsessional patients. Clorgyline, in a double-blind comparison with clomipramine, proved ineffective (47). In other anxiety disorders such as phobic states, MAOIs have been found to be effective (99), so these drugs still show promise.

Benzodiazepines relieve anxiety accompanying obsessions, and antidepressants relieve depression seen with the disorder. Except for clomipramine and the SSRIs, neither group seems to reduce the obsessional thinking. Augmenting treatment response to SSRIs has been tried because of incomplete response. Rauch and colleagues (83, 84) have suggested use of low-dose dopamine antagonists. A recent meta-analysis of 10 randomized controlled trials concluded that the literature supports the use of antipsychotic drugs as an augmentation strategy for treatment-resistant OCD, with a caveat that more and larger trials are needed (92).

In summary, the literature indicates that in vivo exposure is the most effective treatment for compulsive rituals and that several antidepressants (with or without augmentation) are helpful for obsessional ideation/compulsions. Behavior therapy has one distinct advantage over medications: The improvement persists after the treatment ends. Studies agree that clomipramine and the SSRIs are effective only while the medication is being taken.

Electroconvulsive therapy (ECT) has been tried in OCD with generally poor outcomes. However, two studies have reported somewhat favorable results. One study (89) suggested ECT is less effective for depression associated with OCD than for primary depression. In the series, half the OCD patients receiving ECT improved and half did not. The second study (63) reported cautious positive findings in the treatment of OCD with (and without) depression.

Other brain stimulation techniques are being evaluated for treatment of refractory OCD, such as vagal nerve stimulation, transcranial magnetic stimulation, and deep brain stimulation (23, 35, 43, 79). Early findings have been mixed. Small sample sizes and difficulties in methodological design have limited available data addressing the effectiveness of these techniques, which are not approved for treatment of OCD by the Food and Drug Administration (23).

Multiple follow-up studies (8, 21, 40, 57, 98) indicate that various neurosurgical procedures (anterior cingulotomy, limbic leucotomy, anterior capsulotomy, or subcaudate tractotomy) produce symptomatic improvement in OCD superior to that which occurs spontaneously. The more "typical" the obsessive-compulsive illness, one investigator found, the more likely this was true (57). For a small minority of patients, therefore, neurosurgery may warrant consideration. Before undertaking such irreversible treatment, evaluation by two or more psychiatrists is highly desirable. There is also general agreement that, if used at all, surgical intervention should be reserved for those severely ill OCD patients with classical symptoms (especially rituals) who fail to respond to all other reasonable treatments and are totally disabled by their illness.

REFERENCES

1. Jenike, M. A., Baer, L., Minichiello, W. E. (eds.). *Obsessive-Compulsive Disorders: Practical Management*, 3rd edition. St. Louis: Mosby, 1998.

2. Akhtar, S., Wig, N. N., Varma, V. K., Pershad, D., and Verma, S. K. A phenomenological analysis of symptoms in obsessive-compulsive neurosis. Br. J. Psychiat., 127:342–348, 1975.

3. Alsobrook II, J. P., Leckman, J. F., Goodman, W. K., Rasmussen, S. A., and Pauls, D. L. Segregation analysis of obsessive-compulsive disorder using symptom-based factor scores. Am. J. Med. Genet., 88:669–675, 1999.

4. Ananth, J. Clomipramine in obsessive-compulsive disorder: a review. Psychosomat., 24:723–727, 1983.

5. Ananth, J. Clomipramine: an antiobsessive drug. Can. J. Psychiat., 31:253–258, 1986.

6. Ananth, J., Pecknold, J. C., Van Den Steen, M., and Engelsmann, F. Double-blind comparative study of clomipramine and amitriptyline in obsessive neurosis. Prog. Neuropsychopharmacol., 5:257–262, 1981.

7. Baer, L. Behavior therapy for obsessive compulsive disorder in the office-based practice. J. Clin. Psychiat., 54 *Suppl* 15, 30, 1993.

8. Baer, L., Rauch, S. L., Ballantine, Jr. T., Martuza, R., Cosgrove, R., Cassem, E., Giriunas, I., Manzo, P. A., Dimino, C., and Jenike, M. A. Cingulotomy for intractable obsessive-compulsive disorder. Arch. Gen. Psychiat., 52:384–394, 1995.

9. Balslev-Olesen, T., and Geert-Jorgensen, E. The prognosis of obsessive-compulsive neurosis. Acta Psychiat. Scand., 34:232–241, 1959.

10. Baxter Jr, L. R., Schwartz, J. M., Bergman, K. S., Szuba, M. P., Guze, B. H., Mazziotta, J. C., Alazraki, A., Selin, C. E., Ferng, H.-K., Munford, P., and Phelps, M. E. Caudate glucose metabolic rate changes with both drug and behavior therapy for obsessive-compulsive disorder. Arch. Gen. Psychiat., 49:681–689, 1992.

11. Bebbington, P. E. Epidemiology of obsessive-compulsive disorder. Br. J. Psychiat., 173:2–6, 1998.

12. Black, D. W. Efficacy of combined pharmacotherapy and psychotherapy versus monotherapy in the treatment of anxiety disorders. CNS Spectr., 11:29–33, 2006.

13. Black, D. W., Noyes Jr, R., Pfohl, B., Goldstein, R. B., and Blum, N. Personality disorder in obsessive-compulsive volunteers, well comparison subjects, and their first-degree relatives. Am. J. Psychiat., 150:1226–1232, 1993.

14. Burke, K. C., Burke Jr, J. D., Regier, D. A., and Rae, D. S. Age at onset of selected mental disorders in five community populations. Arch. Gen. Psychiat., 47:511–518, 1990.

15. Camarena, B., Aguilar, A., Loyzaga, C., and Nicolini, H. A family-based association study of the 5-HT-1Dbeta receptor gene in obsessive-compulsive disorder. Int. J. Neuropsychopharmacol., 7:49–53, 2004.

16. Carney, R. M. Behavior therapy and the anxiety disorders: some conceptual and methodological issues. Psychiat. Dev., 3:65–81, 1985.

17. Catapano, F., Perris, F., Masella, M., Rossano, F., Cigliano, M., Magliano, L., and Maj, M. Obsessive-compulsive disorder: a 3-year prospective follow-up study of patients treated with serotonin reuptake inhibitors OCD follow-up study. J. Psychiat. Res., 40:502–510, 2006.

18. Cillicilli, A. S., Telcioglu, M., Askin, R., Kaya, N., Bodur, S., and Kucur, R. Twelve-month prevalence of obsessive-compulsive disorder in Konya, Turkey. Compr. Psychiat., 45:367–374, 2004.

19. Cobb, J. Behaviour therapy in phobic and obsessional disorders. Psychiat. Dev., 1:361–365, 1983.

20. Coryell, W. Obsessive-compulsive disorder and primary unipolar depression: comparisons of background, family history, course, and mortality. J. Nerv. Ment. Dis., 169:220–224, 1981.

21. Cosgrove, G. R., and Rauch, S. L. Psychosurgery. Neurosurg. Clin. N. Am., 6:167–176, 1995.

22. Cottraux, J., Mollard, E., Bouvard, M., Marks, I., Sluys, M., Nury, A. M., Douge, R., and Cialdella, P. A controlled study of fluvoxamine and exposure in obsessive-compulsive disorder. Int. Clin. Psychopharmacol., 5:17–30, 1990.

23. Dell'Osso, B., Altamura, A. C., Allen, A., and Hollander, E. Brain stimulation techniques in the treatment of obsessive-compulsive disorder: current and future directions. CNS Spectr., 10:966–79, 983, 2005.

24. DeVeaugh-Geiss, J., Katz, R., Landau, P., Goodman, W., and Rasmussen, S. Clinical predictors of treatment response in obsessive compulsive disorder: exploratory analyses from multicenter trials of clomipramine. Psychopharmacol. Bull., 26:54–59, 1990.

25. Dickel, D. E., Veenstra-VanderWeele, J., Bivens, N. C., Wu, X., Fischer, D. J., Etten-Lee, M., Himle, J. A., Leventhal, B. L., Cook, E. H., Jr., and Hanna, G. L. Association studies of serotonin system candidate genes in early-onset obsessive-compulsive disorder. Biol. Psychiat., 61:322–329, 2007.

26. Dowson, J. The phenomenology of severe obsessive-compulsive neurosis. Br. J. Psychiat., 131:75–78, 1977.

27. Fals-Stewart, W., Marks, A. P., and Schafer, J. A comparison of behavioral group therapy and individual behavior therapy in treating obsessive-compulsive disorder. J. Nerv. Ment. Dis., 181:189–193, 1993.

28. Foa, E. B., Liebowitz, M. R., Kozak, M. J., Davies, S., Campeas, R., Franklin, M. E., Huppert, J. D., Kjernisted, K., Rowan, V., Schmidt, A. B., Simpson, H. B., and Tu, X. Randomized, placebo-controlled trial of exposure and ritual prevention, clomipramine, and their combination in the treatment of obsessive-compulsive disorder. Am. J. Psychiat., 162:151–161, 2005.

29. Foa, E. B., Steketee, G. S., and Ozarow, B. J. Behavior therapy with obsessive-compulsives: from theory to treatment. In *Obsessive-Compulsive Disorders: Psychological and Pharmacological Treatments*, Mavissakalian, M. (ed.). New York: Plenum, pp. 49–129, 1985.

30. Freud, S. Notes upon a case of obsessional neurosis. In *Standard Edition of the Complete Psychological Works of Sigmund Freud, vol. 10, 153*. London: Hogarth Press, 1955.

31. Gittelson, N. L. The phenomenology of obsessions in depressive psychosis. Br. J. Psychiat., 112:261–264, 1966.

32. Goldstein, K. *After Effects of Brain Injuries in War. Their Evaluation and Treatment.* New York: Grune & Stratton, 1942.

33. Goodwin, D. W., Guze, S. B., and Robins, E. Follow-up studies in obsessional neurosis. Arch. Gen. Psychiat., 20:182–187, 1969.

34. Grados, M. A., Walkup, J., and Walford, S. Genetics of obsessive-compulsive disorders: new findings and challenges. Brain Dev., 25 Suppl 1:S55–S61, 2003.

35. Greenberg, B. D., Malone, D. A., Friehs, G. M., Rezai, A. R., Kubu, C. S., Malloy, P. F., Salloway, S. P., Okun, M. S., Goodman, W. K., and Rasmussen, S. A. Three-year outcomes in deep brain stimulation for highly resistant obsessive-compulsive disorder. Neuropsychopharmacol., 31:2384–2393, 2006.

36. Grimshaw, L. The outcome of obsessional disorder: a follow-up study of 100 cases. Br. J. Psychiat., 111:1051–1056, 1965.

37. Hanna, G. L., Yuwiler, A., and Cantwell, D. P. Whole blood serotonin in juvenile obsessive-compulsive disorder. Biol. Psychiat., 29:738–744, 1991.

38. Hasler, G., Kazuba, D., and Murphy, D. L. Factor analysis of obsessive-compulsive disorder YBOCS-SC symptoms and association with 5-HTTLPR SERT polymorphism. Am. J. Med. Genet. B Neuropsychiat. Genet., 141:403–408, 2006.

39. Hastings, D. W. Follow-up results in psychiatric illness. Am. J. Psychiat., 114:1057–1065, 1958.

40. Hay, P., Sachdev, P., Cumming, S., Smith, J. S., Lee, T., Kitchener, P., and Matheson, J. Treatment of obsessive-compulsive disorder by psychosurgery. Acta Psychiat. Scand., 87:197–207, 1993.

41. Hohagen, F., Winkelmann, G., Rasche-Ruchle, H., Hand, I., Konig, A., Munchau, N., Hiss, H., Geiger-Kabisch, C., Kappler, C., Schramm, P., Rey, E., Aldenhoff, J., and Berger, M. Combination of behaviour therapy with fluvoxamine in comparison with behaviour therapy and placebo. Results of a multicentre study. Br. J. Psychiat. Suppl., 35:71–78, 1998.

42. Hunter, R., and Macalpine, I. *Three Hundred Years of Psychiatry, 1535–1860.* London: Oxford University Press, 1963.

43. Husted, D. S., and Shapira, N. A. A review of the treatment for refractory obsessive-compulsive disorder: from medicine to deep brain stimulation. CNS Spectr., 9:833–847, 2004.

44. Ingram, I. M. Obsessional illness in mental hospital patients. J. Ment. Sci., 107:382–402, 1961.

45. Insel, T. R. Similar and dissimilar manifestations of obsessive-compulsive neurosis in monozygotic twins. Am. J. Psychiat., 131:1171–1175, 1965.

46. Insel, T. R. Obsessive-compulsive disorder. Psychiat. Clin. N. Am., 8:105–117, 1985.

47. Insel, T. R., Murphy, D. L., Cohen, R. M., Alterman, I., Kilts, C., and Linnoila, M. Obsessive-compulsive disorder: a double-blind trial of clomipramine and clorgyline. Arch. Gen. Psychiat., 40:605–612, 1983.

48. Insel, T. R., and Winslow, J. T. Neurobiology of obsessive compulsive disorder. Psychiat. Clin. N. Am., 15:813–824, 1992.

49. Jain, V. K., Swinson, R. P., and Thomas, J. G. Phenelzine in obsession neurosis. Br. J. Psychiat., 117:237–238, 1970.

50. James, W. A., and Lippmann, S. B. Clomipramine for obsessive-compulsive disorder: prescribing guidelines. South. Med. J., 84:1243–1245, 1991.

51. Jaspers, K. *General Psychopathology.* Chicago: University of Chicago Press, 1963.

52. Jenike, M. A. Rapid response of severe obsessive-compulsive disorder to tranylcypromine. Am. J. Psychiat., 138:1249–1250, 1981.

53. Jenike, M. A. Obsessive compulsive disorder: a question of a neurologic lesion. Compr. Psychiat., 25:298–304, 1984.

54. Jenike, M. A., and Rausch, S. L. Managing the patient with treatment-resistant obsessive compulsive disorder: current strategies. J. Clin. Psychiat., 55 *Suppl 3*:11–17, 1994.

55. Karno, M., Golding, J. M., Sorenson, S. B., and Burnam, M. A. The epidemiology of obsessive-compulsive disorder in five US communities. Arch. Gen. Psychiat., 45:1094–1099, 1988.

56. Khanna, S., and Channabasavanna, S. M. Phenomenology of obsessions in obsessive-compulsive neurosis. Psychopathol., 21:12–18, 1988.

57. Kringlen, E. Obsessional neurotics: a long-term follow-up. Br. J. Psychiat., 111:709–722, 1965.

58. Langfeldt, G. Studier av Tvangsfernomenenes forelomist, genese, klinik og prognose. Norsk Laegeforen, 13:822–850, 1938.

59. Leckman, J. F., and Cohen, D. J. Recent advances in Gilles de la Tourette syndrome: implications of clinical practice and future research. Psychiat. Dev., 1:301–316, 1983.

60. Lewis, A. J. Problems of obsessional illness. Proc. Roy. Soc. Med., 29:325–336, 1936.

61. Lo, W. H. A follow-up study of obsessional neurotics in Hong Kong Chinese. Br. J. Psychiat., 113:823–832, 1967.

62. Luff, M. C., and Garrod, M. The after results of psychotherapy in 500 adult cases. Br. Med. J., 11:54–59, 1935.

63. Maletzky, B., McFarland, B., and Burt, A. Refractory obsessive compulsive disorder and ECT. Convuls. Ther., 10:34–42, 1994.

64. Marks, I. M. Review of behavioral psychotherapy, I: obsessive-compulsive disorders. Am. J. Psychiat., 138:584–592, 1981.

65. Marks, I. M., Hodgson, R., and Rachman, S. Treatment of chronic obsessive-compulsive neurosis by in-vivo exposure. A two-year follow-up and issues in treatment. Br. J. Psychiat., 127:349–364, 1975.

66. Matsunaga, H., Kiriike, N., Matsui, T., Miyata, A., Iwasaki, Y., Fujimoto, K., Kasai, S., and Kojima, M. Gender differences in social and interpersonal features and personality disorders among Japanese patients with obsessive-compulsive disorder. Compr. Psychiat., 41:266–272, 2000.

67. McGuffin, P., and Mawson, D. Obsessive-compulsive neurosis: two identical twin pairs. Br. J. Psychiat., 137:285–287, 1980.

68. Moore, J. *Of Religious Melancholy*. London: Published by Her Majesty's Special Command, 1692.

69. Nestadt, G., Lan, T., Samuels, J., Riddle, M., Bienvenu, O. J., III, Liang, K. Y., Hoehn-Saric, R., Cullen, B., Grados, M., Beaty, T. H., and Shugart, Y. Y. Complex segregation analysis provides compelling evidence for a major gene underlying obsessive-compulsive disorder and for heterogeneity by sex. Am. J. Hum. Genet., 67:1611–1616, 2000.

70. Nestadt, G., Samuels, J., Riddle, M., Bienvenu III, J., Liang, K.-Y., LaBuda, M., Walkup, J., Grados, M., and Hoehn-Saric, R. A family study of obsessive-compulsive disorder. Arch. Gen. Psychiat., 57:358–363, 2000.

71. Orloff, L. M., Battle, M. A., Baer, L., Ivanjack, L., Pettit, A. R., Buttolph, M. L., and Jenike, M. A. Long-term follow-up of 85 patients with obsessive-compulsive disorder. Am. J. Psychiat., 151:441–442, 1994.

72. Parkin, R. Obsessive-compulsive disorder in adults. Int. Rev. Psychiat., 9:73–82, 1997.

73. Pato, M. T., Schindler, K. M., and Pato, C. N. The genetics of obsessive-compulsive disorder. Curr. Psychiat. Rep., 3:163–168, 2001.

74. Pato, M. T., Zohar-Kadouch, R., Zohar, J., and Murphy, D. L. Return of symptoms after discontinuation of clomipramine in patients with obsessive-compulsive disorder. Am. J. Psychiat., 145:1521–1525, 1988.

75. Pauls, D. L., Alsobrook II, J. P., Goodman, W., Rasmussen, S., and Leckman, J. F. A family study of obsessive-compulsive disorder. Am. J. Psychiat., 152:76–84, 1995.

76. Pauls, D. L., Leckman, J. F., and Cohen, D. J. Evidence against a genetic relationship between Tourette's syndrome and anxiety, depression, panic and phobic disorders. Br. J. Psychiat., 164:215–221, 1994.

77. Pigott, T. A., and Seay, S. M. A review of the efficacy of selective serotonin reuptake inhibitors in obsessive-compulsive disorder. J. Clin. Psychiat., 60:101–106, 1999.

78. Pollitt, J. Natural history of obsessional states: a study of 150 cases. Br. Med. J., 1:194–198, 1957.

79. Prasko, J., Paskova, B., Zalesky, R., Novak, T., Kopecek, M., Bares, M., and Horacek, J. The effect of repetitive transcranial magnetic stimulation (rTMS) on symptoms in obsessive compulsive disorder. A randomized, double blind, sham controlled study. Neuro. Endocrinol. Lett., 27:327–332, 2006.

80. Rasmussen, S. A., and Eisen, J. L. Epidemiology of obsessive compulsive disorder. J. Clin. Psychiat., 51 Suppl:10–13, 1990.

81. Rasmussen, S. A., Eisen, J. L., and Pato, M. T. Current issues in the pharmacologic management of obsessive compulsive disorder. Clin. Psychiat., 54:4–9, 1993.

82. Rasmussen, S. A., and Tsuang, M. T. The epidemiology of obsessive compulsive disorder. J. Clin. Psychiat., 45:450–457, 1984.

83. Rauch, S. L., Baer, L., and Jenike, M. A. Treatment-resistant obsessive-compulsive disorder: practical strategies for management. In *Challenges in Clinical Practice: Pharmacologic and Psychosocial Strategies*. New York: Guilford, pp. 201–218, 1996.

84. Rauch, S. L., and Jenike, M. A. Management of treatment resistant obsessive-compulsive disorder: concepts and strategies, Berend, B., Hollander, E., Marazitti, D., Zohar, J. (eds.). Chichester, England: John Wiley, pp. 227–244, 1994.

85. Ravizz, L., Barzega, G., Bellino, S., Bogetto, F., and Maina, G. Drug treatment of obsessive-compulsive disorder (OCD): long-term trial with clomipramine and selective serotonin reuptake inhibitors (SSRIs). Psychopharmacol. Bull., 32:167–173, 1996.

86. Rennie, T. A. C. *Prognosis in the Psychoneurosis: Benign and Malignant Developments, Current Problems in Psychiatric Diagnosis*. New York: Grune & Stratton, 1953.

87. Robins, L. N., Helzer, J. E., Weissman, M. M., Orvaschel, H., Gruenberg, E., Burke, J. D., and Regier, D. A. Lifetime prevalence of specific psychiatric disorders in three sites. Arch. Gen. Psychiat., 41:949–958, 1984.

88. Rosenberg, C. M. Familial aspects of obsessional neurosis. Br. J. Psychiat., 113:405–413, 1967.

89. Rüdin, G. Ein Beitrag zur Frage der Zwangskrankheit, insbesondere ihrer heriditaren Beziehungen. Arch. Psychiat. Nervenkr., 191:14–54, 1953.

90. Schildre, P. Depersonalization. In *Introduction to Psychoanalytic Psychiatry*, Nervous and Mental Disease Monograph, Series 50, 1928.

91. Shugart, Y. Y., Samuels, J., Willour, V. L., Grados, M. A., Greenberg, B. D., Knowles, J. A., McCracken, J. T., Rauch, S. L., Murphy, D. L., Wang, Y., Pinto, A., Fyer, A. J., Piacentini, J., Pauls, D. L., Cullen, B., Page, J., Rasmussen, S. A., Bienvenu, O. J., Hoehn-Saric, R., Valle, D., Liang, K. Y.,

Riddle, M. A., and Nestadt, G. Genomewide linkage scan for obsessive-compulsive disorder: evidence for susceptibility loci on chromosomes 3q, 7p, 1q, 15q, and 6q. Mol. Psychiat., *11*:763–770, 2006.

92. Skapinakis, P., Papatheodorou, T., and Mavreas, V. Antipsychotic augmentation of serotonergic antidepressants in treatment-resistant obsessive-compulsive disorder: a meta-analysis of the randomized controlled trials. Eur. Neuropsychopharmacol., *17*:79–93, 2007.

93. Steketee, G., and Frost, R. O. Obsessive-compulsive disorder. In *Comprehensive Clinical Psychology, Vol. 6. Adults: Clinical Formulation and Treatment*, Salkovskis, P. (ed.). New York: Pergamon, 1998.

94. Stengel, E. A study of some clinical aspects of the relationship between obsessional neurosis and psychotic reaction types. J. Ment. Sci., *91*:129, 1945.

95. Swedo, S. E., Pietrini, P., Leonard, H. L., Schapiro, M. B., Rettew, D. C., Goldberger, E. L., Rapoport, S. I., Rapoport, J. L., and Grady, C. L. Cerebral glucose metabolism in childhood-onset obsessive-compulsive disorder. Arch. Gen. Psychiat., *49*:690–694, 1992.

96. Taylor, J. *Duktor Dubitantium, or the Role of Conscience.* London: Royston, 1660.

97. Thoren, P., Asberg, M., Cronholm, B., Jornestedt, L., and Traskman, L. Clomipramine treatment of obsessive-compulsive disorder. I. A controlled clinical trial. Arch. Gen. Psychiat., *37*:1281–1285, 1980.

98. Tippin, J., and Henn, F. A. Modified leukotomy in the treatment of intractable obsessional neurosis. Am. J. Psychiat., *139*:1601–1603, 1982.

99. Tyrer, P., Candy, J., and Kelly, D. Phenelzine in phobic anxiety: a controlled trial. Psychol. Med., *3*:120–124, 1973.

100. Vallejo, J., Olivares, J., Marcos, T., Bulbena, A., and Menchón, J. M. Clomipramine versus phenelzine in obsessive-compulsive disorder. A controlled clinical trial. Br. J. Psychiat., *161*:665–670, 1992.

101. van Balkom, A. J., de Haan, E., van Oppen, P., Spinhoven, P., Hoogduin, K. A., and van Dyck, R. Cognitive and behavioral therapies alone versus in combination with fluvoxamine in the treatment of obsessive compulsive disorder. J. Nerv. Ment. Dis., *186*:492–499, 1998.

102. Winokur, G., Clayton, P. J., and Reich, T. *Manic Depressive Illness.* St. Louis: C.V. Mosby, 1969.

103. Wolff, M., Alsobrook, J. P., and Pauls, D. L. Genetic aspects of obsessive-compulsive disorder. Psychiat. Clin. North Am., *23*:535–544, 2000.

104. American Psychiatric Association. *Diagnostic and Statistical Manual of Mental Disorders*, 4th edition, text revision. Washington, DC: Author, 2000.

7

Eating Disorders

The major eating disorders are anorexia nervosa and bulimia nervosa. Anorexia nervosa is characterized by peculiar attitudes toward eating and weight that lead to obsessive refusal to eat, profound weight loss, and, when the disorder occurs in girls, persistent amenorrhea. Bulimia refers to a behavior of gorging of food, typically followed by induced vomiting or purging. Bulimia is seen in many patients with anorexia nervosa, but it is the predominant clinical feature in bulimia nervosa (34). Current diagnostic criteria for anorexia nervosa and bulimia nervosa are presented in Tables 7.1 and 7.2.

Historical Background

In 1689 Richard Morton published a monograph entitled *Phthisiologia or a Treatise of Consumptions*. One of its early chapters, "Nervous Phthisis," contains case histories of the illness we recognize today as anorexia nervosa. An example follows:

> Mr. Duke's Daughter is S. Mary Axe, in the Year 1684 and the Eighteenth Year of her Age, in the Month of July fell into a total Suppression of her Monthly Courses from a multitude of Cares and Passions of her Mind, but without any Symptoms of the Green-Sickness following upon it. From which time her Appetite began to abate, and her Digestion to be bad; her Flesh also began to be flaccid and

191

TABLE 7.1 Diagnostic Criteria for Anorexia Nervosa

A. Refusal to maintain body weight at or above a minimally normal weight for age and height (e.g., weight loss leading to maintenance of body weight less than 85% of that expected; or failure to make expected weight gain during period of growth, leading to body weight less than 85% of the expected)
B. Intense fear of gaining weight or becoming fat, even though underweight
C. Disturbance in the way in which one's body weight or shape is experienced, undue influence of body weight or shape on self-evaluation, or denial of the seriousness of the current low body weight
D. In postmenarcheal females, amenorrhea, that is, the absence of at least three consecutive menstrual cycles (A woman is considered to have amenorrhea if her periods occur only following hormone, e.g., estrogen, administration.)

Adapted from diagnostic criteria in the *DSM-IV-TR* (81).

TABLE 7.2 Diagnostic Criteria for Bulimia Nervosa

A. Recurrent episodes of binge eating. An episode of binge eating is characterized by both of the following:

  (1) Eating, in a discrete period of time (e.g., within any 2-hour period), an amount of food that is definitely larger than most people would eat during a similar period of time and under similar circumstances
  (2) A sense of lack of control over eating during the episode (e.g., a feeling that one cannot stop eating or control what or how much one is eating)

B. Recurrent inappropriate compensatory behavior in order to prevent weight gain, such as self-induced vomiting; misuse of laxatives, diuretics, enemas, or other medications; fasting; or excessive exercise
C. The binge eating and inappropriate compensatory behaviors both occur, on average, at least twice a week for 3 months.
D. Self-evaluation is unduly influenced by body shape and weight.
E. The disturbance does not occur exclusively during episodes of anorexia nervosa.

Adapted from diagnostic criteria in the *DSM-IV-TR* (81).

loose, and her Looks pale, with other symptoms usual in Universal Consumption of the Habit of the Body and by the extreme and memorable cold weather which happened the Winter following, this Consumption did seem to be not a little improved; for that she was wont by her studying at Night, and continual poring upon Books, to expose herself both Day and Night to the Injuries of the Air, which was at that time extremely cold, not without some manifest Prejudice to the System of her Nerves. The Spring following, by the Prescription of some Empirik, she took a Vomit, and after that I know not what Steel

Medicine, but without any Advantage. So from that time loathing all sorts of Medicaments, she wholly neglected the care of herself for two full Years, till at last being brought to the last degree of Marasmus, or Consumption, and thereupon subject to frequent Fainting-Fitts, she apply'd herself to me for Advice.

I do not remember that I did ever in all my practice see one, that was conversant with the Living so much wasted with the greatest degree of Consumption (like a Skeleton only clad with Skin) yet there was no Fever, but on the contrary a Coldness of the whole Body; no cough, or Difficulty of Breathing nor an appearance of any other distemper of the Lungs, or of any other Entrail; No Looseness, or any other sign of a Colliquation, or Preternatural Expence of the Nutritious Juices. Only her Appetite was diminished, and her Digestion uneasy, with Fainting-Fitts, which did frequently return upon her. Which symptoms I did endeavor to relieve by the outward Application of Aromatick Bags made to the Region of the Stomach, and by Stomach-Plaisters, as also by the internal use of bitter Medicines, Chalybeates, and Juleps made of Cephalick and Antihysterick Waters, sufficiently impregnated with Spirit of Salt Armoniack, and Tincture of Castor, and other things of that Nature. Upon the use of which she seemed to be much better; but being quickly tired with Medicines, she beg'd that the whole Affair might be committed again to Nature, whereupon, consuming every day more and more, she was after three Months taken with a Fainting-Fitt, and died.

Another vivid and accurate description was presented in 1908 by Dejerine and Gauckler (14):

It sometimes happens that a physician has patients—they are more apt to be women—whose appearance is truly shocking. Their eyes are brilliant. Their cheeks are hollow, and their cheek bones seem to protrude through the skin. Their withered breasts hang from the walls of their chest. Every rib stands out. Their shoulder blades appear to be loosened from their frame. Every vertebra shows through the skin. The abdominal wall sinks in below the floating ribs and forms a hollow like a basin. The thighs and the calves of their legs are reduced to a skeleton. One would say it was the picture of an immured nun, such as the old masters have portrayed. These women appear to be fifty or sixty years old. Sometimes they seem to be sustained by some unknown miracle of energy; their voices are strong and their steps firm. On the other hand, they often seem almost at the point of death, and ready to draw their last breath.

Are they tuberculous or cancerous patients, or muscular atrophies in the last stages, these women whom misery and hunger have reduced to this frightful gauntness? Nothing of the kind. Their lungs are healthy, there is no sign of any organic affection. Although they look so old they are young women, girls, sometimes children. They may belong to good families, and be surrounded by every care. These patients are what are known as mental anorexics, who, without having any physical lesions, but by the association of various troubles, all having a psychic origin, have lost a quarter, a third, and sometimes a half of their weight. The affection which has driven them to this point may have lasted months, sometimes years. Let it go on too long and death will occur, either from inanition or from secondary tuberculosis. However, it is a case of nothing but a purely psychic affection of which the mechanisms are of many kinds.

Gull and Lasègue described the syndrome independently in 1873 (33, 54). The English term for the illness has been "anorexia nervosa," the French *l'anorexie hysterique,* and the German *Pubertaetsmagersucht.* Of these, the last, literally meaning "adolescent pursuit of thinness" is probably most precise. It is this relentless pursuit of thinness that especially distinguishes anorexia nervosa from other illnesses associated with loss of weight.

Older historical accounts of patients wasting to the point of death do not usually provide enough information to permit distinguishing between cases of anorexia nervosa, tuberculosis, or panhypopituitarism. Some early photographs of alleged pituitary disease, illustrating markedly wasted patients, probably represent cases of anorexia nervosa (see section "Differential Diagnosis").

Epidemiology

Anorexia nervosa is not a common illness. A recent review of the prevalence of eating disorders provided an estimated population prevalence of 1%, and the incidence rate is approximately 10 per 100,000 population per year (41). Bulimia nervosa is somewhat more common than anorexia nervosa (41). The incidence of both anorexia nervosa and bulimia nervosa appear to have increased during the middle of the last century (24, 41, 73). Most large teaching hospitals admit several cases each year.

Anorexia nervosa occurs much more frequently in females than in males. Probably 90% of cases are females (21, 24, 46, 51, 73). A similar female preponderance is seen in bulimia nervosa (21, 41). Anorexia nervosa has long been characterized as an illness of mainly middle-class and upper-class Caucasian girls (46). Analysis of referrals to a national specialist treatment center for anorexia nervosa provided solid evidence of a higher social class bias; representation of lower social classes had apparently increased in the previous decade, however (58). Reviews of ethnicity in anorexia nervosa have identified equal rates in Caucasians and Hispanics and lower rates among African Americans and Asians.

Eating disorders are apparently overrepresented among professional dance and modeling students and competitive athletes, usually developing after the individuals have begun their training (1, 19, 45, 51, 67). Several studies have suggested that homosexual males may have increased risk for eating disorders (25, 38, 39, 69). A chart review study of 135 male eating disorder patients treated at the Massachusetts General Hospital in Boston identified homosexuality or bisexuality in 42% of 62 male bulimia nervosa patients (10). One report suggested that adoptees may also be a high-risk group for eating disorders (42). Although early reports identified associations of sexual abuse and bulimia nervosa, more recent work suggests that a history of sexual abuse may be a nonspecific risk factor for psychiatric disorders (49, 50).

Clinical Picture

An eating disorder typically begins with concern about mild obesity and often dieting, followed by negative attitudes toward eating. A disgust for food that is far stronger than hunger develops. As weight loss progresses, patients may lose their hunger. However thin, they still consider themselves fat and continue to lose weight. These patients may lose so much weight that they resemble survivors of concentration camps, but with several differences. Patients with anorexia nervosa are usually alert and cheerful. In addition, they may be overactive. They often engage in strenuous exercise, sometimes in an open effort to keep from gaining weight.

From the onset of the illness, odd behavior relating to food may be seen. Although starving themselves, patients may hoard food secretly or throw it away. To reduce weight, they may abuse laxatives, enemas, and diuretics. Patients may gorge themselves (bulimia), then induce vomiting voluntarily. In some patients, this feature may be the dominant clinical problem (24, 27, 60, 61, 68).

Amenorrhea may begin before, with, or after the disturbance of appetite (2, 50, 61). It is present in most cases. A few patients first develop anorexia nervosa after bearing children, indicating that an undeveloped reproductive system is not an essential feature of the illness. Other physical findings are bradycardia and lanugo (soft, downy body hair).

Physiological abnormalities have been noted in patients with anorexia nervosa (24, 35, 47, 61). Most investigators believe that starvation produces these abnormalities, which include abnormal glucose tolerance; increased serum cholesterol; increased serum carotene levels; diminished urinary 17-ketosteroids, estrogens, and gonadotropins; elevated serum cortisol; low leptin levels; reduced thyroxine and triiodothyronine; and low basal metabolic rate (24, 35, 47, 61). A striking "immaturity" in the pattern of luteinizing hormone secretion has been described that resembles the hormone functioning of prepubertal girls but usually returns to normal after remission of the anorexia nervosa (30, 61). Male anorexia nervosa patients are reported to have low testosterone levels (51, 76).

Numerous studies have examined the personality profiles of patients with eating disorders. Obsessive-compulsive features, perfectionism, neuroticism, negative emotionality, avoidance, harm avoidance, low self-directedness, and low cooperativeness have been described in association with eating disorders (11). Characteristics especially associated with anorexia nervosa are obsessionality, persistence, perfectionism, self-constraint, and low novelty seeking (11, 37, 51, 52, 78). Features specifically associated with bulimia nervosa are impulsivity, intolerance, immaturity, novelty seeking, and borderline personality traits (11, 18, 50, 52, 71). Even among patients who establish sustained healthy eating patterns, characteristics of high harm avoidance, low cooperativeness, and low self-directedness appear to persist (52).

Biological Findings

The cause of eating disorders is not known, though hypotheses involving endocrine, hypothalamic, and psychosocial factors abound (46, 70). Most investigators assume a multifactorial etiology (50, 51). Imaging studies show reduced brain volumes in both anorexia and bulimia nervosa. When normal weight is regained, brain volume resolves partially, but not completely (74). In anorexia nervosa, imaging studies have demonstrated hypometabolism of the frontal cortex before eating and hyperarousal after eating (64, 65), as well as hyperactivity of the caudate, temporal cortex, lentiform nucleus, and brain stem; these abnormalities normalize with effective treatment (15). Bulimia nervosa appears to involve loss of normal asymmetry of brain activity in frontal and prefrontal areas; these abnormalities fail to correct after long-term recovery (36, 79). In both anorexia and bulimia nervosa, reduced serotonin transporter availability in various brain structures is associated with duration of illness and is not restored with recovery from the illness (3–5, 28, 48). Any of the above brain findings in eating disorders could represent effects of starvation, brain damage over the course of the illness, or brain differences predisposing to the illness (74).

Natural History

The age of onset of anorexia nervosa ranges from pre-puberty to young adulthood, with the mean in the mid-teens (55). Bulimia nervosa typically presents only slightly later on average (55, 56). The onset of eating disorders may be abrupt. Some patients describe possible precipitating events to the illness such as the death of a relative or a broken engagement (31, 50, 63). On the other hand, many patients can give no reason for the onset of their abnormal eating behaviors. The illness may involve one lengthy episode lasting many months or years, or it may be marked by remissions and exacerbations.

A review of 119 studies encompassing a total of 5,590 patients with anorexia nervosa concluded that as many as half of patients may experience full or nearly full recovery, and one-third more may improve (75). One in five patients, however, follows a chronic, unremitting course (50, 51, 75). A recent follow-up study found that nearly half of patients were still having some episodes at 12 years, and 40% had a poor outcome (27). Although little research has been conducted on the long-term course of bulimia nervosa, one study found a somewhat more favorable outcome for bulimia than for anorexia nervosa (26). A typical time course for both anorexia nervosa and bulimia nervosa encompasses substantial improvement during treatment, worsening in the first 2 years after treatment, and further improvement with stabilization in subsequent years (26, 27).

Some patients with anorexia nervosa have persistent difficulties even after the initial massive weight loss has been resolved. These problems include amenorrhea and irregular menses, sexual maladjustment, large weight fluctuations, and persistent disturbed eating behaviors (27, 50, 75).

More favorable prognosis appears to be related to earlier age at onset (24, 27, 75) and to healthy family functioning (63). Poorer prognosis appears to be related to later age at onset, longer duration of illness, disturbed relationship with parents, vomiting, bulimia, laxative abuse, and greater severity of obsessional and depressive symptoms (17, 24, 27, 63, 75). Few studies have compared outcomes of male and female patients with anorexia, but available data suggest that males fare at least as well as females (6).

There has been disagreement about whether anorexia nervosa is a specific illness or a manifestation of other illnesses (59). The vast majority of patients with eating disorders have high rates of psychiatric comorbidity, most often major depression, but also anxiety and substance use disorders (21, 27, 50, 55, 73). Even in patients without mood disorders, depressive symptoms are common during the course of the eating disorder (27, 50, 55, 73). Occasionally patients' descriptions of previous periods of anorexia nervosa are reminiscent of episodes of depression. Dexamethasone suppression of cortisol secretion is impaired in some patients with anorexia nervosa. Curiously, weight gain in these patients does not appear to normalize their cortisol response to dexamethasone suppression (20, 72). These observations raise questions about whether some cases of anorexia nervosa may be manifestations of an underlying affective illness. It has been argued, however, that the fact that eating disorders do not regularly evolve into major depression or other disorders supports their validity as a diagnostic category (24).

Complications

The most obvious complication of anorexia nervosa is death from starvation. The illness is fatal in 5%–10% of adult cases, with an expected death rate approximately 10 times that of a comparable population group (21, 27, 32, 51). Thus, anorexia nervosa should not be regarded lightly. One-half of deaths are due to eating-disorder complications, especially cardiac complications. One-fourth of deaths among these patients are by suicide (17, 40, 47). The fatality rate in bulimia nervosa is lower than the fatality rate in anorexia nervosa (32, 51).

Long-term sequelae of anorexia nervosa are osteopenia and, particularly among adolescents, growth retardation (21, 47). Among the more common complications of bulimia nervosa are dental erosion from repeated exposure of teeth to gastric acid and painless swelling of the parotid glands (51). Gastric rupture and esophageal tears from binging and purging are fortunately rare (51). Eating disorders tend to improve during pregnancy, and most patients who suffer from these disorders have normal pregnancies. Women with eating disorders, however, have more infertility, Caesarian sections, gestationally small babies, premature delivery, and perinatal mortality than other women (21, 24).

Patients with anorexia nervosa apparently develop psychoses no more often than do persons in the general population (27, 66). When psychotic features do develop, they usually appear to be part of co-existing major mood or schizophrenic disorders (13, 44).

Family Studies

Eating disorders appear to run in families. Family studies have demonstrated that family members of individuals with anorexia and bulimia nervosa have a 10- to 20-fold greater likelihood of having these disorders when compared to relatives of unaffected controls (9, 51). Studies in numerous countries have yielded heritability estimates of 28% to 84% for eating disorders (7, 21, 24). Twin studies have demonstrated a concordance rate of 55% in monozygotic twins and 5% in dizygotic twins for anorexia nervosa; less dramatic monozygotic/ dizygotic twin concordance differences have been described for bulimia nervosa (46% vs. 26%) (8, 24). Although eating disorders do not appear to be co-inherited with obsessive-compulsive disorder, there is evidence of co-transmission of anorexia nervosa with obsessive-compulsive personality traits (51).

Differential Diagnosis

Anorexia nervosa is characterized by unceasing pursuit of thinness and should not be confused with weight loss occurring in the course of illness such as major depression or schizophrenia. Starvation, when it has causes other than anorexia nervosa, is usually accompanied by apathy and inactivity rather than by the alertness and hyperactivity characteristic of anorexia nervosa. Hypopituitarism is seldom associated with the severe cachexia of anorexia nervosa or the strikingly high level of physical activity. Levels of urinary gonadotropins and serum growth hormone are consistently lower in hypo-pituitarism than in anorexia nervosa (12, 29).

Differential diagnosis of anorexia nervosa and bulimia nervosa includes consideration of medical illness, especially gastrointestinal diseases: celiac disease, inflammatory bowel disease, bowel adenocarcinoma, and gastro-intestinal motility disorders such as achalasia (16, 22, 57). Evidence of psychiatric problems should not preclude appropriate investigation to exclude medical sources of digestive symptoms (16). Gastrointestinal dis-turbances, especially gastric emptying abnormalities, are frequent among patients with eating disorders, but they usually improve with restoration of healthy eating (16, 57).

Clinical Management

Treatment of patients with anorexia nervosa is far from satisfactory, and there is little agreement about the best form. Engaging the patient in treatment is a necessary first step (80). Patients with anorexia nervosa are usually unconcerned about their weight loss and seek treatment only at the insistence of concerned family or friends. Patients with bulimia nervosa, however, are often more motivated to seek treatment for symptoms that trouble them (43).

Indicators of need for hospitalization are self-destructiveness and suicide risk, severe interpersonal problems, body weight below 75% of expected, severe symptoms not relieved with outpatient treatment, psychiatric comorbidity requiring hospitalization, and medical complications (21, 24, 43, 50). The early goals in anorexia nervosa therapy are to stabilize medical complications and restore body weight to safer levels. Rarely, constant observation on a locked psychiatric floor and tube feeding is required (24). Multidisciplinary treatment teams that include the medical practitioner, a nutritionist, and a mental health specialist are best suited to manage eating disorders (77).

No medication has been demonstrated to promote weight gain in anorexia nervosa. Although preliminary findings suggested potential for fluoxetine in preventing relapse among patients after adequate weight is restored (24, 80), a recent randomized, double-blind placebo-controlled clinical trial did not demonstrate such benefit. For bulimia nervosa, on the other hand, numerous double-blind, placebo-controlled trials of fluoxetine have demonstrated effectiveness in reduction of binging frequency (50). Although fluoxetine may also reduce associated depressive and anxiety symptoms, its effectiveness is independent of depression (62). Doses larger than those typically used for treatment of depression are required in bulimia nervosa patients (50, 80).

Psychotherapy is an important component of treatment. Numerous randomized, controlled trials have found cognitive-behavioral therapy to be effective (21, 24). The combination of cognitive-behavioral therapy with fluoxetine may be the most beneficial strategy for management of bulimia nervosa (43, 62). Family-based interventions have recently been found useful, especially for adolescents with anorexia nervosa (23, 53).

REFERENCES

1. Abraham, S. Characteristics of eating disorders among young ballet dancers. Psychopathol., 29:223–229, 1996.
2. American Psychiatric Association. *Diagnostic and Statistical Manual of Mental Disorders*, 4th edition, text revision. Washington, DC: Author, 2000.
3. Bailer, U. F., Frank, G. K., Henry, S. E., Price, J. C., Meltzer, C. C., Weissfeld, L., Mathis, C. A., Drevets, W. C., Wagner, A., Hoge, J., Ziolko, S. K., McConaha, C. W., and Kaye, W. H. Altered brain serotonin 5-HT1A receptor binding after recovery from anorexia nervosa measured by positron emission tomography and [carbonyl11C]WAY-100635. Arch. Gen. Psychiat., 62:1032–1041, 2005.
4. Bailer, U. F., Price, J. C., Meltzer, C. C., Mathis, C. A., Frank, G. K., Weissfeld, L., McConaha, C. W., Henry, S. E., Brooks-Achenbach, S., Barbarich, N. C., and Kaye, W. H. Altered 5-HT(2A) receptor binding after recovery from bulimia-type anorexia nervosa: relationships to harm avoidance and drive for thinness. Neuropsychopharmacol., 29:1143–1155, 2004.
5. Barbarich, N. C., Kaye, W. H., and Jimerson, D. Neurotransmitter and imaging studies in anorexia nervosa: new targets for treatment. Curr. Drug Targets CNS Neurol. Disord., 2:61–72, 2003.
6. Bean, P., Loomis, C. C., Timmel, P., Hallinan, P., Moore, S., Mammel, J., and Weltzin, T. Outcome variables for anorexic males and females one year after discharge from residential treatment. J. Addict. Dis., 23:83–94, 2004.
7. Bulik, C. M. Exploring the gene-environment nexus in eating disorders. J. Psychiat. Neurosci., 30:335–339, 2005.
8. Bulik, C. M., Sullivan, P. F., Wade, T. D., and Kendler, K. S. Twin studies of eating disorders: a review. Int. J. Eat. Disord., 27:1–20, 2000.
9. Bulik, C. M., and Tozzi, F. Genetics in eating disorders: state of the science. CNS Spectr., 9:511–515, 2004.
10. Carlat, D. J., Camargo, C. A., Jr., and Herzog, D. B. Eating disorders in males: a report on 135 patients. Am. J. Psychiat., 154:1127–1132, 1997.
11. Cassin, S. E., and von Ranson, K. M. Personality and eating disorders: a decade in review. Clin. Psychol. Rev., 25:895–916, 2005.
12. Couzinet, B., Young, J., Brailly, S., Le Bouc, Y., Chanson, P., and Schaison, G. Functional hypothalamic amenorrhoea: a partial and reversible gonadotrophin deficiency of nutritional origin. Clin. Endocrinol., 50:229–235, 1999.
13. Deckelman, M. C., Dixon, L. B., and Conley, R. R. Comorbid bulimia nervosa and schizophrenia. Int. J. Eat. Disord., 22:101–105, 1997.
14. Dejerine, J., and Gauckler, E. Le Réeducation des faux gastropathies. Presse Méd., 16:2–25, 1908.
15. Delvenne, V., Goldman, S., De, M., V, Simon, Y., Luxen, A., and Lotstra, F. Brain hypometabolism of glucose in anorexia nervosa: normalization after weight gain. Biol. Psychiat., 40:761–768, 1996.
16. Desseilles, M., Fuchs, S., Ansseau, M., Lopez, S., Vinckenbosh, E., and Andreoli, A. Achalasia may mimic anorexia nervosa, compulsive eating disorder, and obesity problems. Psychosomat., 47:270–271, 2006.

17. Deter, H. C., Schellberg, D., Kopp, W., Friederich, H. C., and Herzog, W. Predictability of a favorable outcome in anorexia nervosa. Eur. Psychiat., 20:165–172, 2005.

18. Diaz-Marsa, M., Carrasco, J. L., and Saiz, J. A study of temperament and personality in anorexia and bulimia nervosa. J. Pers. Disord., 14:352–359, 2000.

19. Dotti, A., Fioravanti, M., Balotta, M., Tozzi, F., Cannella, C., and Lazzari, R. Eating behavior of ballet dancers. Eat. Weight Disord., 7:60–67, 2002.

20. Duclos, M., Corcuff, J. B., Roger, P., and Tabarin, A. The dexamethasone-suppressed corticotrophin-releasing hormone stimulation test in anorexia nervosa. Clin. Endocrinol., 51:725–731, 1999.

21. Ebeling, H., Tapanainen, P., Joutsenoja, A., Koskinen, M., Morin-Papunen, L., Jarvi, L., Hassinen, R., Keski-Rahkonen, A., Rissanen, A., and Wahlbeck, K. A practice guideline for treatment of eating disorders in children and adolescents. Ann. Med., 35:488–501, 2003.

22. Eberman, L. E., and Cleary, M. A. Celiac disease in an elite female collegiate volleyball athlete: a case report. J. Athl. Train., 40:360–364, 2005.

23. Eisler, I., Simic, M., Russell, G. F., and Dare, C. A randomised controlled treatment trial of two forms of family therapy in adolescent anorexia nervosa: a five-year follow-up. J. Child Psychol. Psychiat., 48:552–560, 2007.

24. Fairburn, C. G., and Harrison, P. J. Eating disorders. Lancet, 361:407–416, 2003.

25. Fichter, M. M., and Daser, C. Symptomatology, psychosexual development and gender identity in 42 anorexic males. Psychol. Med., 17:409–418, 1987.

26. Fichter, M. M., and Quadflieg, N. Twelve-year course and outcome of bulimia nervosa. Psychol. Med., 34:1395–1406, 2004.

27. Fichter, M. M., Quadflieg, N., and Hedlund, S. Twelve-year course and outcome predictors of anorexia nervosa. Int. J. Eat. Disord., 39:87–100, 2006.

28. Frank, G. K., Kaye, W. H., Meltzer, C. C., Price, J. C., Greer, P., McConaha, C., and Skovira, K. Reduced 5-HT2A receptor binding after recovery from anorexia nervosa. Biol. Psychiat., 52:896–906, 2002.

29. Gianotti, L., Broglio, F., Ramunni, J., Lanfranco, F., Gauna, C., Benso, A., Zanello, M., Arvat, E., and Ghigo, E. The activity of GH/IGF-I axis in anorexia nervosa and in obesity: a comparison with normal subjects and patients with hypopituitarism or critical illness. Eat. Weight Disord., 3:64–70, 1998.

30. Gold, M. S., Pottash, A. C., Martin, D., Extein, I., and Howard, E. The 24-hour LH test in the diagnosis and assessment of response to treatment of patients with anorexia nervosa. Int. J. Psychiat. Med., 11:245–250, 1981.

31. Gowers, S. G., North, C. D., Byram, V., and Weaver, A. B. Life event precipitants of adolescent anorexia nervosa. J. Child Psychol. Psychiat., 37:469–477, 1996.

32. Gucciardi, E., Celasun, N., Ahmad, F., and Stewart, D. E. Eating Disorders. BMC. Womens Health, 4 Suppl 1:S21, 2004.

33. Gull, W. W. Anorexia nervosa (apepsia hysterica). Br. Med. J., 2:5–27, 1873.

34. Gwirtsman, H. E. Bulimic disorders: pharmacotherapeutic and biological studies. Psychopharmacol. Bull., 29:109–114, 1993.

35. Haas, V., Onur, S., Paul, T., Nutzinger, D. O., Bosy-Westphal, A., Hauer, M., Brabant, G., Klein, H., and Muller, M. J. Leptin and body weight regulation in patients with anorexia nervosa before and during weight recovery. Am. J. Clin. Nutr., 81:889–896, 2005.

36. Hagman, J. O., Buchsbaum, M. S., Wu, J. C., Rao, S. J., Reynolds, C. A., and Blinder, B. J. Comparison of regional brain metabolism in bulimia nervosa and affective disorder assessed with positron emission tomography. J. Affect. Disord., 19:153–162, 1990.

37. Halmi, K. A., Sunday, S. R., Strober, M., Kaplan, A., Woodside, D. B., Richter, M., Treasure, J., Berrettini, W. H., and Kaye, W. H. Perfectionism in anorexia nervosa; variation by clinical subtype, obsessionality, and pathological eating behavior. Am. J. Psychiat., 157:1799–1805, 2000.

38. Hepp, U., Milos, G., and Braun-Scharm, H. Gender identity disorder and anorexia nervosa in male monozygotic twins. Int. J. Eat. Disord., 35:239–243, 2004.

39. Herzog, D. B., Norman, D. K., Gordon, C., and Pepose, M. Sexual conflict and eating disorders in 27 males. Am. J. Psychiat., 141:989–990, 1984.

40. Hoek, H. W. Incidence, prevalence and mortality of anorexia nervosa and other eating disorders. Curr. Opin. Psychiat., 19:389–394, 2006.

41. Hoek, H. W., and Van Hoeken, D. Review of the prevalence and incidence of eating disorders. Int. J. Eat. Disord., 34:383–396, 2003.

42. Holden, N. L. Adoption and eating disorders: a high-risk group? Br. J. Psychiat., 158:829–833, 1991.

43. Hsu, L. K. Eating disorders: practical interventions. J. Am. Med. Womens Assoc., 59:113–124, 2004.

44. Hudson, J. I., Pope, Jr. H. G., and Jonas, J. M. Psychosis in anorexia nervosa and bulimia. Br. J. Psychiat., 145:420–423, 1984.

45. Hughes, C. S., and Hughes, S. The female athlete syndrome. Anorexia nervosa–reflections on a personal journey. Orthop. Nurs., 23:252–260, 2004.

46. Jacobi, C., Hayward, C., de Zwaan, M., Kraemer, H. C., and Agras, W. S. Coming to terms with risk factors for eating disorders: application of risk terminology and suggestions for a general taxonomy. Psychol. Bull., 130:19–65, 2004.

47. Katzman, D. K. Medical complications in adolescents with anorexia nervosa: a review of the literature. Int. J. Eat. Disord., 37 Suppl:S52–S59, 2005.

48. Kaye, W. H., Frank, G. K., Bailer, U. F., and Henry, S. E. Neurobiology of anorexia nervosa: clinical implications of alterations of the function of serotonin and other neuronal systems. Int. J. Eat. Disord., 37 Suppl:S15–S19, 2005.

49. Kendler, K. S., Bulik, C. M., Silberg, J., Hettema, J. M., Myers, J., and Prescott, C. A. Childhood sexual abuse and adult psychiatric and substance use disorders in women: an epidemiological and cotwin control analysis. Arch. Gen. Psychiat., 57:953–959, 2000.

50. Klein, D. A., and Walsh, B. T. Eating disorders. Int. Rev. Psychiat., 15:205–216, 2003.

51. Klein, D. A., and Walsh, B. T. Eating disorders: clinical features and pathophysiology. Physiol. Behav., 81:359–374, 2004.

52. Klump, K. L., Strober, M., Bulik, C. M., Thornton, L., Johnson, C., Devlin, B., Fichter, M. M., Halmi, K. A., Kaplan, A. S., Woodside, D. B., Crow, S., Mitchell, J., Rotondo, A., Keel, P. K., Berrettini, W. H., Plotnicov, K., Pollice, C., Lilenfeld, L. R., and Kaye, W. H. Personality characteristics of women before and after recovery from an eating disorder. Psychol. Med., 34:1407–1418, 2004.

53. Kotler, L. A., Boudreau, G. S., and Devlin, M. J. Emerging psychotherapies for eating disorders. J. Psychiat. Pract., 9:431–441, 2003.

54. Lasègue, E. C. De l'anorexia hystérique. Arch. Gen. Med., 21:385, 1873.

55. Lewinsohn, P. W., Striegel-Moore, R. H., and Seeley, J. R. Epidemiology and natural course of eating disorders in young women from adolescence to young adulthood. J. Am. Acad. Child Adolesc. Psychiat., 39:1284–1292, 2000.

56. Matsumoto, H., Takei, N., Kawai, M., Saito, F., Kachi, K., Ohashi, Y., Takeuchi, H., and Mori, N. Differences of symptoms and standardized weight index between patients with early-onset and late-onset anorexia nervosa. Pediat. Drugs, 3:91–99, 2001.

57. McClain, C. J., Humphries, L. L., Hill, K. K., and Nickl, N. J. Gastrointestinal and nutritional aspects of eating disorders. J. Am. Coll. Nutr., 12:466–474, 1993.

58. McClelland, L., and Crisp, A. Anorexia nervosa and social class. Int. J. Eat. Dis., 29:150–156, 2001.

59. McElroy, S. L., Kotwal, R., Keck, P. E., Jr., and Akiskal, H. S. Comorbidity of bipolar and eating disorders: distinct or related disorders with shared dysregulations? J. Affect. Disord., 86:107–127, 2005.

60. Milos, G., Spindler, A., Schnyder, U., and Fairburn, C. G. Instability of eating disorder diagnoses: prospective study. Br. J. Psychiat., 187:573–578, 2005.

61. Mitan, L. A. Menstrual dysfunction in anorexia nervosa. J. Pediatr. Adolesc. Gynecol., 17:81–85, 2004.

62. Mitchell, J. E., de Zwaan, M., and Roerig, J. L. Drug therapy for patients with eating disorders. Curr. Drug Targets CNS Neurol. Disord., 2:17–29, 2003.

63. North, C., Gowers, S., and Byram, V. Family functioning and life events in the outcome of adolescent anorexia nervosa. Br. J. Psychiat., 171:545–549, 1997.

64. Nozoe, S., Naruo, T., Nakabeppu, Y., Soejima, Y., Nakajo, M., and Tanaka, H. Changes in regional cerebral blood flow in patients with anorexia nervosa detected through single photon emission tomography imaging. Biol. Psychiat., 34:578–580, 1993.

65. Nozoe, S., Naruo, T., Yonekura, R., Nakabeppu, Y., Soejima, Y., Nagai, N., Nakajo, M., and Tanaka, H. Comparison of regional cerebral blood flow in patients with eating disorders. Brain Res. Bull., 36:251–255, 1995.

66. Oldham, J. M., Skodol, A. E., Kellman, H. D., Hyler, S. E., Doidge, N., Rosnick, L., and Gallaher, P. E. Comorbidity of axis I and axis II disorders. Am. J. Psychiat., 152:571–578, 1995.

67. Ravaldi, C., Vannacci, A., Zucchi, T., Mannucci, E., Cabras, P. L., Boldrini, M., Murciano, L., Rotella, C. M., and Ricca, V. Eating disorders and body image disturbances among ballet dancers, gymnasium users and body builders. Psychopathol., 36:247–254, 2003.

68. Reba, L., Thornton, L., Tozzi, F., Klump, K. L., Brandt, H., Crawford, S., Crow, S., Fichter, M. M., Halmi, K. A., Johnson, C., Kaplan, A. S., Keel, P., LaVia, M., Mitchell, J., Strober, M., Woodside, D. B., Rotondo, A., Berrettini, W. H., Kaye, W. H., and Bulik, C. M. Relationships between features associated with vomiting in purging-type eating disorders. Int. J. Eat. Disord., 38:287–294, 2005.

69. Robinson, P. H., and Holden, N. L. Bulimia nervosa in the male: a report of nine cases. Psychol. Med., 16:895–903, 1986.

70. Romans, S. E., Gendall, K. A., Martin, H. L., and Mullen, P. E. Child sexual abuse and later disordered eating: a New Zealand epidemiological study. Int. J. Eat. Dis., 29:380–392, 2001.

71. Rosenvinge, J. H., Martinussen, M., and Ostensen, E. The comorbidity of eating disorders and personality disorders: a meta-analytic review of studies published between 1983 and 1998. Eat. Weight Dis., 5:52–61, 2000.

72. Schweitzer, I., Szmukler, G. I., Maguire, K. P., Harrison, L. C., Tuckwell, V., and Davies, B. M. The dexamethasone suppression test in anorexia nervosa. The influence of weight, depression, adrenocorticotrophic hormone and dexamethasone. Br. J. Psychiat., 157:713–717, 1990.

73. Soundy, T. J., Lucas, A. R., Suman, V. J., and Melton, L. J., III. Bulimia nervosa in Rochester, Minnesota from 1980 to 1990. Psychol. Med., 25:1065–1071, 1995.

74. Stamatakis, E. A., and Hetherington, M. M. Neuroimaging in eating disorders. Nutr. Neurosci., 6:325–334, 2003.

75. Steinhausen, H. C. The outcome of anorexia nervosa in the 20th century. Am. J. Psychiat., 159:1284–1293, 2002.

76. Wabitsch, M., Ballauff, A., Holl, R., Blum, W. F., Heinze, E., Remschmidt, H., and Hebebrand, J. Serum leptin, gonadotropin, and testosterone concentrations in male patients with anorexia nervosa during weight gain. J. Clin. Endocrinol. Metab, 86:2982–2988, 2001.

77. Walsh, J. M., Wheat, M. E., and Freund, K. Detection, evaluation, and treatment of eating disorders the role of the primary care physician. J. Gen. Intern. Med., 15:577–590, 2000.

78. Wonderlich, S. A., Lilenfeld, L. R., Riso, L. P., Engel, S., and Mitchell, J. E. Personality and anorexia nervosa. Int. J. Eat. Disord., 37 Suppl:S68–S71, 2005.

79. Wu, J. C., Hagman, J., Buchsbaum, M. S., Blinder, B., Derrfler, M., Tai, W. Y., Hazlett, E., and Sicotte, N. Greater left cerebral hemispheric metabolism in bulimia assessed by positron emission tomography. Am. J. Psychiat., 147:309–312, 1990.

80. Zhu, A. J., and Walsh, B. T. Pharmacologic treatment of eating disorders. Can. J. Psychiat., 47:227–234, 2002.

81. American Psychiatric Association. Diagnostic and Statistical Manual of Mental Disorders, 4th edition, text revision. Washington, DC: Author, 2000.

8

Somatization Disorder
(Hysteria)

The diagnosis of hysteria was applied to cases of unexplained physical complaints for many centuries. Building upon the earlier work of Briquet in France (10), Savill in England (68), and Purtell and colleagues in Boston (20, 62), investigators at Washington University in Saint Louis (4, 16–18, 29, 31, 33–35, 37–39, 60) carried out a series of studies and proposed that this diagnosis be replaced by two labels: "Briquet's syndrome" (after the French psychiatrist who described a large series of such patients) and "conversion symptoms." This proposal was designed to eliminate the pejorative implications associated with the diagnosis of hysteria and to avoid the complications of inconsistent use of terminology.

Toward the same ends, *DSM-III* introduced the category of somatoform disorders in place of hysteria generally, with somatization disorder being substituted for Briquet syndrome. The categorization of conversion symptoms was not fully clarified.

The importance of distinguishing between Briquet syndrome and conversion symptoms continued to be emphasized by the Washington University group. They argued that the former is typically a polysymptomatic disorder that begins early in life (usually in the teens, rarely after the 20s), chiefly affects women, and is characterized by recurrent, multiple somatic complaints often described dramatically. Characteristic features, all unexplained by other known clinical disorders, include varied pains, anxiety symptoms, gastrointestinal disturbances, urinary symptoms, menstrual difficulties, sexual and marital maladjustment, nervousness, mood disturbances, and "pseudoneurological" symptoms (the last often used synonymously with the term "conversion symptoms"). Repeated visits to physicians and clinics, the use of a large number of medications—often at the same time—prescribed by different physicians, and frequent hospitalizations and operations produce a florid medical history (33, 34).

In keeping with this view, somatization disorder continues to be the term for Briquet syndrome in *DSM-IV-TR*. (In citing historical research on this disorder, this chapter will apply a convention of using the terminology of the study's original authors to help readers appreciate the context of the research.) The specific diagnostic criteria for somatization disorder are presented in Table 8.1.

TABLE 8.1 Diagnostic Criteria for Somatization Disorder

A. A history of many physical complaints beginning before age 30 years that occur over a period of several years and result in treatment being sought or significant impairment in social, occupational, or other important areas of functioning

B. Each of the following criteria must have been met, with individual symptoms occurring at any time during the course of the disturbance:

   (1) *Four pain symptoms:* a history of pain related to at least four different sites or functions (e.g., head, abdomen, back, joints, extremities, chest, rectum, during menstruation, during sexual intercourse, or during urination)

   (2) *Two gastrointestinal symptoms:* a history of at least two gastrointestinal symptoms other than pain (e.g., nausea, bloating, vomiting other than during pregnancy, diarrhea, or intolerance of several different foods)

   (3) *One sexual symptom:* a history of at least one sexual or reproductive symptom other than pain (e.g., sexual indifference, erectile or ejaculatory dysfunction, irregular menses, excessive menstrual bleeding, vomiting throughout pregnancy)

   (4) *One pseudoneurological symptom:* a history of at least one symptom or deficit suggesting a neurological condition not limited to pain (conversion symptoms such as impaired coordination or balance, paralysis or localized weakness, difficulty swallowing or lump in throat, aphonia, urinary retention, hallucinations, loss of touch or pain sensation, double vision, blindness, deafness, seizures; dissociative symptoms such as amnesia; or loss of consciousness other than fainting)

C. Either (1) or (2):

   (1) After appropriate investigation, each of the symptoms in Criterion B cannot be fully explained by a known general medical condition or the direct effects of a substance (e.g., a drug of abuse, a medication).

   (2) When there is a related general medical condition, the physical complaints or resulting social or occupational impairment are in excess of what would be expected from the history, physical examination, or laboratory findings.

D. The symptoms are not intentionally produced or feigned (as in factitious disorder or malingering).

Adapted from diagnostic criteria in the *DSM-IV-TR* (92).

It should be emphasized, however, that the diagnostic criteria for somati-zation disorder in *DSM-IV-TR* are less stringent than those for Briquet syn-drome and were proposed to offer a shortcut to the diagnosis (89). As yet, we have few data about the validity of these criteria for somatization disorder from systematic, controlled follow-up and family studies. The findings thus far indicate that the two sets of criteria (for Briquet syndrome and somatization disorder) select overlapping but somewhat different populations (18, 25).

The Saint Louis group proposed that the term "conversion symptom" be reserved for *unexplained symptoms suggesting neurological disease* such as amnesia, unconsciousness, paralysis, "spells," aphonia, urinary retention, dif-ficulty walking, anesthesia, and blindness—the so-called pseudoneurological or "grand hysterical" symptoms (50). "Unexplained" means only that the history, neurological examination, and diagnostic tests have failed to reveal a satisfactory explanation for the symptoms. Thus used, the term "conversion symptom" has no etiologic implication; it refers, in a descriptive way only, to a limited group of symptoms. In order to give the term greater specificity, unexplained pains and other unexplained medical symptoms that do not suggest neurological disease are not included in the definition. If other unex-plained medical symptoms such as headaches, backaches, and abdominal pains were included, conversion symptom would mean any unexplained med-ical symptom and thus would lose any precision it has (33, 34).

Sometimes a related syndrome occurs as a sudden, short-lived epidemic (mass hysteria), characteristically in a school population and most frequently affecting female students (52, 72). Blackouts, dizziness, weakness, headaches, hyperventilation, nausea, and abdominal pain are the usual symptoms. Suggestion and fear are thought to be major factors in the pathogenesis of these episodes. Long-term follow-up of the affected children has not been reported, though the short-term prognosis appears to be very good.

To recapitulate: Conversion symptoms comprise a limited group of indivi-dual symptoms suggesting neurological disease. Somatization disorder or Briquet syndrome refers to a polysymptomatic syndrome that typically includes conversion symptoms.

One major criticism of the definition of Briquet syndrome or somatiza-tion disorder is that practically everyone experiences many symptoms char-acteristic of the syndrome. It is true that most people have experienced headaches, fatigue, anorexia, nausea, diarrhea, vomiting, nervousness, and varied pains. But when responding to a physician, few report such symptoms. Most people interpret the physician's questions to mean significant symp-toms; they report only symptoms that are recent, recurrent, or otherwise troublesome. Furthermore, the physician evaluates the patient's responses, ignoring symptoms that are not recent, recurrent, or disabling. He or she pays attention to symptoms that led the patient to consult a physician, take medicines, or alter usual routines. In addition, there are some symptoms that will be considered significant regardless of qualifying features, such as blindness and paralysis. These criteria—ones that physicians ordinarily use to evaluate symptoms—are the same as those applied in the studies of Briquet syndrome or somatization disorder cited above. By these criteria, very few people report enough symptoms, otherwise unexplained medically, to warrant these diagnoses.

Historical Background

The concept of hysteria, which probably originated in Egypt, is at least 4,000 years old. The name *hysteria* has been in use since the time of Hippocrates. The original Egyptian approach to hysteria was perhaps the most fanciful. Believing that physical displacement of the uterus caused the varied symptoms, physicians treated the patient by trying to attract the "wandering uterus" back to its proper site. Sweet-smelling substances were placed in the region of the vagina to attract the errant organ; unpleasant materials were ingested or inhaled to drive it away from the upper body (78).

Although Egyptian and Greek physicians applied the diagnosis whenever they believed that unusual symptoms were caused by a displaced uterus, the available records do not provide explicit diagnostic criteria. This state of affairs persisted, although various speculations about pathogenesis have been offered over the centuries (71). In particular, witchcraft, demonology, and sorcery were associated with hysteria in the Middle Ages (78). Mysterious symptoms, spells, and odd behavior were frequently considered manifestations of supernatural, evil influences. Hysterical patients were sometimes perceived as either the active evil spirit (witch, sorceress, or demon) or as the passive victim of such an evil being. Since the Middle Ages there have been speculations of many kinds about the cause of hysteria. Such speculations have included ideas about neurological weakness, neurological degeneration, the effects of various toxins, and disturbances of what Mesmer called "animal magnetism."

Hysteria became Freud's central concern during the early years of psychoanalysis (9). That interest had developed while Freud was working in Paris with Charcot, who was treating hysteria with hypnosis. The psychoanalytic concept of conversion as an ego defense mechanism, referring to unconscious conversion of "psychic energy" into physical symptoms, ultimately led to the identification of conversion symptoms with hysteria in psychoanalytic practice. Many psychoanalysts considered hysteria a simulation of illness designed to work out unconscious conflicts, partially through attention-getting and "secondary gain," a term that refers to possible advantages of illness such as sympathy and support, including financial support, from relatives and friends and being excused from various duties (91).

This view led easily to the attitude, widely held by physicians though seldom stated openly, that hysteria is a term of opprobrium to be applied whenever the patient's complaints are not explained or when the demands appear excessive. The most fully developed version of this view is the concept of the hysterical personality. Here, the emphasis is on immature, histrionic, manipulative, seductive, and attention-getting behavior regardless of the presenting complaint of present illness. In the absence of specific diagnostic criteria and systematic studies, however, use of the term has been inconsistent and confusing. Many clinicians believe that conversion symptoms, somatization disorder, and hysterical personality are different, although any combination of these three is frequently present in the same individual (14, 15, 42).

The syndromatic approach to the diagnosis of hysteria began in 1859 when the French physician Pierre Briquet published his monograph, *Traits clinique et thérapeutique á l'hystérie* (10, 48, 49). Similar descriptions of the syndrome were provided in 1909 by the English physician Savill (68) and in 1951 by the American psychiatrists Purtell, Cohen, and Robins (62). In recent decades a series of studies by Guze and colleagues has refined and clarified the concept of hysteria as a syndrome (33, 34, 36, 60, 60, 85), and in a systematic study of women diagnosed as "having a hysterical personality or as being hysterics," Blinder (6) confirmed the clinical description and familiar characteristics described below.

Epidemiology

A study in an urban community (82) indicated the prevalence of somatization disorder to be 0.4%. Assuming that nearly all of the cases occurred in women, and correcting for the sex distribution of the sample, the prevalence in urban women was just under 1% according to this report. A recent (2004) meta-analysis by Creed and Barsky revealed a prevalence of 0.4% (range, 0.03%–0.84%) in a population-based sample (23). In studies of hospitalized, post-partum women whose pregnancies and deliveries were without complication, the prevalence of the syndrome was between 1% and 2% (29, 55).

A history of conversion symptoms, on the other hand, is commonly found when systematic interviewing is done among hospitalized, normal, postpartum women (29), hospitalized medically ill women (86), and male and female psychiatric outpatients (38). On average, about one-quarter of such patients give a history of conversion symptoms.

All authors, except those describing psychiatric problems encountered in the military, report that the great majority of patients with the diagnosis of hysteria (using a variety of diagnostic criteria) are women (24, 40, 44, 65, 75). Nearly all men with symptoms resembling hysteria in women have had histories of associated compensation factors such as litigation following injuries, consideration for veterans' and other pensions, disability payments, or serious legal difficulties (67).

There is a generally held view that hysteria and conversion symptoms are more common among less sophisticated people. One group of investigators found that higher education (1 or more years of college) was significantly less common in patients with conversion symptoms—with or without Briquet syndrome—than in patients without conversion symptoms. This was also true for patients with Briquet syndrome compared to other psychiatric patients as a group (38). Several investigators have reported that "hysterical neurosis, conversion type" is much more frequent in nonwhites than in whites and is highest in the lowest socioeconomic classes (75, 76).

Of interest is the work of British psychiatrist Carothers whose anthropological studies led to a theory that "psychopathy and hysteria" may be manifestations of the persistence in modern society of preliterate "magical" modes of thinking. On the basis of this theory, Carothers concluded that sociopathy should predominate in men, hysteria in women (see below) (13).

Indeed, although a history of conversion symptoms may be elicited from patients with any psychiatric disorder, two conditions are most often associated with such a history: Briquet syndrome and sociopathy. A report indicates that women with Briquet syndrome are significantly more likely to show an earlier birth order than are women with other psychiatric disorders (53).

In summary, a history of conversion symptoms can be found among psychiatric patients of either sex suffering from any psychiatric disorder. However, such a history is most likely to be associated with somatization disorder in women or sociopathy in men. Somatization disorder is much less common than conversion symptoms; it is seen less infrequently among men; and, like conversion symptoms, it is infrequently associated with higher education.

Clinical Picture

When first seen by a psychiatrist, the typical patient with somatization disorder is a married woman in her 30s. Her history is often delivered in a dramatic, complicated fashion. She usually presents with multiple vague complaints to her general physician, and a straightforward history of the present illness is difficult, if not impossible, to elicit. Frequently, the physician has difficulty deciding when the current illness began or even why the patient presented. Table 8.2 presents the most common symptoms reported by patients with somatization disorder. Not only do they report large numbers of these and other symptoms, but also the symptoms are distributed widely throughout all or nearly all organ systems. It is this range of symptoms in addition to their number that defines somatization disorder.

TABLE 8.2 The Frequency of Symptoms in Hysteria

Symptom	%	Symptom	%	Symptom	%
Dyspnea	72	Weight loss	28	Joint pain	84
Palpitation	60	Sudden fluctuations	16	Extremity pain	84
Chest pain	72	in weight		Burning pains in rectum,	28
Dizziness	84	Anorexia	60	vagina, mouth	
Headache	80	Nausea	80	Other bodily pain	36
Anxiety attacks	64	Vomiting	32	Depressed feelings	64
Fatigue	84	Abdominal pain	80	Phobias	48
Blindness	20	Abdominal bloating	68	Vomiting all 9 months	20
Paralysis	12	Food intolerances	48	of pregnancy	
Anesthesia	32	Diarrhea	20	Nervous	92
Aphonia	44	Constipation	64	Had to quit working	44
Lump in throat	28	Dysuria	44	because felt bad	
Fits or	20	Urinary retention	8	Trouble doing anything	72
convulsions		Dysmenorrhea	4	because felt bad	
Faints	56	(prepremarital only)		Cried a lot	60
Unconsciousness	16	Dysmenorrhea	8	Felt life was hopeless	28
Amnesia	8	(prepregnancy only)		Always sickly (most of life)	40
Visual blurring	64	Dysmenorrhea (other)	48	Thought of dying	48
Visual	12	Menstrual irregularity	48	Wanted to die	36
hallucination		Excessive menstrual	48	Thought of suicide	28
Deafness	4	bleeding		Attempted suicide	12
Olfactory	16	Sexual indifference	44		
hallucination		Frigidity (absence of	24		
Weakness	84	orgasm)			
		Dyspareunia	52		
		Back pain	88		

Adapted from M. Perley and S. B. Guze (60).

The dramatic, colorful, exaggerated description of symptoms is best conveyed by quoting patients, though it should be noted that not all patients show this trait to the same degree. The following quotations are from Purtell et al. (62):

Vomiting: "I vomit every ten minutes. Sometimes it lasts for two to three weeks at a time. I can't even take liquids. I even vomit water. I can't stand the smell of food."

Food intolerance: "I can't eat pastries. Always pay for it. I can't eat steak now. I throw up whole milk. I always throw up the skins of tomatoes. Pudding made with canned milk makes me sick. I have to use fresh milk."

A trance: "I passed out on the bathroom floor during my period and was still on the floor when they found me the next morning."

Weight change: "I can lose weight just walking down the street. I can hold my breath and lose weight. I was down to 65 pounds at one time."

Dysmenorrhea: "I can't work. Every month I am in bed for several days. I have had to have morphine hypos. There is a throbbing pain in the legs as if the blood doesn't circulate. Can't go to the bathroom as I faint. It's murder! I want to die. It affects my nervous system."

Sexual indifference: "Have never been interested." "It's not a normal thing to me. Disgusting. My husband has never bothered me." "It's just a part of my married life. I have to do it." "I was only disappointed. Never really enjoyed it, but I had to please my husband." "I have no feelings. It's just a duty."

Dyspareunia: "Every time I had intercourse I swelled up on one side. It's sore and burns, and afterwards is very painful." "I hate it. I have a severe pain on the right side and have to go to bed for a day."

Presenting complaints: "I am sore all over. I can't explain it. I have been sick all my life. Now I am alone since my husband died, and the doctor said I must come for help. It has taken $10,000 to keep me alive. This is my 76th hospitalization." "I have been taking care of my invalid mother and I get very little rest or sleep." "My father came here for a checkup on his diabetes and insisted that I come along. I had a nervous breakdown in 1943 and have never gotten around to being really well."

The gynecologist, the neurologist, and the psychiatrist are likely to see somatization-disorder patients with more focused complaints: the gynecologist because of menstrual pain, irregularity, lapses, or dyspareunia; the neurologist because of headaches, "spells," or other conversion symptoms; the psychiatrist because of suicide attempts, depression, or marital discord. But even these specialists find it difficult to obtain straightforward histories from patients with somatization disorder.

Among the characteristic recurrent or chronic symptoms in hysteria, pains are very prominent: headaches, chest pain, abdominal pain, back pain, and joint pain. Abdominal, pelvic, and back pain in association with menstrual or sexual difficulties account for frequent gynecologic surgery: dilatation and curettage, uterine suspension, and salpingo-oophorectomy. Abdominal pain, back pain, dysuria, and dyspareunia account for frequent catheterization and cystoscopy. Abdominal pain, indigestion, bowel difficulties, and vomiting are associated with frequent gastrointestinal X-ray examinations and rectal and gallbladder surgery.

Repeated hospitalization and surgery are characteristic of these conditions (20). Because of the dramatic and persistent symptoms, patients are hospitalized for observation, tests, X-rays, and treatment of a wide variety of medical and surgical conditions that may be mimicked by somatization disorder.

Nervousness and somatic anxiety symptoms (palpitation, dyspnea, chest pain, dizziness, fatigue, tremulousness) are frequent. When chest pain is prominent, it often leads to a diagnosis of heart disease, too often supported only by nonspecific deviations in the EKG. The same nervousness and anxiety symptoms, especially when associated with globus (lump in throat) or weight loss, frequently lead to thyroid studies and the diagnosis of thyroid abnormalities. Before the advent of modern laboratory methods for evaluating thyroid function, thyroidectomy was performed for suspected hyperthyroidism, particularly in older patients. Moodiness, irritability, depression, suicidal ideation, and suicide attempts are common and lead to psychiatric hospitalization (22). Hysteria accounts for a significant minority of suicide attempts (69) but rarely leads to suicide (64).

Menstrual symptoms and sexual indifference or frigidity are so characteristic that a diagnosis of Briquet syndrome or somatization disorder should be made with care if the menstrual and sexual histories are normal. Marital discord related to sexual indifference and frigidity frequently leads to separation and divorce (36).

Recent studies emphasize a point recognized in the past—that somatization disorder is a "psychoform" condition as much as a "somatoform" one (45, 56, 59, 70, 83). Patients are as prone to report a wide range of psychological or emotional symptoms as they are to report physical ones.

The question of malingering frequently arises in discussions about these patients. Although often suspected, malingering is difficult to prove. Nevertheless, malingering and factitious lesions are striking features in some cases (63). Factitious fever produced by heating thermometers with matches or friction, skin lesions produced by self-injections, and hemoptysis and hematuria produced by pricking fingers and adding blood to sputum or urine may take months or years to recognize. An occasional patient will confide that a given symptom or sign was produced artificially in the past but will insist that it is now real.

These syndromes may be present in many patients demonstrating full or partial manifestations of dissociative identity disorder (formerly termed multiple personality disorder) (7, 59). Though multiple personality disorder is considered a rare phenomenon, the reported frequency increased dramatically in the last 25 years (59), perhaps as a result of widespread attention in the professional and popular news media (8, 32). Similarly, Briquet syndrome or somatization disorder can often be diagnosed in patients meeting the criteria for borderline personality disorder. In fact, evidence from a number of recent studies suggests that many cases of these two overlapping syndromes and both borderline and multiple personality disorders may all be manifestations of a single condition, the various manifestations of which may vary in prominence and severity over time and with different circumstances (7, 32, 41, 59, 83).

The long-recognized association of antisocial personality and Briquet syndrome within the same individual and within families (4, 11, 12, 16–18, 37, 39, 74, 86), discussed below, may tie together a number of different clinical features, and one is reminded of the old tale of several blind men drawing different conclusions about an elephant from the different parts of the animal's body each touches.

Another characteristic feature of somatization disorder is the tendency of many patients to give inconsistent histories (35); thus, symptoms that lead to hospitalization on one occasion are denied on another (54). Though this inconsistency has not been studied systematically, it may be related to the patient's perception of the physician's response to her and her desire to influence the physician's judgment about her illness.

Patients with somatization disorder do not often confide all their symptoms in a single interview, and thus it is usually necessary to obtain sufficient information by consulting medical records, questioning collateral sources, and observing the evolution of symptom complaints over time (51). These patients may incorrectly attribute their symptoms to medical illness, obscuring the pattern of multiple medically unexplained symptoms characteristic of somatization disorder (19, 51). The difficulties in obtaining information needed for the diagnosis commonly lead to underrecognition of the disorder in clinical practice. To detect cases, a high index of suspicion for the diagnosis must be maintained and systematic effort made to track down the necessary information (26, 30, 77).

The association between somatization disorder and sociopathy is of great interest. The familial aspect of this association will be discussed below (see section "Family Studies"), but there is a clinical aspect as well. Many delinquent or antisocial adolescent girls develop somatization disorder as adults (66); many somatization-disorder patients give a history of delinquent or antisocial behavior earlier in life (39, 47); the medical histories of delinquent children indicate an increased prevalence of medical contacts (46); and many convicted women felons present with a mixed picture of sociopathy and somatization (16, 17). Thus, school delinquency, repeated fighting, running away from home, poor work record, poor marital history, sexual promiscuity, heavy drinking, and police trouble are events found in the histories of many, though not all, such women (74). It may be pertinent that Eysenck has concluded from his studies of personality that both hysterics and psychopaths are "extroverted neurotics," a possible reason for associating the two conditions (28).

During periods of emotional stress, somatization disorder patients' speech patterns can deteriorate into disorganized and confused discourse that may simulate cognitive processes of psychosis. These speech patterns in somatization disorder can, however, be differentiated from the formal disturbances of logic and syntax observed in schizophrenia and mania (3, 27, 90). North and colleagues systematized abnormal speech patterns into specific elements (e.g., circumstantialy, vagueness, and loss of goal) collectively termed "nonpsychotic formal thought disorder" (57, 58). Blind raters systematically categorizing elements of speech samples according to nonpsychotic thought disorder criteria successfully differentiated patients with somatization disorder and antisocial personality disorder from each other and from controls with neither disorder.

Natural History

As already noted, it is not easy to determine when the illness began. The vague and often inconsistent history makes the chronology of symptoms difficult to establish. The patient may insist that she has always been "sick" and may describe early difficulties that are hard to evaluate. These patients may also suffer from other illnesses, and, therefore, descriptions of childhood or adolescent disorders that allegedly were diagnosed as rheumatic fever, appendicitis, poliomyelitis, or typhoid fever can be most difficult to judge.

The symptoms fluctuate in severity, but the characteristic features persist: recurrent pains, conversion symptoms, nervousness and depression, sexual and marital discord, repeated hospitalization, and repeated surgery (36). Although systematic follow-up until death of a series of patients has not yet been reported, there is no indication that more than a minority of patients experience marked improvement or permanent remission. Twenty to thirty years of symptoms are typical, and patients who have had the illness for over 40 years are not unusual (61). There is no evidence of excess mortality (24).

On the other hand, the long-term course of the patient with conversion symptoms is determined by the underlying illness rather than by the nature of the symptoms themselves. Because conversion symptoms may be seen in a wide variety of medical, neurologic, and psychiatric disorders (31, 40, 81), patients with these symptoms have a variable prognosis and course.

Complications

The most frequent and important complications of somatization disorder are repeated surgical procedures, drug dependence, marital separation or divorce, and suicide attempts. The first two are presumably preventable if physicians learn to recognize the disorder and manage patients properly. Knowledge that somatization disorder may be an alternate explanation for various pains and other symptoms can help surgeons withhold or postpone cases where objective indications are equivocal or missing. Habit-forming or addictive drugs should be avoided for recurrent or persistent pain. Whether the physician can modify marital discord through psychotherapy is uncertain, but recognizing the frequency of separation and divorce, the physician can certainly direct attention to these problems. The same may be said about suicide attempts, but there the physician can approach patients with hysteria knowing that the risk of complicated suicide is low.

Family Studies

Studies using the Briquet syndrome criteria suggest that the disorder runs in families (4, 21, 84). It was found in one study that about 20% of first-degree (siblings, parents, children) female relatives of index cases met the criteria for the same condition, a 10-fold increase over the prevalence in the general population of women, lending strong support to the validity of the concept of hysteria as an illness. A second study, using "blind" examiners, showed lower numbers and only a 3.5-fold increase in first-degree female relatives compared to similar relatives of index women with a range of other psychiatric disorders (35), but it again confirmed the familial aggregation of cases.

Family studies also indicate that a significant association exists between somatization disorder and antisocial personality. First-degree male relatives of women selected by the Briquet syndrome criteria show an increased prevalence of sociopathy and alcoholism (4, 35, 84). The first-degree female relatives of convicted male felons also show an increased prevalence of Briquet syndrome (37). The findings, in conjunction with the observation that many female sociopaths present with, or develop, the full Briquet syndrome or meet the criteria for somatization disorder (17), have suggested that at least some cases of somatization disorder (Briquet syndrome) and sociopathy share a common etiology.

The widely recognized observation that somatization disorder is predominantly a disorder of women, whereas sociopathy is predominantly a disorder of men, raises the interesting possibility that, depending on the sex of the individual, the same etiologic and pathogenetic factors may lead to different, although sometimes overlapping, clinical pictures. As suggested above, future studies may also show a familial aggregation involving borderline and dissociative disorders as well as somatization disorder and antisocial personality. It may be established that many individuals with any or all of these four clinical conditions are suffering from a common disorder whose overt manifestations vary in accordance with gender and a variety of clinical and social circumstances.

Two studies (11, 12, 79) of adopted children whose biological parents showed antisocial behavior revealed greater-than-normal frequency in female offspring of Briquet syndrome or somatization disorder or other multiple unexplained somatic complaints, thus supporting the hypothesis that these are related disorders. One of these studies was carried out in the United States; the other in Sweden.

Differential Diagnosis

Three psychiatric conditions must, at times, be considered in the differential diagnosis of somatization disorder: panic disorder, major depressive disorder, and schizophrenia. As already noted, the characteristic symptoms of somatization disorder include many that are also seen in panic disorder and depression. If the patient is a young woman with menstrual and sexual difficulties who presents with a full range of anxiety or depressive symptoms, she may nearly meet the diagnostic criteria. Age of onset, details of the symptom picture, course, and mental status will usually help clarify the diagnostic problem. A number of patients with schizophrenia also meet the diagnostic criteria for Briquet syndrome or somatization disorder. Also, an occasional patient with these latter conditions who does not show definite evidence of schizophrenia when first seen will, in time, develop the typical clinical picture of schizophrenia (85). While family studies suggest that some patients may meet the diagnostic criteria for both sociopathy and hysteria (which are thought to be related), similar types of studies on schizophrenia do not reveal an overlap (sociopathy/hysteria), suggesting a lack of familial association. Unlike the situation in which the same patients may meet diagnostic criteria for sociopathy and hysteria, a situation in which family studies suggest that the disorders are associated, the overlap with schizophrenia is not accompanied by evidence of a familial association.

Clinical Management

The diagnosis of somatization disorder (based on Briquet syndrome criteria) provides two advantages. (Whether the *DSM-IV-TR* criteria will prove to be as satisfactory awaits more experience.) For patients with the full diagnostic picture, the physician can predict in over 90% of cases that the characteristic symptoms will continue through time and that other illnesses, which in retrospect could account for the original clinical picture, will not become evident. For patients who do not present with the full diagnostic picture, especially for those who have conversion symptoms and little else, the physician knows that in a substantial number of cases other disorders will become evident that do, in retrospect, account for the original clinical picture (60, 80). Many, perhaps most, of the patients whose symptoms resemble somatization disorder, but fail to meet the explicit diagnostic criteria, will remain undiagnosed at follow-up. Enough of them, however, will turn out to have other serious medical, neurological, or psychiatric disorders to justify the kind of diagnostic open-mindedness that can lead to early recognition of the other illnesses.

Patients with somatoform conditions are difficult to treat (5, 54, 87, 88). The typical clinical picture of recurrent, multiple, vague symptoms combined with doctor-shopping and frequent requests for time and attention can frustrate many physicians. Few of these patients referred for psychiatric treatment persist with such treatment (36). Thus, the burden of caring for them continues to rest with other physicians. A controlled, randomized study indicates, however, that psychiatric consultation may be helpful in reducing the extent and cost of medical care (73). Frustration with "somatizing patients" eventually led to a review (43) of the literature reporting the effectiveness of cognitive-behavioral therapy (CBT). While CBT was considered "effective for somatization" (not necessarily somatization disorder/Briquet syndrome patients), some questioned its lasting effectiveness (1). These questions and the cost of treating somatizing patients eventually led to a NIH-funded research project designed to study patients meeting the formal criteria for somatization disorder in a randomized, single-blind efficacy study of CBT (versus care as usual) (2). The results of this formal first study were encouraging because a significant number were rated as "much" to "very much" improved with CBT (as opposed to augmented medical care) and the patients reported an increase in functioning (with corresponding decrease in symptoms and health care costs). Replication will be necessary.

Until there is general acceptance of a particular therapeutic intervention, the physician's major goal should be to avoid the complications described earlier. Success will depend on winning the patient's confidence without allowing her symptomatic behavior to exhaust the physician's sympathy. The patient and family can be told that the patient tends to experience symptoms that suggest other disorders, but that they are not medically serious. On this basis, the physician can approach each new complaint circumspectly and conservatively, especially with regard to elaborate or expensive diagnostic studies. As the physician grows familiar with the patient, the physician will become increasingly confident in his or her clinical judgments. Remembering that somatization disorder can "explain" many puzzling symptoms, the physician, always looking for objective evidence of other disorders, can avoid unnecessary hospitalization and surgery.

The physician should strive to substitute discussions of the patient's life problems, personality, and concerns for a quick-triggered response of ordering additional tests and X-rays or yet another medication. At the same time, the physician must recognize the limitations resulting from our lack of knowledge about the causes and mechanisms of the disorder.

REFERENCES

1. Allen, L. A., Escobar, J. I., Lehrer, P. M., Gara, M. A., and Woolfolk, R. L. Psychosocial treatments for multiple unexplained physical symptoms: a review of the literature. Psychosom. Med., 64:939–950, 2002.
2. Allen, L. A., Woolfolk, R. L., Escobar, J. I., Gara, M. A., and Hamer, R. M. Cognitive-behavioral therapy for somatization disorder: a randomized controlled trial. Arch. Intern. Med., 166:1512–1518, 2006.
3. Andreasen, N. C., and Grove, W. M. Thought, language, and communication in schizophrenia: diagnosis and prognosis. Schizophr. Bull., 12:348–359, 1986.

4. Arkonac, O., and Guze, S. B. A family study of hysteria. N. Engl. J. Med., *268*:239–242, 1963.

5. Bird, J. The behavioral treatment of hysteria. Br. J. Psychiat., *134*:129–137, 1979.

6. Blinder, M. G. The hysterical personality. Psychiat., *29*:227–235, 1966.

7. Bliss, E. L. A symptom profile of patients with multiple personalities, including MMPI results. J. Nerv. Ment. Dis., *172*:197–202, 1984.

8. Boor, M. The multiple personality epidemic. Additional cases and inferences regarding diagnosis, etiology, dynamics, and treatment. J. Nerv. Ment. Dis., *170*:302–304, 1982.

9. Breuer, J., and Freud, S. *Studies in Hysteria* (Brill, A. A., trans.). New York: Journal of Nervous and Mental Disease Monograph, 1936.

10. Briquet, P. *Traité clinique et thérapeutique â l'hystére.* Paris: J-B Bailliére & Fils, 1859.

11. Cadoret, R. J. Psychopathology in adopted-away offspring of biologic parents with antisocial behavior. Arch. Gen. Psychiat., *35*:176–184, 1978.

12. Cadoret, R. J., Cunningham, L., Loftus, R., and Edwards, J. Studies of adoptees from psychiatrically disturbed biological parents: III. Medical symptoms and illnesses in childhood and adolescence. Am. J. Psychiat., *133*:1316–1318, 1976.

13. Carothers, J. C. Hysteria, psychopathy and the magic word. Mankind Q., *16*:93–103, 1975.

14. Chodoff, P. The diagnosis of hysteria: an overview. Am. J. Psychiat., *131*:1073–1078, 1974.

15. Chodoff, P., and Lyons, H. Hysteria, the hysterical personality and "hysterical" conversion. Am. J. Psychiat., *114*:734–740, 1958.

16. Cloninger, C. R., and Guze, S. B. Female criminals: their personal, familial, and social backgrounds. The relation of these to the diagnoses of sociopathy and hysteria. Arch. Gen. Psychiat., *23*:554–558, 1970.

17. Cloninger, C. R., and Guze, S. B. Psychiatric illness and female criminality: the role of sociopathy and hysteria in the antisocial woman. Am. J. Psychiat., *127*:303–311, 1970.

18. Cloninger, C. R., Martin, R. L., Guze, S. B., and Clayton, P. J. A prospective follow-up and family study of somatization in men and women. Am. J. Psychiat., *143*:873–878, 1986.

19. Cloninger, C. R. and Dokucu, E. M. Somatoform and dissociative disorders. In *The Medical Basis of Psychiatry*, 3rd edition, Fatemi, S. H., Clayton, P. J. (eds.). Totowa, NJ: Humana, pp. 181–194, 2008.

20. Cohen, M., Robins, E., Purtell, J., Altmann, M., and Reid, D. Excessive surgery in hysteria. JAMA, *151*:977–986, 1953.

21. Coryell, W. A blind family history study of Briquet's syndrome. Arch. Gen. Psychiat., *37*:1266–1269, 1980.

22. Coryell, W., and Norten, S. G. Briquet's syndrome (somatization disorder) and primary depression: comparison of background and outcome. Compr. Psychiat., *22*:249–256, 1981.

23. Creed, F., and Barsky, A. A systematic review of the epidemiology of somatisation disorder and hypochondriasis. J. Psychosom. Res., *56*:391–408, 2004.

24. de Figuieredo, J. M., Baiardi, J. J., and Long, D. M. Briquet syndrome in a man with chronic intractable pain. Johns Hopkins Med. J., 147:102–106, 1980.

25. DeSouza, C., and Othmer, E. Somatization disorder and Briquet's syndrome. An assessment of their diagnostic concordance. Arch. Gen. Psychiat., 41:334–336, 1984.

26. duGruy, F., Columbia, L., and Dickinson, P. Somatization in a family practice. J. Fam. Pract., 25:45–51, 1987.

27. Edell, W. S. Role of structure in disordered thinking in borderline and schizophrenic disorders. J. Pers. Assess., 51:23–41, 1987.

28. Eysenck, H. The Dynamics of Anxiety and Hysteria. New York: Praeger, 1957.

29. Farley, J., Woodruff, R. A., and Guze, S. B. The prevalence of hysteria and conversion symptoms. Br. J. Psychiat., 114:1121–1125, 1968.

30. Fink, P., Ewald, H., Jensen, J., Sørensen, L., Engberg, M., Holm, M., and Mink-Jørgensen, P. Screening for somatization and hypochondriasis in primary care and neurological in-patients: a seven-item scale for hypochondriasis and somatization. J. Psychosomat. Res., 46:261–273, 1999.

31. Gatfield, P. D., and Guze, S. B. Prognosis and differential diagnosis of conversion reactions (a follow-up study). Dis. Nerv. Syst., 23:1–8, 1962.

32. Greaves, G. B. Multiple personality. 165 years after Mary Reynolds. J. Nerv. Ment. Dis., 168:577–596, 1980.

33. Guze, S. B. The diagnosis of hysteria: what are we trying to do? Am. J. Psychiat., 124:491–498, 1967.

34. Guze, S. B. The role of follow-up studies: their contribution to diagnostic classification as applied to hysteria. Semin. Psychiat., 2:392–402, 1970.

35. Guze, S. B., Cloninger, C. R., Martin, R. L., and Clayton, P. J. A follow-up and family study of Briquet's syndrome. Br. J. Psychiat., 149:17–23, 1986.

36. Guze, S. B., and Perley, M. J. Observations on the natural history of hysteria. Am. J. Psychiat., 119:690–695, 1963.

37. Guze, S. B., Wolfgram, E. D., McKinney, J. K., and Cantwell, D. P. Psychiatric illness in the families of convicted criminals: a study of 519 first-degree relatives. Dis. Nerv. Syst., 28:651–659, 1967.

38. Guze, S. B., Woodruff, R. A., and Clayton, P. J. A study of conversion symptoms in psychiatric outpatients. Am. J. Psychiat., 128:643–646, 1971.

39. Guze, S. B., Woodruff, R. A., and Clayton, P. J. Hysteria and antisocial behavior: further evidence of an association. Am. J. Psychiat., 127:957–960, 1971.

40. Hafeiz, H. B. Hysterical conversion: a prognostic study. Br. J. Psychiat., 136:548–551, 1980.

41. Hudziak, J. J., Boffelli, T. J., Kreisman, J. J., Battaglia, M. M., Stanger, C., Guze, S. B., and Kriesman, J. J. A clinical study of borderline personality disorder: the significance of Briquet's syndrome (hysteria), somatization disorder, antisocial personality disorder, and substance abuse disorders. Am. J. Psychiat., 153:1598–1606, 1996.

42. Kimble, R., Williams, J. G., and Agra, S. A comparison of two methods of diagnosing hysteria. Am. J. Psychiat., 132:1197–1199, 1975.

43. Kroenke, K., and Swindle, R. Cognitive-behavioral therapy for somatization and symptom syndromes: a critical review of controlled clinical trials. Psychother. Psychosom., 69:205–215, 2000.

44. Kroll, P., Chamberlain, K. R., and Halpern, J. The diagnosis of Briquet's syndrome in a male population. J. Nerv. Ment. Dis., 167:171–174, 1979.

45. Lenze, E. L., Miller, A., Munir, Z., Pornoppadol, C., and North, C. S. Psychiatric symptoms endorsed by somatization disorder patients in a psychiatric clinic. Ann. Clin. Psychiat., 11:73–79, 1999.

46. Lewis, D. O., and Shanok, S. S. Medical histories of delinquent and non-delinquent children: an epidemiologic study. Am. J. Psychiat., 134:1020–1025, 1977.

47. Lilienfeld, S. O., VanValkenburg, C., Larnitz, K., and Akiskal, H. S. The relationship of histrionic personality disorder to antisocial personality and somatization disorders. Am. J. Psychiat., 143:718–722, 1986.

48. Mai, F. M., and Merskey, H. Briquet's Treatise on Hysteria. A synopsis and commentary. Arch. Gen. Psychiat., 37:1401–1405, 1980.

49. Mai, F. M., and Merskey, H. Historical review. Briquet's concept of hysteria: an historical perspective. Can. J. Psychiat., 26:57–63, 1981.

50. Marsden, C. D. Hysteria: a neurologist's view. Psychol. Med., 16:277–288, 1986.

51. Martin, R. L. Problems in the diagnosis of somatization disorder: effects on research and clinical practice. Psychiat. Ann., 18:357–362, 1988.

52. Mohr, P. D., and Bond, M. J. A chronic epidemic of hysterical blackouts in a comprehensive school. Br. Med. J., 284:961–962, 1982.

53. Morrison, J. R. Early birth order in Briquet's syndrome. Am. J. Psychiat., 140:1596–1598, 1983.

54. Murphy, G. E. The clinical management of hysteria. JAMA, 247:2559–2564, 1982.

55. Murphy, G. E., Robins, E., Kuhn, N., and Christiansen, R. F. Stress, sickness and psychiatric disorder in a "normal" population: a study of 101 young women. J. Nerv. Ment. Dis., 134:228–236, 1962.

56. North, C. S. Somatoform disorders. In Adult Psychiatry, 2nd edition, Rubin, E. H., Zorumski, C. F. (eds.). Malden, MA: Blackwell, pp. 261–274, 2005.

57. North, C. S., Hansen, K., Wetzel, R. D., Compton, W., Napier, M., and Spitznagel, E. L. Non-psychotic thought disorder: objective clinical identification of somatization and antisocial personality in language patterns. Compr. Psychiat., 38:171–178, 1997.

58. North, C. S., Kienstra, D. M., Osborne, V. A., Dokucu, M. E., Vassilenko, M., Hong, B., Wetzel, R. D., and Spitznagel, E. L. Interrater reliability and coding guide for nonpsychotic formal thought disorder. Percept. Mot. Skills, 103:395–411, 2006.

59. North, C. S., Ryall, J. M., Ricci, D. A., and Wetzel, R. D. Multiple Personalities, Multiple Disorders: Psychiatric Classification and Media Influence. New York: Oxford, 1993.

60. Perley, M. J., and Guze, S. B. Hysteria—the stability and usefulness of clinical criteria. N. Engl. J. Med., 266:421–426, 1962.

61. Pribor, E. F., Smith, D. S., and Yutzy, S. H. Somatization disorder in elderly patients. Am. J. Geriat. Psychiat., 2:109–117, 1994.

62. Purtell, J. J., Robins, E., and Cohen, M. E. Observations on the clinical aspects of hysteria: a quantitative study of 50 patients and 156 control subjects. JAMA, 146:902–909, 1951.

63. Reis, R. K. Single case study. DSM-III differential diagnosis of Munchausen's syndrome. J. Nerv. Ment. Dis., 168:629–632, 1980.

64. Robins, E., Murphy, G. E., Wilkinson, R. H., Jr., Gassner, S., and Kayes, J. Some clinical considerations in the prevention of suicide based on a study of 134 successful suicides. Am. J. Publ. Health, 49:888–899, 1959.

65. Robins, E., Purtell, J. J., and Cohen, M. E. "Hysteria" in men. N. Engl. J. Med., 246:677–685, 1952.

66. Robins, L. N. *Deviant Children Grown Up: A Sociological and Psychiatric Study of Sociopathic Personality.* Baltimore: Williams & Wilkins, 1966.

67. Rounsaville, B. J., Harding, P. S., and Weissman, M. M. Single case study. Briquet's syndrome in a man. J. Nerv. Ment. Dis., 167:364–367, 1979.

68. Savill, T. D. *Lectures on Hysteria and Allied Vasomotor Conditions.* London: H.J. Glaisher, 1909.

69. Schmidt, E. H., O'Neal, P., and Robins, E. Evaluation of suicide attempts as guide to therapy. Clinical and follow-up study of 109 patients. JAMA, 155:547–557, 1954.

70. Simon, G. E., and VonKorff, M. Somatization and psychiatric disorder in the NIMH Epidemiologic Catchment Area study. Am. J. Psychiat., 148:1494–1500, 1991.

71. Slater, E. Diagnosis of "hysteria." Br. Med. J., 29:1395–1399, 1965.

72. Small, G. W., and Nicoli Jr, A. M. Mass hysteria among schoolchildren. Early loss as a predisposing factor. Arch. Gen. Psychiat., 39:721–724, 1982.

73. Smith, G. R., Monson, R. A., and Ray, D. C. Psychiatric consultation in somatization disorder. N. Engl. J. Med., 314:1407–1413, 1986.

74. Spalt, L. Hysteria and antisocial personality. A single disorder? J. Nerv. Ment. Dis., 168:456–464, 1980.

75. Stefansson, J. G., Messina, J. A., and Meyerwitz, S. Hysterical neurosis, conversion type: clinical and epidemiological considerations. Acta Psychiat. Scand., 53:119–138, 1976.

76. Swartz, M., Blazer, D., Woodbury, M., George, L., and Landerman, R. Somatization disorder in a US southern community: use of a new procedure for analysis of medical classification. Psychol. Med., 16:595–609, 1986.

77. Tomasson, K., Kent, D., and Coryell, W. Somatization and conversion disorders: comorbidity and demographics at presentation. Acta Psychiat. Scand., 84:288–293, 1991.

78. Veith, I. *Hysteria: The History of a Disease.* Chicago: University of Chicago Press, 1965.

79. Von Knorring, A.-L. *Adoption Studies on Psychiatric Illness.* Sweden: Umea, 1983.

80. Watson, C. G., and Buranen, C. J. Nerv. Ment. Dis., 167:243–247, 1979.

81. Watson, C. G., and Buranen, C. The frequency and identification of false positive conversion reactions. J. Nerv. Ment. Dis., 167:243–247, 1979.

82. Weissman, M. M., Myers, J. K., and Harding, P. S. Psychiatric disorders in a US urban community: 1975–1976. Am. J. Psychiat., *135*:459–462, 1978.

83. Wetzel, R. D., Guze, S. B., Cloninger, C. R., Martin, R. L., and Clayton, P. J. Briquet's syndrome (hysteria) is both a somatoform and a "psychoform" illness: a Minnesota Multiphasic Personality Inventory study. Psychosomat. Med., *56*:564–569, 1994.

84. Woerner, P. I., and Guze, S. B. A family and marital study of hysteria. Br. J. Psychiat., *114*:161–168, 1968.

85. Woodruff, R. A., Clayton, P. J., and Guze, S. B. Hysteria: studies of diagnosis, outcome, and prevalence. JAMA, *215*:425–428, 1971.

86. Woodruff, R. Hysteria: an evaluation of objective diagnostic criteria by the study of women with chronic medical illness. Br. J. Psychiat., *114*:1115–1119, 1968.

87. Yutzy, S. H. Somatization. In *Psychosomatic Medicine in the 21st Century*, Blumenfield, B., Strain, J. J. (eds.). Baltimore: Lippincott, Williams, and Wilkins, pp. 537–543, 2006.

88. Yutzy, S. H. Somatoform disorders. In *The American Psychiatric Press Textbook of Psychiatry*, 5th edition, Hales, R. E., Yudofsky, S., Gabbard, G. O. (eds.). Washington, DC: American Psychiatric Press, 2008.

89. Yutzy, S. H., Cloninger, C. R., Guze, S. B., Pribor, E. F., Martin, R. L., Kathol, R. G., Smith, G. R., and Strain, J. J. DSM-IV field trial: testing a new proposal for somatization disorder. Am. J. Psychiat., *152*:97–101, 1995.

90. Zanarini, M. C., Gunderson, J. G., and Frankenburg, F. R. Cognitive features of borderline personality disorder. Am. J. Psychiat., *147*:57–63, 1990.

91. Ziegler, F. J., Imboden, J. B., and Meyer, E. Contemporary conversion reactions: clinical study. Am. J. Psychiat., *116*:901–910, 1960.

92. American Psychiatric Association. *Diagnostic and Statistical Manual of Mental Disorders*, 4th edition, text revision. Washington, DC: Author, 2000.

9

Antisocial Personality (Sociopathy)

Antisocial personality (sociopathy or sociopathic personality) refers to a pattern of recurrent antisocial, delinquent, and criminal behavior that begins in childhood or early adolescence and is manifested by disturbances in many areas of life: family relations, schooling, work, military service, and marriage.

Historical Background

Prichard's 1835 monograph, *A Treatise on Insanity and Other Disorders Affecting the Mind*, is often cited as furnishing the first description of what is now called antisocial or sociopathic personality (71). Under the label "moral insanity" he defined the disorder in this way:

> The intellectual faculties appear to have sustained little or no injury, while the disorder is manifested principally or alone in the state of the feelings, temper, or habits. In cases of this description the moral and active principles of the mind are strongly perverted and depraved, the power of self government is lost or impaired and the individual is found to be incapable . . . of conducting himself with decency and propriety, having "undergone a morbid change." As Craft argued (19), Prichard included under this rubric many examples of "temporary mental illness,"

and most of those cases were probably patients with affective disorder. Craft quoted Clouston's 1883 volume (17): "Prichard... vividly described the disease, but I should place most of his cases in my category of simple mania."

Clouston referred also to children "so constituted that they cannot be educated in morality on account of an innate brain deficiency... incapable of knowing... right and wrong.... Such moral idiots I, like others, have met with frequently... and persons with this want of development we may label under moral insanity."

Craft pointed out that Prichard used "moral" in three ways: first, in referring to "moral" treatment, meaning psychological treatment; second, in referring to emotional or affective responses in contrast to intellectual ones; and third, in an ethical sense of right or wrong. Most of the time, Prichard used the term in the first two ways and only incidentally in the last way.

As Craft also noted, Benjamin Rush in 1812 described "derangement of the moral faculties" as follows (78):

The moral faculty, conscience, and sense of deity are sometimes totally deranged. The Duke of Sully has given us a striking instance of this universal moral derangement in the character of a young man who belonged to his suite, of the name of Servin, who, after a life uncommonly distinguished by every possible vice, died, cursing and denying his God. Mr. Haslam has described two cases of it in the Bethlem Hospital, one of whom, a boy of 13 years of age, was perfectly sensible of his depravity, and often asked "why God had not made him like other men."... In the course of my life, I have been consulted in three cases of the total perversion of the moral faculties. One of them was in a young man, the second in a young woman, both of Virginia, and the third was in the daughter of a citizen of Philadelphia. The last was addicted to every kind of mischief. Her mischief and wickedness had no intervals while she was awake, except when she was kept busy in some steady and difficult employment. In all of these cases of innate, preternatural moral depravity, there is probably an original defective organization in those parts of the body which are occupied by the moral faculties of the mind.

It was Craft's conclusion that "Rush appears to give the first description of those with sound reason and good intellect who have an innate or lifelong irresponsibility without shame, being unchanged in affect, or by the consequences or by regard for others." Thus, Craft challenged the appropriateness of crediting Prichard with the first description.

Controversy over the concept of "moral insanity" developed partly in regard to the question of whether the "morally insane" should be committed to mental hospitals or should be considered mentally ill in a court of law. The terms gradually fell into disuse as interest in the whole range of personality disorders grew.

In 1889 Koch (47) introduced the term "psychopathic inferiority" to imply a constitutional predisposition for many deviations of personality, including at least some that are now classified as anxiety disorders. Kraepelin (49), Kahn (45), and Schneider (81) proposed various classifications of personality disorders. Schneider's definition of psychopathic personalities as "all those abnormal personalities who suffer from their abnormalities or cause society to suffer" clearly included much more than "moral imbecility."

The term "psychopathic personality" was used inconsistently, sometimes to refer to the whole spectrum of deviant personalities and sometimes to a subgroup of antisocial or aggressive "psychopaths." Finally, to reduce confusion, the term "sociopathic personality disturbance" was introduced for the latter group and was adopted in 1952 by the American Psychiatric Association's *Diagnostic and Statistical Manual of Mental Disorders*, first edition (*DSM-I*). Nevertheless, many went on using the terms "psychopathy" and "sociopathy" interchangeably, whereas others continued to regard sociopathy as only one form of psychopathy. In a further attempt to reduce confusion, "antisocial personality" was adopted as the official diagnosis for the aggressive or antisocial psychopath or sociopath in later revisions of the *DSM* and the International Classification of Disease (ICD). Sir Aubrey Lewis summarized the history of the concept (52). Over time the antisocial personality disorder diagnosis became widely accepted as the first formally established personality disorder. Unfortunately, because of evidence in the recent past in other countries that psychiatric diagnoses have been applied to political dissenters, some psychiatrists have been reluctant to use this diagnosis, despite the recognition that individuals with the clinical picture of antisocial personality are found all over the world and that only a few are political dissenters.

Epidemiology

Satisfactory data on the prevalence of antisocial personality are lacking. This partly reflects the failure to reach a general agreement about a definition. In the Epidemiologic Catchment Area Study, the prevalence varied between 2.6% and 5.1%, depending upon variation in diagnostic criteria (77). The ratio of males to females in this study varied between 1.62%/1.25% and 9.4%/1.5%. The prevalence of sociopathy in forensic settings and correctional settings has been estimated at 50% (40, 77). In general, we do not know what proportion of sociopaths come to the attention of physicians. Nevertheless, sociopathy is seen frequently in psychiatric facilities, usually because of associated alcohol/other substance abuse/dependence and depression, and because psychiatric care is made a condition of probation/parole. In one series, 15% of male and 3% of female psychiatric outpatients were sociopaths (91).

Indirect estimates of population frequency, based on figures for juvenile delinquency and police trouble of all kinds, suggest that sociopathy is common, probably increasingly so; much more frequent in males than females; more common in urban than rural environments; and most common in low socioeconomic groups (55, 76).

Individuals with sociopathy usually come from grossly disturbed families. Parental separation or divorce, early death, desertion, alcoholism, and criminality are characteristic. Only a small minority of sociopaths, in fact, come from families that are not characterized by one or more of these phenomena (18, 24, 35, 44, 48).

Clinical Picture

Sociopathy begins in childhood or early adolescence (4, 64). The first manifestations may be those of the hyperactive child syndrome (24, 57, 63, 65, 79, 80, 90). An adoption study found evidence for a genetic factor associated with some cases of childhood hyperactivity/attention-deficit disorder and adult antisocial personality (11). Other investigators have demonstrated, however, when early hyperactivity is not accompanied by delinquent or antisocial behavior, it much less often leads to antisocial personality patterns. At the same time, delinquency associated with hyperactivity tends to be more severe than delinquency alone, with a worse prognosis for adult adjustment (67, 88). Restlessness, a short attention span, and unresponsiveness to discipline are common. Frequent fighting, often leading to conflicts with adults, and a history of being a general neighborhood nuisance are also common (14, 75).

A disturbed school history is characteristic of early sociopathy. In fact, a history of satisfactory school adjustment through high school is so unusual that either the diagnosis or the history should be questioned if it is present. Disruption of classes by talking out of turn, failure to pay attention to the teacher, fighting with classmates, arguing with the teacher, and even fighting with the teacher occur. Academic failures, truancy, and suspension often lead to school dropout or permanent expulsion (14, 37, 75).

Running away from home is also common, though it may be limited to a few one-night episodes. Occasionally, adolescents will disappear for weeks or months. During such absences, they may wander around the country, hitch-hiking, doing odd jobs, and bumming around (75).

The job history is characterized by poor performance. Lack of dependability (being late, missing work, quitting without warning), inability to accept criticism and advice, frequent job changes without advancement, and being fired are typical (14, 75). Poor job performance coupled with limited and incomplete education result in low socioeconomic status, low income, and frequent requests for financial assistance from family or society.

Early marriage is typical, especially among women. Very few women with sociopathy, in fact, fail to marry. Their marriages are marked by infidelity, separation, and divorce. Males have similar marital difficulties. Individuals with the disorder tend to marry those with the disorder (15, 33).

Judges used to handle male delinquents by suspending punishment if the delinquent enlisted in the armed services. Generally, however, individuals with sociopathy do not do well in military service. Lack of reliability and inability to conform to military discipline results in AWOL absences, difficulties with superiors, court-martials, and less-than-honorable discharges. The type of discharge is usually determined by the nature of the offenses, the philosophy of the commanding officer, and general military policy at the time.

Sooner or later most individuals with the disorder have trouble with the law. Some investigators, in fact, have required police trouble for the diagnosis of sociopathy (32). Stealing money from mother's purse or father's wallet or from a schoolmate may be an early sign of a budding criminal career. Shoplifting, peace disturbance (usually associated with drunkenness and fighting), various traffic offenses, auto theft, burglary, larceny, rape, robbery, and homicide may all occur. A sociopathic pattern of behavior is found in many convicted male (32, 34, 39) and female (15) felons.

Many individuals with sociopathy engage in lying and the use of aliases, usually as understandable responses to social or legal difficulties, but sometimes without any obvious need to avoid punishment or retaliation. Such behavior has been called "pathological lying." Elaborate stories may be told to confuse or impress relatives. This behavior can take extreme forms such as masquerading as a physician, military officer, or businessperson. In time, relatives, friends, parole officers, and physicians learn to discount a significant amount of what they are told by the individual.

Conversion symptoms (unexplained neurological symptoms) are common in the disorder; in fact, sociopathy is second only to somatization disorder in producing such symptoms (36). Among individuals with sociopathy, conversion symptoms are characteristically associated with obvious social stresses such as police trouble. The full somatization disorder may also be seen in association with sociopathy. Many women with somatization disorder give a history of previous or concurrent sociopathy (15); many young delinquent and antisocial girls develop somatization disorder as adults (15, 56, 75).

Many studies of delinquents and individuals with sociopathy indicate that their average IQ is below normal, but only a minority of delinquents and individuals with sociopathy suffer from significant mental deficiency, with an IQ less than 70 (19, 55). These studies have not all been adequately controlled for socioeconomic status, sibship size, and other variables correlated with intelligence. Low intelligence probably is not an important factor in the etiology of sociopathy.

A charming manner, lack of guilt or remorse, absence of anxiety, and a failure to learn by experience are said to be characteristic of sociopathy. The easygoing, open, and winning style, when present, presumably accounts for the sociopath's success as a confidence man. At best, however, the charm and appeal are superficial; often they are entirely absent.

When seen by psychiatrists, many individuals with sociopathy report anxiety symptoms, depression, and guilt (12, 91). These frequently occur with alcoholism. The guilt and remorse do not seem to lead to reduction of sociopathic behavior, however. This persistence of sociopathic behavior, despite repeated failure and punishment, is the basis for the statement that sociopaths "do not learn from experience." Suicide attempts are not rare, but completed suicide, in the absence of alcoholism or drug dependence, is infrequent (25).

Many people occasionally manifest antisocial or delinquent behavior. But only a minority demonstrates a consistent pattern of recurrent and repeated antisocial, delinquent, and criminal behavior beginning in childhood and lasting well into adulthood. The following case provides a vivid example of such persistent and pervasive behavior, justifying the diagnosis of antisocial personality.

A 28-year-old white man was seen in a hospital's emergency room because of repeated "spells" or "fits" while in jail; he had been arrested for driving while intoxicated, disturbing the peace, and resisting arrest. The patient's problem behavior had begun at about age 7 or 8 when his parents reported to the local school that they could not handle their son because he was "wild" and "couldn't sit still." Similar behavior had been noted by the school, and a request had been made for the parents to meet with the teacher. From that time forward, a recurrent pattern became evident of fighting in school, other discipline troubles, poor academic performance, several periods of suspension, and several periods of truancy.

At the same time, the parents noted that the patient stole money from them and began to stay out late at night, presumably running around with a neighborhood gang. At about age 14, the boy had his first police contact. He and several members of his gang were arrested for stealing from a number of neighborhood stores. Nothing came of this, but at age 17 the patient was arrested for driving a stolen vehicle; he received a suspended sentence. Soon thereafter, he dropped out of school and started to work. His work record was most unsatisfactory, however, because of frequently missing days of work and because he was considered to be a troublemaker by his supervisors. As a result of this pattern, he failed at several jobs. He then enlisted in the army, where his inability to conform to expectations and accept military discipline resulted in a discharge "without honor" after about 10 months.

Soon after leaving the army, he got married, but, as soon as his wife became pregnant, he deserted her. Around that time his parents became aware that he was drinking excessively and experimenting with a variety of illicit street drugs. He and his wife had a stormy marriage with frequent separations and reconciliations. After the birth of three children, they permanently separated. His wife accused him of physical abuse and repeated infidelity, as well as inappropriate physical aggression toward the children (beating).

His work record continued to be erratic, and he was a frequent visitor to local medical clinics and emergency rooms with a variety of physical complaints. On one occasion, he was admitted briefly to a psychiatric unit because of taking an overdose of sleeping pills and some of the other drugs he was using.

In short, this patient's history is typical for antisocial personality. It includes all sorts of interpersonal and social difficulties, including problems and conflicts at school, with parents, on the job, in the army, with his wife and children, and with the police. The diagnostic criteria from *DSM-IV-TR* are presented in Table 9.1.

Biological Findings

Multitudinous studies have attempted to assess "constitutional" factors in sociopathy over many years (84). One of the earlier organic theories was based on more frequent reports of nonspecifically disordered electroencephalograms

TABLE 9.1 Diagnostic Criteria for Antisocial Personality Disorder

---

A. There is a pervasive pattern of disregard for and violation of the rights of others occurring since age 15 years, as indicated by three (or more) of the following:

  (1) Failure to conform to social norms with respect to lawful behaviors as indicated by repeatedly performing acts that are grounds for arrest
  (2) Deceitfulness, as indicated by repeated lying, use of aliases, or conning others for personal profit or pleasure
  (3) Impulsivity or failure to plan ahead
  (4) Irritability and aggressiveness, as indicated by repeated physical fights or assaults
  (5) Reckless disregard for safety of self or others
  (6) Consistent irresponsibility, as indicated by repeated failure to sustain consistent work behavior or honor financial obligations
  (7) Lack of remorse, as indicated by being indifferent to or rationalizing having hurt, mistreated, or stolen from another

B. The individual is at least age 18 years.
C. There is evidence of conduct disorder with onset before age 15 years.
D. The occurrence of antisocial behavior is not exclusively during the course of schizophrenia or a manic episode.

Adapted from diagnostic criteria in the *DSM-IV-TR* (93).

(EEGs) among individuals with sociopathy than controls; however, many, if not most, do not have abnormal EEGs (3, 28). Some authors have reported an association between delinquency, learning disability, and neurological impairment, but this has not been a completely consistent finding (87). Many studies have explored psychophysiological response patterns in sociopathy, and a theory of low autonomic and cortical arousal has been formulated to account for a persistent "stimulus hunger" or for the inability to learn socially approved behavior. The theory is thought to explain the impulsive, excitement-seeking, and antisocial behavior of sociopathy (38, 61, 72, 79). More recent studies have suggested that lowered cerebrospinal fluid 5-hydroxyindoleacetic acid levels, pointing to some alteration in serotonin metabolism, may predict antisocial behavior, alone or in combination with various measures of autonomic arousal (51). The research findings have not been entirely consistent (61), and some authors (60) have emphasized "a wider degree of variability in arousal levels and reactivity than [in] normal individuals." An association between criminal behavior and chromosomal abnormalities has been reported. In particular, XYY karyotype, unusual height, and impulsive crimes have been associated, but not all studies are consistent (2, 22, 43, 66). On the other hand, more cases of the XXY karyotype (Klinefelter syndrome) than of the XYY karyotype were found in a large Finnish series of male criminals referred for psychiatric evaluation (82).

Studies of hormone levels, including androgens and adrenal steroids, have shown inconsistent differences between sociopathic and nonsociopathic subjects (23, 50, 59). In summary, innumerable investigations have been undertaken over many years, but they have yet to reveal an organic etiology or a reliable physiological marker.

Natural History

Sociopathy begins early in life (76). In some cases it may begin before the child starts attending school. Few sociopaths get through high school without recurrent difficulties. If the antisocial and delinquent pattern has not begun by age 15 or 16, it is unlikely to occur. The prognosis may be better when the juvenile delinquency is "socialized," that is, when it occurs in a setting of close group involvement or loyalty (41). Lower social class, being female, and relative youth may adversely affect the clinical picture, but this is not a consistent finding (5).

The disorder is recurrent and varies in severity. Some individuals with sociopathy, generally milder cases, may remit during the late teens or early or mid-20s (46). In other instances, sociopathic behavior persists into early middle age and then remits (1, 6, 89). Some of these individuals never improve. Attempts to explain remission have been based on hypothetical maturing or burning out.

Remission, when it occurs, usually comes only after years of sociopathic behavior, during which education and work achievement have been severely compromised. Individuals with sociopathy rarely recover sufficiently to compensate for the "lost years." Thus, "remission" usually means no more than a marginal social adjustment. Even if sociopathic behavior subsides, alcohol and drug abuse/dependence persist and influence long-term adjustment (58).

Complications

The complications of sociopathy explain why the disorder is legitimately a medical concern. High rates of sexually transmitted disease, extramarital pregnancies, injuries from fights and accidents, alcohol and drug dependence (10, 26, 42, 53, 54), and various medical complications of these conditions mean that individuals with sociopathy often come to the attention of physicians. Furthermore, increased mortality from accidents and homicide contributes to a reduced life expectancy, particularly in early adulthood (32, 74).

Family Studies

As noted, individuals with sociopathy generally come from families with severe social disturbances and disruption. Much of this family pathology consists of sociopathy and alcoholism (68–70). In a study of male felons, most of whom were sociopathic, one-fifth of the first-degree male relatives had sociopathy and one-third were alcoholics (35). In a study of female felons, half of whom had sociopathy, one-third of the male relatives had sociopathy and one-half were alcoholic (16). In a study of children seen in a child guidance clinic (75), one-third of the fathers and one-tenth of the mothers of antisocial children had either sociopathy or alcohol dependence.

Among the attempts to determine whether this familial pattern reflects genetic factors have been investigations of twins and adoptees. Twin studies generally have focused on antisocial behavior, delinquency, or criminality, without distinguishing between individuals with sociopathy and others who show these behavior patterns. Nevertheless, as most criminals apparently have sociopathy (32), this approach appears somewhat justified. In twin studies, the concordance rates with regard to behavior difficulties, delinquency, and criminality have nearly always been higher for monozygotic than dizygotic twins (61, 85). However, the differences have not been as great as those seen in other psychiatric illnesses where a genetic predisposition is suspected. Furthermore, all of the series have been small and the monozygotic-dizygotic difference in some did not reach statistical significance.

Twin studies of psychiatric illness may involve bias in ascertainment of cases because concordant cases may come to the attention of physicians more often than discordant cases. Population twin registries have been proposed as more suitable for unbiased ascertainment. Christiansen was able to obtain a presumably unselected series of criminal twins through access to a register of all Danish twin births (13). He found that monozygotic twins had a significantly higher concordance rate than dizygotic twins (36% versus 12%).

Several follow-up studies of children of criminals and "psychopaths" indicate that these children, when adopted early in life by nonrelatives, are more likely to reveal psychopathic and criminal behavior as adults than are adopted children whose biological parents were not criminals or psychopaths (7–9, 20, 21, 83). The association between sociopathy and somatization disorder within families and in the same individual (discussed in Chapter 8) has been confirmed in other studies (86). In summary, twin and adoptee studies at least suggest a genetic predisposition in some cases of sociopathy.

Differential Diagnosis

The differential diagnosis of sociopathy includes alcohol dependence, drug dependence, somatization disorder, schizophrenia, mania, and brain syndrome. Alcohol and drug abuse are frequent complications of sociopathy, and they aggravate antisocial and criminal patterns. In addition, however, some alcohol and drug abusers who did not show sociopathic behavior in childhood or adolescence before the onset of alcohol or drug dependence do show such behavior as a manifestation of the alcohol or drug dependence. In these cases, the crucial diagnostic feature is the age of onset of antisocial and delinquent behavior; it is usually after age 15 and coincident with, or following, the onset of the alcohol and drug abuse. When sociopathic behavior and alcohol or drug abuse all begin about the same time and before age 15, only follow-up may clarify the diagnosis, and often it is not possible to separate the sociopathy from the alcohol or drug dependence.

The familial and clinical associations between sociopathy and somatization disorder have already been noted. Many women with sociopathy and an occasional man with sociopathy develop the picture of somatization disorder (37, 56). Moreover, there is an increased frequency of antisocial behavior and delinquency in the past histories and family histories of women with somatization disorder who are not sociopathic (37). Finally, somatization disorder and sociopathy cluster in the same families. All these observations suggest that the differential diagnosis between the two conditions may involve the recognition of overlapping manifestations of similar etiologic factors (31).

A small minority of men with schizophrenia give a history of sociopathic patterns in adolescence, and a small number of young people with sociopathy, at follow-up, turn out to have schizophrenia (75), but the prevalence of antisocial personality is not increased in the biological relatives of individuals with schizophrenia compared to the relatives of controls (73). If evidence of schizophrenia has not appeared by the early 20s, however, it is unlikely to develop.

The behavior in early-onset mania may mimic that of sociopathy, especially in women. Occasionally it will be difficult to distinguish mania from sociopathy when the latter is complicated by amphetamine or other drug abuse. Follow-up should clarify the issue. Because mania before age 15 is rare, a history of antisocial and delinquent behavior before that age would suggest sociopathy rather than mania. Although antisocial and criminal behavior may accompany an organic brain syndrome, the latter rarely develops in childhood or early adolescence.

Clinical Management

A major problem in treating sociopathy is the patient's lack of motivation for change. Few sociopaths volunteer for treatment. They are nearly always brought to the physician's attention by pressure from schools, parents, or judges. Moreover, the commonly disturbed family situation and poor socioeconomic circumstances provide little support for any treatment program. Many therapists believe that early institutional therapy offers the only hope for success, but there is no consensus about this (29). Psychotherapy has not achieved impressive results (92). Biological psychiatry provides no offer of any empirically supported treatment intervention (30, 62).

It is particularly difficult to carry out treatment if associated alcoholism or drug dependence cannot be controlled. In many cases, remission of the alcohol or drug abuse is accompanied by a reduction in antisocial and criminal behavior (32). Because sociopathy begins early and individuals at high risk can be readily recognized (27, 75), early case finding and intervention may ultimately offer hope of prevention.

REFERENCES

1. Stoff, D. M., Breiling, J., and Maser, J. D. (eds.). *Handbook of Antisocial Behavior.* New York: John Wiley, 1997.
2. Akesson, H. O., Forssman, H., Wahlstrom, J., and Wallin, L. Sex chromosome aneuploidy among men in three Swedish hospitals for the mentally retarded and maladjusted. Br. J. Psychiat., 125:386–389, 1974.
3. Arthurs, R., and Cahoon, E. A clinical and electroencephalographic survey of psychopathic personality. Am. J. Psychiat., 120:875–877, 1964.
4. Behar, D., and Stewart, M. A. Aggressive conduct disorder of children. The clinical history and direct observations. Acta Psychiat. Scand., 65:210–220, 1982.
5. Behar, D., and Stewart, M. A. Aggressive conduct disorder: the influence of social class, sex and age on the clinical picture. Psychol. Psychiat., 25:119–124, 1984.
6. Bland, R. C., Newman, S. C., and Orn, H. Age and remission of psychiatric disorders. Can. J. Psychiat., 42:722–729, 1997.
7. Cadoret, R. J. Psychopathology in adopted-away offspring of biologic parents with antisocial behavior. Arch. Gen. Psychiat., 35:176–184, 1978.
8. Cadoret, R. J., and Cain, C. Sex differences in predictors of antisocial behavior in adoptees. Arch. Gen. Psychiat., 37:1171–1175, 1980.
9. Cadoret, R. J., Cunningham, L., Loftus, R., and Edwards, J. Studies of adoptees from psychiatrically disturbed biological parents. II. Temperament, hyperactive, antisocial and developmental variables. J. Pediat., 87:301–306, 1975.

10. Cadoret, R. J., O'Gorman, T. W., Troughton, E., and Heywood, E. Alcoholism and antisocial personality: interrelationships, genetics and environmental factors. Arch. Gen. Psychiat., 42:161–167, 1985.

11. Cadoret, R. J., and Stewart, M. A. An adoption study of attention deficit/hyperactivity/aggression and their relationship to adult antisocial personality. Compr. Psychiat., 32:73–82, 1991.

12. Chiles, J. A., Miller, M. L., and Cox, G. B. Depression in an adolescent delinquent population. Arch. Gen. Psychiat., 37:1179–1184, 1980.

13. Christiansen, K. O. Crime in a Danish twin population. Acta Genet. Med. Gemellol., 19:323–326, 1970.

14. Cleckley, H. The Mask of Sanity. New York: Mosby, 1982.

15. Cloninger, C. R., and Guze, S. B. Psychiatric illness and female criminality: the role of sociopathy and hysteria in the antisocial woman. Am. J. Psychiat., 127:303–311, 1970.

16. Cloninger, C. R., and Guze, S. B. Psychiatric illness in the families of female criminals: a study of 288 first-degree relatives. Br. J. Psychiat., 122:697–703, 1973.

17. Clouston, T. S. Clinical Lectures on Mental Diseases. London: Churchill, 1883.

18. Cowie, J., Cowie, V., and Slater, E. Delinquency in Girls. London: Humanities Press, 1968.

19. Craft, M. Ten Studies into Psychopathic Personality. Bristol: John Wright & Sons, 1965.

20. Crowe, R. R. The adopted offspring of women criminal offenders. Arch. Gen. Psychiat., 27:600–603, 1972.

21. Crowe, R. R. An adoption study of antisocial personality. Arch. Gen. Psychiat., 31:785–791, 1974.

22. Editorial. What becomes of the XYY male? Lancet, 2:1297–1298, 1974.

23. Ehrenkranz, J., Bliss, E., and Sheard, M. H. Plasma testosterone: correlation with aggressive behavior and social dominance in man. Psychosomat. Med., 36:468–475, 1974.

24. Farrington, D. P. Childhood origins of teenage antisocial behaviour and adult social dysfunction. J. Roy. Soc. Med., 86:13–17, 1993.

25. Garvey, M. J. Suicide attempts in antisocial personality disorder. Compr. Psychiat., 21:146–149, 1980.

26. Gerstley, L. J., Alterman, A. I., McLellan, A. T., and Woody, G. E. Antisocial personality disorder in patients with substance abuse disorders: a problematic diagnosis? Am. J. Psychiat., 147:173–178, 1990.

27. Glueck, S., and Glueck, E. Predicting Delinquency and Crime. Cambridge, MA: Harvard University Press, 1959.

28. Gottlieb, J. S., Ashby, M. C., and Knott, J. R. Primary behavior disorders and psychopathic personality. Arch. Neurol. Psychiat., 56:381–400, 1946.

29. Gralnick, A. Management of character disorders in a hospital setting. Am. J. Psychother., 33:54–66, 1979.

30. Gunderson, J. G., and Phillips, K. A. Personality disorders. In Comprehensive Textbook of Psychiatry, Volume 2, 4th edition, Kaplan, H. I., Sadock, B. J. (eds.). Baltimore: Williams & Wilkins, pp. 1425–1444, 1995.

31. Guze, S. B. The role of follow-up studies: their contribution to diagnostic classification as applied to hysteria. Semin. Psychiat., 2:392–402, 1970.

32. Guze, S. B., Goodwin, D. W., and Crane, J. B. Criminality and psychiatric disorders. Arch. Gen. Psychiat., 20:583–591, 1969.

33. Guze, S. B., Goodwin, D. W., and Crane, J. B. A psychiatric study of the wives of convicted felons: an example of assortative mating. Am. J. Psychiat., 126:1773–1776, 1970.

34. Guze, S. B., Goodwin, D. W., and Crane, J. B. Criminal recidivism and psychiatric illness. Am. J. Psychiat., 127:832–835, 1970.

35. Guze, S. B., Wolfgram, E. D., McKinney, J. K., and Cantwell, D. P. Psychiatric illness in the families of convicted criminals: a study of 519 first-degree relatives. Dis. Nerv. Syst., 28:651–659, 1967.

36. Guze, S. B., Woodruff, R. A., and Clayton, P. J. A study of conversion symptoms in psychiatric outpatients. Am. J. Psychiat., 128:643–646, 1971.

37. Guze, S. B., Woodruff, R. A., and Clayton, P. J. Hysteria and antisocial behavior: further evidence of an association. Am. J. Psychiat., 127:957–960, 1971.

38. Hare, R. D. *Psychopathy: Theory and Research*. New York: John Wiley & Sons, 1970.

39. Hare, R. D. Diagnosis of antisocial personality disorder in two prison populations. Am. J. Psychiat., 140:887–890, 1983.

40. Hare, R. D., Hart, S. D., and Harpur, T. J. Psychopathy and the DSM-IV criteria for antisocial personality disorder. J. Abnorm. Psychol., 100:391–398, 1991.

41. Henn, F. A., Bardwell, R., and Jenkins, R. L. Juvenile delinquents re-visited. Adult criminal activity. Arch. Gen. Psychiat., 37:1160–1163, 1980.

42. Hesselbrock, V., Meyer, R., and Hesselbrock, M. Psychopathology and addictive disorders. In *Addictive States*, O'Brien, C. P., Jaffe, J. H. (eds.). New York: Raven Press, Ltd., pp. 179–191, 1992.

43. Hook, E. B. Behavioral implications of the human XYY genotype. Science, 179:139–150, 1973.

44. Jonsson, G. Delinquent boys, their parents and grandparents. Acta Psychiat. Scand. Suppl., 195:1–264, 1967.

45. Kahn, E. *Psychopathic Personalities*. New Haven, CT: Yale University Press, 1931.

46. Kelso, J., and Stewart, M. A. Factors which predict the persistence of aggressive conduct disorder. J. Child Psychol. Psychiat., 27:77–86, 1986.

47. Koch, J. L. A. *Leitfaden der Psychiatrie*, 2nd edition. Ravensburg, Germany: Dorn, 1889.

48. Koller, K. M., and Castanos, J. N. Family background in prison groups: a comparative study of parental deprivation. Br. J. Psychiat., 117:371–380, 1970.

49. Kraepelin, E. *Dementia Praecox and Paraphrenia* (Barclay, R. M., Robertson, G. M., trans.). Edinburgh: E. & S. Livingstone, 1919.

50. Kreuz, L. E., and Rose, R. M. Assessment of aggressive behavior and plasma testosterone in a young criminal population. Psychosomat. Med., 34:321–332, 1972.

51. Kruesi, M. J., Hibbs, E. D., Zahn, T. P., Keysor, C. S., Hamburger, S. D., Bartko, J. J., and Rapoport, J. L. A 2-year prospective follow-up study of children and adolescents with disruptive behavior disorders. Arch. Gen. Psychiat., 49:429–435, 1992.

52. Lewis, A. Psychopathic personality: a most elusive category. Psychol. Med., 4:133–140, 1974.

53. Lewis, C. E. Alcoholism, antisocial personality, narcotic addiction: an integrative approach. Psychiat. Dev., 3:223–235, 1984.

54. Lucker, G. W., Kruzich, D. J., Holt, M. T., and Gold, J. D. The prevalence of antisocial behavior among U.S. Army DWI offenders. J. Stud. Alcohol., 52:318–320, 1991.

55. Lundin, W. A. Statistics on Delinquents and Delinquency. Springfield, IL: C. C. Thomas, 1964.

56. Maddocks, P. D. A five-year follow-up of untreated psychopaths. Br. J. Psychiat., 116:511–515, 1970.

57. Mannuzza, S., Klein, R. G., Bessler, A., Malloy, P., and LaPadula, M. Adult outcome of hyperactive boys. Educational achievement, occupational rank, and psychiatric status. Arch. Gen. Psychiat., 50:565–576, 1993.

58. Martin, R. L., Cloninger, C. R., and Guze, S. B. The evaluation of diagnostic concordance in follow-up studies: II. A blind, prospective follow-up of female criminals. J. Psychiat. Res., 15:107–125, 1979.

59. Mattson, A., Schalling, D., Olweus, D. L., Löw, H., and Svensson, J. Plasma testosterone, aggressive behavior, and personality dimensions in young male delinquents. J. Am. Acad. Child Adolesc. Psychiat., 19:476–490, 1980.

60. Mawson, A. R., and Mawson, C. D. Psychopathy and arousal: a new interpretation of the psychophysiological literature. Biol. Psychiat., 12:49–74, 1977.

61. Mednick, S., and Christiansen, K. O. Biosocial Bases of Criminal Behavior. New York: Gardner Press, 1977.

62. Meloy, J. R. Antisocial personality disorder. In Treatment of Psychiatric Disorders, Volume 2, 3rd edition, Gabbard, G. O. (ed.). Washington, DC: American Psychiatric Press, pp. 2251–2273, 2001.

63. Mendelson, W., Johnson, N., and Stewart, M. A. Hyperactive children as teenagers: a follow-up study. J. Nerv. Ment. Dis., 153:273–279, 1971.

64. Mitchell, S., and Rosa, P. Boyhood behaviour problems as precursors of criminality: a fifteen-year follow-up study. J. Child Psychol. Psychiat., 22:19–33, 1981.

65. Morrison, J. Adult psychiatric disorders in parents of hyperactive children. Am. J. Psychiat., 137:825–827, 1980.

66. Nielsen, J., and Henrickson, F. Incidence of chromosome aberrations among males in a Danish youth prison. Acta Psychiat. Scand., 48:87–102, 1972.

67. Offord, D. R., Sullivan, K., Allen, N., and Abrams, N. Delinquency and hyperactivity. J. Nerv. Ment. Dis., 167:734–741, 1979.

68. Oliver, J. E. Successive generations of child maltreatment: social and medical disorders in the parents. Br. J. Psychiat., 147:484–490, 1985.

69. Oliver, J. E. Successive generations of child maltreatment. The children. Br. J. Psychiat., 153:543–553, 1988.

70. Oliver, J. E. Intergenerational transmission of child abuse: rates, research, and clinical implications. Am. J. Psychiat., 150:1315–1324, 1993.

71. Prichard, J. C. A Treatise on Insanity and Other Disorders Affecting the Mind. London: Sherwood, Gilbert, and Piper, 1835.

72. Raine, A., Venables, P. H., and Williams, M. Relationships between central and autonomic measures of arousal at age 15 years and criminality at age 24 years. Arch. Gen. Psychiat., 47:1003–1007, 1990.

73. Rimmer, J., and Jacobsen, B. Antisocial personality in the biological relatives of schizophrenics. Compr. Psychiat., 21:258–262, 1980.

74. Robins, L., and O'Neal, P. Mortality, mobility, and crime: problem children thirty years later. Am. Soc. Rev., 23:162–171, 1958.

75. Robins, L. N. *Deviant Children Grown Up: A Sociological and Psychiatric Study of Sociopathic Personality*. Baltimore: Williams & Wilkins, 1966.

76. Robins, L. N. *The Consequences of Conduct Disorder in Girls. Development of Antisocial and Prosocial Behavior*. New York: Academic Press, 1986.

77. Robins, L. N., and Regier, D. A. *Psychiatric Disorders in America: The Epidemiologic Catchment Area Study*. New York: The Free Press, 1991.

78. Rush, B. *Medical Inquiries and Observations upon the Diseases of the Mind*. Philadelphia: Kimber and Richardson, 1812.

79. Satterfield, J. H. The hyperactive child syndrome: a precursor of adult psychopathy. In *Psychopathic Behavior*, Hare, R. D., Schalling, D. (eds.). New York: John Wiley & Sons, pp. 329–346, 1978.

80. Satterfield, J. H., Hoppe, C. M., and Schell, A. M. A prospective study of delinquency in 110 adolescent boys with attention deficit disorder and 88 normal adolescent boys. Am. J. Psychiat., 139:795–798, 1982.

81. Schneider, K. *Psychopathic Personalities*. London: Cassell, 1958.

82. Schröder, J., de la Chapelle, A., Hakola, P., and Virkkunen, M. The frequency of XYY and XXY men among criminal offenders. Acta Psychiat. Scand., 63:272–276, 1981.

83. Schulsinger, F. Psychopathy: heredity and environment. Int. J. Ment. Health, 1:190–206, 1972.

84. Shah, S. Z., and Roth, L. H. Biological and psychophysiological factors in criminality. In *Handbook of Criminology*, Glazer, D. (ed.). Chicago: Rand McNally, pp. 101–173, 1974.

85. Slater, E., and Cowie, V. *The Genetics of Mental Disorders*. London: Oxford University Press, 1971.

86. Spalt, L. Hysteria and antisocial personality. A single disorder? J. Nerv. Ment. Dis., 168:456–464, 1980.

87. Spreen, O. The relationship between learning disability, neurological impairment, and delinquency. Results of a follow-up study. J. Nerv. Ment. Dis., 169:791–799, 1981.

88. Stewart, M. A., Cummings, C., Singer, S., and deBlois, C. S. The overlap between hyperactive and unsocialized aggressive children. J. Child Psychol. Psychiat., 22:35–45, 1981.

89. Sutker, P., and Allain, A. N. Antisocial personality disorder. In *Comprehensive Handbook of Psychopathology*, 3rd edition, Sutker, P. B., Adams, L. J. (eds.). New York: Kluwer Academic/Plenum Publishers, pp. 445–490, 2001.

90. Weiss, G., Hechtman, L., Milroy, T., and Perlman, T. Psychiatric status of hyperactives as adults: a controlled prospective 15-year follow-up of 63 hyperactive children. J. Am. Acad. Child Adolesc. Psychiat., 24:211–220, 1985.

91. Woodruff, Jr. R. A., Guze, S. B., and Clayton, P. J. The medical and psychiatric implications of antisocial personality (sociopathy). Dis. Nerv. Syst., 32:712–714, 1971.

92. Woody, G. E., McClellan, A. T., Luborsky, L., and O'Brien, C. P. Sociopathy and psychotherapy outcome. Arch. Gen. Psychiat., 42:1081–1086, 1985.

93. American Psychiatric Association. *Diagnostic and Statistical Manual of Mental Disorders*, 4th edition, text revision. Washington, DC: Author, 2000.

10

Borderline Personality Disorder

Borderline personality disorder (BPD) is a diagnosis in evolution, as science is actively accruing evidence to demonstrate the validity of diagnostic criteria. The cardinal features of BPD—as it is currently understood—are emotional crises, self-mutilation, and chronic suicidality. Patients may present with multiple wrist and forearm scars from self-inflicted lacerations. If permitted, they may call their psychiatrist every day with suicidal threats or multiple times a day with intolerable emotional states. These features are not the only characteristics of BPD, and they are not pathognomonic—but their presence suggests consideration of the presence of this disorder. Four major areas of psychiatric disturbance are characteristic of BPD: affective instability, cognitive problems, impulsivity, and intense and unstable personal relationships (48).

Borderline personality does not signify borderline schizophrenia. The name "borderline" was originally applied, however, because at the time it was thought to represent a marginal form of schizophrenia.

Borderline personality disorder is one of four disorders classified in the Cluster B category of personality disorders, with the other three being antisocial, histrionic, and narcissistic personality disorders (4). Cluster B personality disorders are a collection of disorders that share pervasive and longstanding patterns of dramatic, emotional, erratic, and impulsive behaviors. Borderline personality disorder in particular is known for its

TABLE 10.1 Criteria for Borderline Personality Disorder *(DSM-IV-TR)*

A pervasive pattern of instability of interpersonal relationships, self-image, and affects, and marked impulsivity beginning by early adulthood and present in a variety of contexts, as indicated by five (or more) of the following:

(1) Frantic efforts to avoid real or imagined abandonment

   Note: Do not include suicidal or self-mutilating behavior covered in Criterion 5.

(2) A pattern of unstable and intense interpersonal relationships characterized by alternating between extremes of idealization and evaluation
(3) Identity disturbance: markedly and persistently unstable self-image or sense of self
(4) Impulsivity in at least two areas that are potentially self-damaging (e.g., spending, sex, substance abuse, reckless driving, binge eating)

   Note: Do not include suicidal or self-mutilating behavior covered in Criterion 5.

(5) Recurrent suicidal behavior, gestures, or threats, or self-mutilating behavior
(6) Affective instability due to a marked reactivity of mood (e.g., intense episodic dysphoria, irritability, or anxiety usually lasting a few hours and only rarely more than a few days)
(7) Chronic feelings of emptiness
(8) Inappropriate, intense anger or difficulty controlling anger (e.g., frequent displays of temper, constant anger, recurrent physical fights)
(9) Transient, stress-related paranoid ideation or severe dissociative symptoms

Adapted from diagnostic criteria in the *Diagnostic and Statistical Manual of Mental Disorders,* fourth edition text revision. Washington, DC: American Psychiatric Association, 2000.

chronic instability of emotions, self-image, and interpersonal relationships. Current diagnostic criteria for BPD are presented in Table 10.1.

The first hint of a "borderline" disorder in the evolving editions of the diagnostic manual of the American Psychiatric Association appeared in 1968 in the second edition, which placed "borderline schizophrenia" within a subcategory of schizophrenia, latent type (93). Borderline personality disorder eventually became an official diagnosis in the manual's third edition in 1980. At that time, BPD was clearly separated from schizophrenia and schizotypal personality disorder. Spitzer and colleagues (93) formally organized the observations of Kernberg (39) and Gunderson and Singer (32) to develop the currently accepted diagnostic criteria for BPD.

Despite many years of research characterizing important aspects of this disorder, its conceptualization is still evolving, in the midst of continuing controversy surrounding the categorization and validity of the borderline personality syndrome. The disorder's name, signifying the entity as a borderline area of another class of psychopathology, reflects confusion about its validity dating to its first origins. A recent apt observation by Paris is that "the 'border' on which BPD lies is between multiple trait dimensions and intersecting diagnostic spectra" (p. 468) (65).

Although progress toward validation of the diagnosis has been made (110), the current definition of BPD does not appear to meet the accepted criteria for diagnostic validity and reliability established nearly 40 years ago (74), especially because of problems of widely inconsistent symptom presentations and phenomenological overlap with other disorders (65). This chapter will identify and discuss the specific areas of diagnostic validity needing further work.

For the reader it should be noted that BPD has been a topic of great interest to researchers and clinicians particularly in the last 30 years. The data-based references in this chapter are cited for what they contribute to the developing knowledge base. The reader should not conclude that the amount of research or findings, or even the inclusion of this diagnosis in this text, signifies validity of the current definition of the disorder.

Historical Background

The diagnosis of BPD has relatively recent historic origins in the psychiatric literature. In the early part of the last century, concepts of "borderland neuroses and psychoses" (15) and "borderline" neuroses (94) arose within the context of clinical observations by therapists of patients undergoing psychoanalysis. Descriptions of "borderline" disorders over the next several decades characterized these patients as suffering from narcissism, hypersensitivity, feelings of inferiority and insecurity, delusion-like projection, masochism, personal rigidity, impaired interpersonal and general reality testing, and negative therapeutic response (95). Many of these patients hailed from chaotic and dysfunctional family backgrounds. Three out of four patients reported childhood histories of longstanding and repeated abuse and neglect.

For more than half a century, the classification of this "borderline syndrome" languished in an ill-defined region between neurotic and psychotic illness (29, 95). During this time, many labels were applied to patients sharing the above characteristics: ambulatory schizophrenia, simple schizophrenia, latent schizophrenia, subclinical schizophrenia, occult schizophrenia, abortive schizophrenia, preschizophrenia, early schizophrenia, pseudopsychopathic schizophrenia, pseudoneurotic schizophrenia, borderland schizophrenia, atypical psychosis, latent psychosis, borderline psychosis, schizophrenic character, psychotic character, "as-if" personality, infantile personality, and hysteroid dysphoria (32, 40, 95, 96). Research eventually led to the development of nine diagnostic criteria based on characteristic features, shown in Table 10.1. These nine criteria have been demonstrated to differentiate severe borderline personality from schizophrenia (93).

Investigators have long contemplated the relationship of mood dysregulation with BPD (86). Akiskal and colleagues recommended classification of borderline disorders with "subaffective" characterologic syndromes, including cyclothymic, dysthymic, and bipolar II disorders (2). Alternatively, Soloff's group identified mood regulation as a core constitutional and biological feature of borderline personality (88), placing mood features with BPD rather than BPD into a mood disorders category. The rapidly changing affective states inherent in borderline personality prompted characterization of these patients as chronically "stable in their instability" (79). A name briefly proposed, "unstable personality disorder," epitomized the this affective instability as a prime feature of the borderline syndrome defined as a personality disorder (93).

Confirming the aforementioned mood, neurotic, and psychotic symptoms in his patients with borderline disorders, Hoch described an even broader array of psychiatric complaints in them. His patients exhibited "panneurosis, pananxiety, and pansexuality together with symptoms of schizophrenia" (p. 1) (32) and "widespread symptoms mimicking the classical neuroses: compulsions, phobias, depressions and so forth, all occurring in a jumble and in such intensity as to cripple the patient's functioning" (p. 349) (95). Tracing the history of the psychiatric classification of these patients, Stone (95) was struck by the range of diagnostic categories of their symptoms. His synopsis of the state of the field reads like the proverbial blind men describing different parts of the elephant:

> . . . there is considerable debate, and many psychiatrists see borderline personality as actually a subset of biologic depressive illness. Some see it as a variant of other, better-characterized traditional diagnoses, such as hysteria, sociopathy, or alcoholism since, rarely, patients who appear to be borderlines with alcoholism can become quite normal with sustained sobriety, and sociopaths in tightly closed social systems may become indistinguishable from borderlines. Descriptive subtypes range from the border with the psychoses, in which the patient is chaotic, explosive, or irrational ("schizotypal"), to the border with the neuroses, in which the patient is a depressed, empty clinger with a desperate need for companionship in order just to feel real (the "anaclitic" type). Because some patients lack a sense of their own realness, they adapt like chameleons to the environment of the moment ("as-if personality").

Independently, Guze (33) reported that many patients with BPD also met diagnostic criteria for sociopathy, alcoholism, drug dependence, hysteria, primary or secondary affective illness, or schizophrenic illness. Guze and his colleagues were troubled by the extensive comorbidity observed with borderline personality. This extensive comorbidity has kindled doubt over the ultimate validity of this disorder (25, 33, 35). The critical question is whether these many psychiatric disorders actually coexist with BPD, or whether they merely represent mirages emerging from the plethora of psychiatric symptoms these patients present. The confusing nature of the numerous, varied, and unstable symptom presentations of BPD undoubtedly contribute to the continuing controversy surrounding the unsettled classification of this disorder (111).

Epidemiology

Use of the diagnosis of BPD has varied widely, yielding vastly differing estimates of the prevalence of the disorder in separate locales (124). Diagnostic imprecision may have contributed to an apparent increase in prevalence of BPD to "epidemic" proportions during the years after its introduction into formal diagnostic criteria in 1980 (57, 124). Borderline personality disorder is presently the most frequently used diagnosis among the personality disorders. Current estimates, based on meticulous application of established criteria, indicate that as many as 2% of the general population may have BPD, with women representing three-fourths of cases (48).

Borderline personality disorder is found in many settings and populations. Prevalence of the disorder in primary care settings has been estimated at 6% (30). The prevalence is much higher, 15%–20%, in psychiatric inpatient settings (108). A study of 370 treated substance abusers diagnosed BPD in 18% of patients (104). Borderline personality disorder is also reported in association with eating disorders, specifically with bulimia, but not with anorexia nervosa (54, 75). Borderline personality disorder has also been described among patients with anxiety disorders and depression (16, 62). Comorbidity of BPD with other psychiatric disorders may represent a marker for general severity of psychopathology (16, 55, 62).

Borderline personality disorder is not just an American construct. Evidence of this syndrome has been documented in countries around the world, including England (103), France (14), Spain (102), Germany (46), The Netherlands (104), Norway (100), Sweden (44), Switzerland (56), Turkey (81), Brazil (20), New Zealand (13), Japan (16, 55), China (122), India (69), Siberia (80), and Egypt (7).

Clinical Picture

Patients with BPD can present with many symptoms representing multiple diagnostic categories. They complain of symptoms of psychosis, mania, depression, anxiety, dissociation, sociopathy, substance abuse, eating disorders (especially bulimia), and other impulse control disorders. Given the diagnostic complexity of these patients' presentations, the illness can be difficult to understand and to manage. In a study of a psychiatric emergency service, 18 patients with BPD had many more psychiatric complaints and problems than 102 other psychiatric patients visiting the same service. More patients with BPD than those with other psychiatric disorders had suicide attempts, anger and irritability, anhedonia, depression, hypomania, grandiose or omnipotent tendencies, dissociation, sexual promiscuity, destructiveness to property, exploitation of others, alcohol abuse, and transient psychotic episodes without formal thought disorder (68). In a university psychiatry clinic, 9 female patients with Cluster B personality disorders (most representing BPD) described more depressive, manic, anxious, and psychotic symptoms than did 101 other female patients diagnosed with mood, anxiety, and schizophrenic disorders from the same clinic—the same pattern observed among the 32 patients from the same study diagnosed with somatization disorder (47). This pattern of endorsement of many symptoms of diverse psychiatric disorders by patients not suffering from those disorders prompted the emergence of a new term, "psychoform," to describe this classic clinical presentation (47, 59).

The psychoform pattern of reporting many complaints of symptoms of multiple psychiatric disorders in BPD is supported by findings of psychological profiles of these patients recorded using the Minnesota Multiphasic Personality Inventory (MMPI). MMPI testing of 26 patients with BPD demonstrated a characteristic "floating" profile in which all the clinical scale scores were in abnormally elevated ranges (defined as T score > 70). The schizophrenia and psychasthenia scales showed the highest elevations (87). The validity scales of most of the MMPI profiles for these patients revealed a style of exaggerated symptom reporting. This study further confirmed that these patients complain vociferously that virtually everything is wrong with their minds.

Not surprisingly, studies have recorded high rates of apparent psychiatric comorbidity in these polysymptomatic patients. Upon finding a 91% diagnostic comorbidity rate in 180 inpatients with BPD, Fyer and colleagues concluded that BPD must represent a heterogeneous category with unclear boundaries, overlapping with many different disorders rather than with any one specific disorder (25). Around the same time, Swartz's group found high rates of current-year psychiatric comorbidity among 21 BPD inpatients and outpatients. Comorbid diagnoses were major depression (81%), generalized anxiety disorder (86%), panic disorder (62%), dysthymia (52%), alcohol abuse/dependence (24%), and drug abuse/dependence (19%) (97). The Swartz et al. study identified a threshold of at least 11 of 24 current-year psychiatric symptoms that predicted the BPD diagnosis with sensitivity and specificity exceeding 85%.

These symptoms represent a broad range of psychopathology—panic, anxiety, depression, suicidality, irritability, impulsivity, interpersonal difficulties, brief psychotic phenomena—further illustrating the psychoform character of BPD. This extensive pattern of psychopathology expressed by patients with BPD was well characterized in the title of a recent article authored by Paris: "The nature of borderline personality disorder: multiple dimensions, multiple symptoms, but one category" (65).

Hudziak and colleagues later found that 100% of 87 patients with BPD in their study met lifetime criteria for one or more additional psychiatric diagnoses. Remarkably, these patients averaged five diagnoses each (35). Around the same time, Zanarini's group described high lifetime comorbidity rates among 379 BPD inpatients: virtually all (98%) had mood disorders, and 73% had "complex" comorbidity (defined as both mood and anxiety disorders with substance abuse and/or an eating disorder) (111). Compared to patients with other personality disorders, the patients with BPD also had significantly higher rates of major depression, bipolar II disorder, panic disorder, generalized anxiety disorder, phobias, posttraumatic stress disorder, obsessive-compulsive disorder, somatization disorder, and eating disorders. Similarly, Zimmerman and Mattia documented current comorbid disorders in 98% of 49 outpatients with BPD, and the average number of comorbid diagnoses was 3.4 (123). Compared to 350 psychiatric outpatients without BPD, the patients with BPD in this study had significantly greater current prevalence of major depression, bipolar I and II disorders, panic disorder, posttraumatic stress disorder, phobic disorders, obsessive-compulsive disorder, eating disorders, and somatoform disorders. Table 10.2 lists the specific comorbidity rates of patients with BPD in the above three studies, further demonstrating the uniformly psychoform nature of these patients' complaints.

Symptoms among patients with BPD present not only with a wide range but also with remarkable severity. The Beck Depression Inventory and Hamilton Rating Scale for Anxiety, documenting symptoms of major depression and anxiety disorders, were administered to 283 psychiatric outpatients, and 38 of these patients diagnosed with BPD by structured interview were compared with the others. Only 13 of the 38 patients with BPD were free of major depression, yet even this BPD subgroup presented their depression symptoms on these self-rating instruments more severely than did 139 patients without BPD who were diagnosed with major depression, and they also rated their anxiety symptoms more severely than did 134 patients without BPD who were diagnosed with anxiety disorders (16). Zanarini and her colleagues have commented, "It may be that it is their eagerness to confide in others about their

TABLE 10.2 Studies of Diagnostic Comorbidity in Patients with Borderline Personality
Disorder

Comorbid Disorder Prevalence (%)	Hudziak et al. (Lifetime) (35)	Zanarini et al. (Lifetime) (111)	Zimmerman & Mattia (Current) (123)
Major depression	87	83	61
Dysthymia	44	39	12
Manic episode	19	–	9
Bipolar II disorder	–	10	9
Somatization disorder	45	16	–
Any somatoform disorder	–	39	20
Panic disorder	51	48	31
Generalized anxiety disorder	55	14	14
Simple phobia	31	32	20
Agoraphobia	7	12	2
Social phobia	11	46	42
Alcohol abuse/dependence	49	52	12
Drug abuse/dependence	27	46	3
Antisocial personality disorder	23	–	–
Posttraumatic stress disorder	28	56	36
Obsessive compulsive disorder	7	16	20
Eating disorder	16	53	17

dysphoria rather than their actual level of dysphoria which sets borderline patients apart" (p. 164) (119).

The broad psychiatric comorbidity in BPD extends not only to mood, anxiety, and psychotic disorders but also to other personality disorders. A chart review study of 180 inpatients with BPD revealed that 92% met criteria for at least one other personality disorder, and nearly one-half met criteria for two or more other personality disorder diagnoses (25). Similarly, Nurnberg's group found that 82% of BPD outpatients without concurrent major psychiatric disorders had at least one additional personality disorder diagnosis (60). The mean number of additional personality disorder diagnoses was 3.7, although no single accompanying personality disorder predominated. Zanarini's group described sex differences in personality disorder comorbidity among 504 inpatients with personality disorders (112). Comorbid paranoid, passive-aggressive, narcissistic, and antisocial personality disorders were more prevalent among male patients with BPD.

Individual psychological and behavioral features that are considered characteristic of BPD are sometimes also observed in other disorders. It is the occurrence of these features collectively within a single disorder, however, that defines BPD. Patients with BPD struggle with chronic loneliness and emptiness, feelings of inferiority and insecurity, intolerance of anxiety, dependency, helplessness, distrust, poor emotional control, impulsivity, over-reactivity to external stressors, projection (e.g., when feeling hostile, accusing others of hostile feelings), "splitting" (i.e., describing self or others as all good or all bad), extreme idealization and devaluation of others, identity disturbance, narcissistic preoccupation with self, special and entitled feelings, lack of empathy for others, extreme attention-seeking, demanding and manipulative behaviors, and wrist-slashing and other self-mutilation (12, 68).

Described as easily bored, stimulation-seeking, and impulsive, patients with BPD are prone to engage in impulsive, potentially self-damaging behaviors such as gambling, excessive spending, binge eating, substance abuse, unsafe sex, or reckless driving. Their self-image may be unstable with dramatic shifts in their goals, values, and roles. Often in the context of emotional storms, they may abruptly change their career plans, friends, or sexual identity. Patients with BPD overreact to interpersonal stresses, erupting into dramatic episodes of despair, panic, or rage. Many patients with BPD have difficulty controlling their anger and may display intense anger outbursts, especially when they feel others are abandoning them. During stressful episodes, they may exhibit dissociative symptoms or brief psychotic-like symptoms (e.g., feelings of unreality of self or the world, body image distortion, visual hallucinations, paranoid feelings, and ideas of reference) (12, 68).

The interpersonal relationships of patients with BPD are characteristically intense and unstable. Their interactions with health care professionals are often quite difficult. These patients often demand a great deal of time or special treatment. They may idealize relationships, quickly becoming emotionally involved, then rapidly switching to devalue other persons when their demands are not met, at the same time making accusations of abandonment or lack of concern. Patients with BPD have an uncanny propensity for stimulating conflict and disagreement among their health care providers over their care.

Recurrent suicidal behavior is a classic presentation of BPD, particularly during periods of stress. One study found that 73% of inpatients diagnosed with BPD had previously made at least one suicide attempt, and their average number of attempts was 3.4 (91). Suicide attempts in these patients were associated not with comorbid major depression, but with antisocial personality disorder. Among the suicide attempters, 20% had antisocial personality, compared to 4% of nonattempters.

One hallmark feature of BPD is self-mutilation, occurring in 90% or more of patients. Although self-mutilation often occurs as part of recurrent suicidal behavior, many patients with BPD engage in self-mutilation during episodes of emotional distress not associated with suicidality (31, 105). Most commonly, patients present with self-inflicted lacerations of the anterior forearms and self-inflicted burns, often in the context of interpersonal stresses. Physical examination may reveal multiple superficial scars of the wrists or anterior upper extremities, or a collection of circular burn scars from lighted cigarettes. One patient had hundreds of visible scars from self-inflicted lacerations extending from her wrists to axillae. Self-mutilation is not pathognomonic for BPD, however; it is observed in many other disorders as well.

Clues to the diagnosis of BPD may be detected in speech patterns, collectively termed "nonpsychotic thought disorder" (58), reflecting the cognitive styles of these patients. They exhibit "all-or-nothing" logic and overreactive tendencies, which are expressed in overgeneralized and inappropriately globalized statements. Their verbal expressions are peppered with words and phrases that denote extremes (e.g., "the worst," "never," "always," "nobody," "everybody"). Their speech is characteristically circumstantial and overly inclusive, yet simultaneously vague, impressionistic, imprecise, and lacking important detail. They describe their many symptoms inefficiently and with irrelevancies, apparently unable to provide the specific information requested of them. The history-taking process in these patients can be arduous (22, 42).

Biological Findings

The neurobiology of BPD is poorly understood, but many abnormalities have been identified in several lines of research. Hyper-responsiveness of the hypothalamic-pituitary-adrenal axis has been implicated (72). Another area under investigation is abnormal serotonergic transmission, which may be linked to the disinhibition of aggression that can occur with BPD (48). Structural and functional neuroimaging studies have identified abnormalities in brain areas mediating serotonergic functions. Findings of reduced volumes in the orbitofrontal and dorsolateral prefrontal cortex, hippocampus, and amygdala; deactivation of anterior cingulate cortex; and hyperactivity in the amygdala in BPD all point to a potential role for serotonin in this disorder (21, 34, 53, 78, 99, 106). In theory, ineffectual prefrontal inhibitory control of amygdala activity may lead to states of emotional overdrive in the amygdala. Collectively, abnormal findings in these systems may represent neurobiological correlates of emotional states in BPD (48).

Natural History

The literature describes BPD as typically manifesting during early adulthood with pervasive chronic affective instability and impulsivity. In some patients, behaviors associated with the disorder such as self-mutilation and dramatic suicide gestures begin in adolescence or childhood (110). The clinical course of BPD is frequently described as "stormy" (61), reflecting the chronically turbulent episodes of emotional crises and affective instability characteristic of this disorder. Psychosocial functioning is characteristically significantly impaired in work settings, social relationships, and leisure activities (85).

The association between BPD and patient reports of childhood abuse/neglect histories has long been recognized, and the extent of childhood abuse and neglect in BPD has increasingly been appreciated in the last two decades (121). Zanarini's group found that 91% of 358 patients with BPD reported a history of childhood abuse, and 92% reported childhood neglect (117). A subgroup of 29 BPD inpatients examined by these investigators described particularly severe forms of abuse and neglect, which correlated with severity of their BPD symptoms. The severe abuse reported by these inpatients had typically occurred in both childhood and adolescence on at least a weekly basis, for a minimum of 1 year, by two or more perpetrators, and involving penetration and use of force or violence. Most patients with BPD who describe abuse histories do not report this level of severity of abuse, however. A large longitudinal study controlling for parental psychopathology and level of education found that even verbal abuse and neglect in childhood are associated with the development of borderline and several other personality disorders in adolescence and early adulthood (36, 37). Taken together, however, collective findings from these studies do not demonstrate the association between childhood abuse and BPD to be particularly robust (65).

Although the relationship between reported childhood abuse and BPD has been repeatedly documented, there is insufficient evidence to implicate causality of childhood abuse in the generation of BPD. Zanarini and her colleagues initially assumed such negative early experiences to be instrumental in the generation of borderline psychopathology, but these authors more recently revised their etiological model to account for important contributions of constitutional temperament interacting with early environmental challenges of a range of severity (110).

The validity of memories of childhood abuse reported by patients with BPD has been challenged (63), especially memories claimed to be recovered after having been forgotten or "repressed." Questions have been raised as to whether reported childhood abuse memories may more accurately represent exaggerated reporting behaviors characteristics of many of these patients, distorted perceptions of interpersonal events (63), or even products of therapist suggestion (10, 71). It is likely, however, that patients with BPD actually do have more frequent histories of exposure to adverse environments through their families of origin, in association with the elevated rates of antisocial personality disorder and substance abuse demonstrated among biological relatives of patients with BPD. The clinician is generally not in a position to draw conclusions about the veracity of patient reports of childhood mistreatment, and maintaining an open mind is likely to be in the patient's best interest. Regardless of the validity of the reports of abuse by these patients, the importance to the clinician of the knowledge of these apparent associations is to prompt the clinician to include borderline psychopathology in the differential diagnosis among patients who report childhood abuse and neglect histories.

The long-term course of BPD can be quite variable. The disorder's course is not as bleak as it once was considered (28, 82, 110, 113). Some patients achieve a stable equilibrium, especially as they develop maturity in the fourth and fifth decades of life. With maturity, some remarkable patients may manage to overcome the grip of the illness on their lives. Social impairment and suicide risk are greatest during the early adult years and tend to diminish with age.

Initial follow-up studies of small samples of patients with BPD collectively pointed to relatively discouraging prospects for recovery (114). Schizophrenia did not develop in these patients. Many, however, had other personality disorder diagnoses in addition to BPD. Two large, more recent systematic outcome studies of patients with BPD with longer follow-up periods suggest more optimistic outcomes. In a study of 100 hospitalized patients with BPD, Paris and colleagues found that 75% no longer met BPD criteria 15 years later (66). These investigators successfully followed 64 of the 100 patients for another 12 years; at an average of 27 years after the index admission, further improvement was evident, and only 5 patients still met BPD criteria (67). A 10-year follow-up study by Zanarini's group of 275 BPD inpatients reported an 88% remission rate with few recurrences (118). Rapid resolution was typical for impulsive symptoms (self-mutilation and manipulative suicide efforts) and interpersonal difficulties (demanding and entitled behaviors and resistance to treatment), but dysphoria (loneliness, emptiness, anger) and abandonment and dependency issues tended to be chronic.

The disappearance of BPD in the majority of patients over time has invited questions about the validity of the original BPD diagnosis in these patients, and even about the validity of the diagnostic category in general (65), because personality disorders are defined as being generally stable and enduring conditions (4). Remission of BPD in these studies, however, was defined as no longer meeting full diagnostic criteria, which more accurately aligns with the *DSM-IV-TR* definition of "partial remission" (p. 2) (4) of a disorder than with full remission, which entails the disappearance of all signs and symptoms of the disorder. Closer examination of the findings from the above follow-up studies, however, reveals that while the patients' impulsive and suicidal behaviors tended to improve, their affective instability was chronic and, true to the classic conceptualization of personality disorders, the patients' functional impairment persisted (65).

Complications

Borderline personality disorder has been described as a disorder that can be as severe and functionally disabling as major Axis I psychiatric disorders. A follow-up study of hospitalized patients with BPD determined their outcomes to be worse than those of mania or schizoaffective disorder, approaching the chronicity and severity of schizophrenia (70). Functional impairment in BPD has been described as rivaling that of major depression in domains of work, social relationships, and leisure functioning (85). Nearly two-thirds (64%) of patients previously hospitalized for BPD had not been able to work for at least 1 year (92). A 3- to 10-year follow-up study of 86 borderline patients admitted to a day hospital program documented only 24% employed full time, full disability in 34%, and only 27% married or cohabitating (76). A 6-year prospective follow-up study of patients with BPD found their social functioning to be even more impaired than among other personality-disordered patients, especially in vocational achievement (114).

Functional impairment in BPD can be quite variable. Some patients work or attend school as well as manage to maintain friendships and leisure activities. At the other end of the spectrum, others cannot maintain stable employment and must rely on disability benefits to support themselves. Some patients with BPD enjoy close, supportive relationships with their families, others have continuously stormy relationships with them, and a few terminate all contact with their families of origin (110).

Suicidal behaviors may represent chronic problems among patients with BPD. Clinicians may be inclined to dismiss frequent suicide gestures as manipulative and posing little risk for suicide. Patients with chronic or repeated suicidality, however, do present significant risk for eventual completed suicide, although compared to the chronic suicide threats and gestures characteristic of these patients, completed suicide is proportionately infrequent (110). A 27-year follow-up study of 64 patients with BPD found that 9% had died by suicide (67). The suicide rate in BPD has been estimated at 400 times the rate of suicide in the general population (61). Early hospital discharge against the patient's wishes or for violating the treatment contract were noted to be associated with completed suicide in two different studies (41, 43). It is unclear from these studies, however, whether the suicides in these patients were specifically associated with psychiatric comorbidities of BPD that are also associated with suicide in other patients, such as major depression and substance use disorders. The frequent suicide gestures in patients with BPD can also result in accidental fatality even when the patient did not intend to die.

Among 84 inpatients with BPD in one study, nearly one-half had made at least one attempt with clear intent to die, and two-thirds of these attempters had made at least one medically serious, potentially lethal, suicide attempt (91). Intent to die was not associated with severity of borderline traits or major depression, but degree of medical lethality was associated with the number of lifetime attempts. Studies have been inconsistent in concluding whether comorbid substance abuse is associated with suicide in BPD (43, 67). Previous suicide attempts by patients with BPD are also found to be associated with completed suicide (43). Therefore, a history of multiple failed suicide attempts among patients with BPD is no guarantee—and no predictor—that subsequent suicide attempts will not be lethal (9).

Family Studies

Most studies of psychiatric illness in the families of patients with BPD have relied on patients reporting about family members or chart reviews of recorded family histories. Such "family history" studies are widely considered inferior to direct interviews of the family members themselves (family studies). Family history studies, including those relying on chart review, have identified high prevalence rates of mood disorders among family members of patients with BPD (92) that are similar to those documented among relatives of patients with mood disorders (26, 52), and disputably higher than rates described in relatives of patients with schizophrenia (52, 84). High prevalence rates of BPD (12%) are described in relatives of hospitalized patients with BPD, 10 times higher than in relatives of patients hospitalized for schizophrenia or bipolar disorder (52). Relatives of patients with BPD may also have higher rates of histrionic and antisocial personality disorders than relatives of patients with schizophrenia and bipolar disorders (70), more impulsivity than relatives of patients with other personality disorders or with schizophrenia (84), and two to three times the rates of alcohol disorders compared to relatives of patients with schizophrenia or bipolar disorder (52). Comorbid mood disorders are associated with greater prevalence of alcohol use disorders in family members (26). No excess of schizophrenia or schizotypal personality disorder has been identified in families of patients with BPD (70). Eccentric or peculiar behavior is frequently observed among relatives of BPD inpatients, however (92). Patients with BPD are more likely to be adopted than patients with schizophrenia or bipolar disorder (70), further limiting available family information.

Direct psychiatric interviews of family members in a small study of 11 outpatients with BPD without comorbid mood disorders revealed the prevalence of mood and personality disorders among their 54 relatives to be similar to rates in families of patients with mood disorders, and higher than in relatives of controls with no psychiatric illness (73). This suggests that BPD may run in families with mood disorders.

Genetic contribution to BPD has been most conclusively demonstrated in a single study of twins from a registry that demonstrated a significantly higher rate of BPD concordance among monozygotic (35%) compared to dizygotic (7%) twin pairs (101). Multivariate genetic analyses have further shown that a group of traits suggesting emotional dysregulation, including instability of emotions, thinking patterns, sense of self, and interpersonal relationships, has a heritability estimate of 47% (48).

Differential Diagnosis

The differential diagnosis of BPD encompasses depressive and anxiety disorders, bipolar disorders, schizoaffective disorder, schizophrenia, bulimia, substance use disorders, somatization disorder, and other personality disorders, especially of the Cluster B grouping of personality disorders (61). This is because patients with BPD report many symptoms of other disorders.

Pope and colleagues demonstrated that differences in family histories, treatment response, and outcomes distinguish BPD from schizophrenia and mood disorders (70). Zanarini's group examined 22 borderline personality features identified by the Revised Diagnostic Interview for Borderline Patients, and found that while 18 features discriminated BPD from other personality disorders, only 7 were relatively specific to BPD: psychotic-like thought, self-mutilation, manipulative suicide efforts, abandonment issues, demanding and entitlement behaviors, stormy course of treatment, and elicitation of negative therapist responses (119). Several studies have observed that the general psychoform pattern of reporting multiple psychiatric symptoms across many diagnostic classes is a major feature differentiating BPD from other psychiatric disorders (65, 111, 112, 120, 123).

The characteristic pattern in which BPD patients report extensive symptoms of many psychiatric disorders that do not add up to consistent diagnostic entities (i.e., multiple psychoform symptoms) has invited questions about the validity of the diagnosis of BPD. Many patients with somatization disorder, however, similarly describe multiple symptoms of many psychiatric categories (47, 59, 107), but this pattern has not reduced the well-established validity of this diagnosis. The key to distinguishing somatization disorder from BPD is to identify the classic pattern of multiple medically unexplained complaints throughout the body's organ systems in somatization disorder patients that is not a defining characteristic of BPD. Many patients with BPD display somatoform symptoms such as unexplained vomiting (38) and may utilize medical treatment excessively (77), but not to the degree that defines somatization disorder. It is not unusual for patients to meet criteria for both disorders (35, 111).

In the last quarter of a century, scientific investigation has emphasized the relationship between dissociative disorders and BPD. The validity of dissociative disorders, however, has been extensively debated. The defining elements of dissociative disorders are disruption in the usually integrated functions of consciousness, memory, identity, or perception of the environment (3). Dissociative disorders, like somatization and borderline personality disorder, classically present with many symptoms in multiple psychiatric categories (17, 23, 59). Therefore, overlap of these disorders is not unexpected. Most patients with multiple personality disorder (recently renamed as dissociative identity disorder) also have somatization disorder, borderline personality disorder, or both (59), complicating attempts to differentiate multiple personality disorder from borderline and somatoform disorders. Patients with multiple personality disorder have been observed to complain of symptoms even more profusely than patients with only borderline or somatization disorder (23, 45, 83). In a study of 60 female BPD inpatients, those with dissociation reported higher rates of self-mutilation, childhood abuse, current depressive symptoms, and psychiatric treatment utilization (11). Lauer and colleagues (45) found no differences between patients with BPD and multiple personality disorder in family history, childhood history, psychiatric comorbidity, and symptom complaints aside from more dissociative symptoms among multiple personality disorder patients. They concluded that multiple personality disorder may simply represent a severe manifestation or variant (an "epiphenomenon") of BPD.

Because the psychoform presentation of BPD can mimic virtually any psychiatric disorder, independent evidence of the characteristic patterns of other disorders should be sought to confirm or rule out these other diagnoses in patients thought to have BPD. Conversely, because patients with other psychiatric disorders may transiently exhibit BPD features during illness episodes, it is advisable to refrain from making the diagnosis of BPD until a history of early onset of the behavior and a longstanding course of BPD independent of other psychiatric illness can be established.

Clinical Management

Patients with BPD in treatment have been described as challenging and demanding. Zanarini and colleagues identified specific features of these patients' behavior that frightens or annoys therapists: accusations that the therapist is mean and uncaring, demanding behaviors, and frequent suicide threats and gestures that may appear manipulative (110). Some patients seem to worsen during treatment. Zanarini and colleagues described these patients as having "a toxic reaction to" therapy (p. 522) (110).

General principles of BPD treatment involve exercising flexibility, establishing rules for dealing with crises and suicidality, achieving agreement about patient and therapist roles and responsibilities, mutually setting limits on topics of discussion, carefully maintaining professional boundaries that are often tested by the intense interpersonal styles of patients with BPD, and consulting with colleagues as needed (1, 6, 61). Managing and reducing behavioral dyscontrol, intense dysphoria, and suicidal behaviors are early goals of treatment. Longer-term goals are to improve functioning, productivity, and emotional stability (48).

Few controlled studies of treatment for BPD have been carried out, and these studies have suffered from high dropout rates, potential for placebo effects, and emphasis on less severe and predominantly female populations, limiting interpretation and generalizability of the findings (48, 98).

It is generally agreed at present that psychotherapy should be considered a first-line treatment for BPD (110). Supportive psychotherapy with an active problem-solving emphasis is recommended in conjunction with adjunctive, symptom-targeted pharmacotherapy (5, 48). Assumptions that childhood adversity is the sole source of these patients' distress and disability provide a nonproductive premise for the basis of psychotherapy in these patients (110). Focusing on early maltreatment by others can derail these patients from healthy objectives of gaining insight into and changing their behavior and further alienate these patients from family members who might otherwise provide helpful social support.

Dialectical behavior therapy, a specialized derivative of cognitive therapy developed for patients with chronic suicidality or BPD, teaches problem-solving skills, emotional regulation strategies, distress tolerance, and interpersonal skills in outpatient settings (49). This form of therapy has proved effective in nonrandomized and randomized controlled trials for patients with chronic suicidality or BPD (48, 50, 51). Two other specialized therapies, mentalization-based (8) and schema-focused (27) therapies, have also shown promise in therapeutic trials. These specialized therapies are intensive and likely to be most useful for the most severe and chronic cases (110).

Medications should be considered adjunctive to psychotherapy rather than the mainstay of treatment for BPD (110). Despite this recommendation, however, aggressive pharmacotherapy is too often seen (115, 116) and undoubtedly involves a tendency to mistake the unstable moods of these patients for the sustained mood swings of bipolar disorder and to misconceptualize BPD as representing a form of bipolar disorder (65, 110). Hospitalization and pharmacotherapy have little benefit beyond providing a brief stopgap in the long-term management of emotional crises and suicidality in patients with BPD. Psychiatric hospitalization has not been demonstrated to prevent suicide in patients with BPD, and it sometimes has untoward effects (64). Habitual reliance on hospitalization and pharmacotherapy in the long-term management of BPD can lead to escalation of maladaptive behaviors in these patients (48).

Pharmacotherapy may be most beneficial in early phases of psychotherapy by calming intense emotions and allowing the patient to reflect and develop cognitive strategies for coping (48, 65). Although pharmacotherapy aims to reduce unstable moods, impulsive behavior, and distorted thinking and perceptions (1, 61), the benefit from antidepressant, mood stabilizer, and antipsychotic medications commonly prescribed for BPD may represent no more than nonspecific or sedating characteristics of these agents (110).

Although antidepressants and low-dose antipsychotic medications have long been used in treatment of BPD, results have been modest or mixed at best. Patients with BPD sometimes worsen on antidepressants (18, 89, 90). Antidepressant effects appear to be independent of comorbid mood disorders (88), and typically residual symptoms continue (18). Newer antidepressants have more favorable safety profiles than older antidepressants in borderline patients, especially those at risk for impulsive suicide attempts, but the benefit of these medications has not been tested in controlled, randomized studies.

In small placebo-controlled studies, mood stabilizers have been shown to reduce interpersonal sensitivity and irritability and anger (24), and antipsychotics to reduce anxiety, paranoia, anger, and hostility (109). The mechanism of improvement is unclear, likely related in part to nonspecific sedative effects. The use of antipsychotic medication for agitation and psychotic-like features, however, is usually reserved for the most severe cases and should be weighed against the risk of significant adverse effects such as neuroleptic malignant syndrome, tardive dyskinesia, sudden death, metabolic syndrome, and other side effects of antipsychotic agents. Newer antipsychotic medications are preferable to the older agents in attempting to manage psychotic-like symptoms for their lower propensity for tardive dyskinesia, but their use may be complicated by metabolic syndrome. Because many patients with BPD complain of profuse anxiety, benzodiazepines are often used (and requested by many of these patients), but their use must be carefully monitored for risk of misuse or addiction (1). No clear medication choice has emerged for long-term management of BPD (18).

A review of 13 studies of electroconvulsive therapy for depression in patients with BPD found that it can be effectively administered in these patients, although outcomes may not be as favorable as in depressed patients without BPD (19). Rigorous randomized treatment studies with follow-up are needed.

Unfortunately, the characteristic extensive, varied, and shifting psychiatric symptoms reported by patients with BPD complicate diagnosis and treatment of this condition (111). Because other psychiatric disorders may complicate BPD and are potentially treatable, clinicians are reminded to complete the psychiatric evaluation for other psychiatric disorders (123). Management of BPD can be expected to be less tumultuous when comorbid disorders are quiescent or absent.

REFERENCES

1. (No authors listed). Borderline personality: new recommendations. Harv. Ment Health Lett., 18:4–6, 2002.

2. Akiskal, H. S. Subaffective disorders: dysthymic, cyclothymic and bipolar II disorders in the "borderline" realm. Psychiat. Clin. N. Am., 4:25–46, 1981.

3. American Psychiatric Association. *Diagnostic and Statistical Manual of Mental Disorders*, 4th edition. Washington, DC: Author, 1994.

4. American Psychiatric Association. *Diagnostic and Statistical Manual of Mental Disorders*, 4th edition, text revision. Washington, DC: Author, 2000.

5. American Psychiatric Association. *Practice Guideline for the Treatment of Patients with Borderline Personality Disorder*. Washington, DC: Author, 2001.

6. Aronson, T. A. A critical review of psychotherapeutic treatments of the borderline personality. Historical trends and future directions. J. Nerv. Ment. Dis., 177:511–528, 1989.

7. Asaad, T., Okasha, T., and Okasha, A. Sleep EEG findings in ICD-10 borderline personality disorder in Egypt. J. Affect. Dis., 71:11–18, 2002.

8. Bateman, A. W., and Fonagy, P. Mentalization-based treatment of BPD. J. Personal. Disord., 18:36–51, 2004.

9. Black, D. W., Blum, N., Pfohl, B., and Hale, N. Suicidal behavior in borderline personality disorder: prevalence, risk factors, prediction, and prevention. J. Pers. Dis., 18:226–239, 2004.

10. Boakes, J. False complaints of sexual assault: recovered memories of childhood sexual abuse. Med. Sci. Law, 39:112–120, 1999.

11. Brodsky, B. S., Cloitre, M., and Dulit, R. A. Relationship of dissociation to self-mutilation and childhood abuse in borderline personality disorder. Am. J. Psychiat., 152:1788–1792, 1995.

12. Butler, A. C., Brown, G. K., Beck, A. T., and Grisham, J. R. Assessment of dysfunctional beliefs in borderline personality disorder. Behav. Res. Ther., 40:1231–1240, 2002.

13. Carter, J. D., Joyce, P. R., Mulder, R. T., Sullivan, P. F., and Luty, S. E. Gender differences in the frequency of personality disorders in depressed outpatients. J. Pers. Dis., 13:67–74, 1999.

14. Chabrol, H., Chouicha, K., Montovany, A., and Callahan, S. Symptoms of DSM IV borderline personality disorder in a nonclinical population of adolescents: study of a series of 35 patients. Encephale, 27:120–127, 2001.

15. Clark, L. P. Some practical remarks upon the use of modified psychoanalysis in the treatment of borderland neuroses and psychoses. Psychoanal. Rev., 6:306–308, 1919.

16. Comtois, K. A., Cowley, D. S., Dunner, D. L., and Roy-Byrne, P. P. Relationship between borderline personality disorder and Axis I diagnosis in severity of depression and anxiety. J. Clin. Psychiat., 60:752–758, 1999.

17. Coons, P. M. The differential diagnosis of multiple personality: a comprehensive review. Psychiat. Clin. N. Am., 7:51–67, 1984.

18. Cornelius, J. R., Soloff, P. H., Perel, J. M., and Ulrich, R. F. Continuation pharmacotherapy of borderline personality disorder with haloperidol and phenelzine. Am. J. Psychiat., 150:1843–1848, 1993.

19. DeBattista, C., and Mueller, K. Is electroconvulsive therapy effective for the depressed patient with comorbid borderline personality disorder? J. ECT, 17:91–98, 2001.

20. Del Ben, C. M., Rodrigues, C. R., and Zuardi, A. W. Reliability of the Portuguese version of the structured clinical interview for DSM-III-R (SCID) in a Brazilian sample of psychiatric outpatients. Braz. J. Med. Biol. Res., 29:1675–1682, 1996.

21. Driessen, M., Herrmann, J., Stahl, K., Zwaan, M., Meier, S., Hill, A., Osterheider, M., and Petersen, D. Magnetic resonance imaging volumes of the hippocampus and the amygdala in women with borderline personality disorder and early traumatization. Arch. Gen. Psychiat., 57:1115–1122, 2000.

22. Drob, S., Stewart, S., and Bernard, H. The problem of reinterpretive distortions in group psychotherapy with borderline patients. Group, 6:14–22, 1982.

23. Fink, D., and Golinkoff, M. MPD, borderline personality disorder and schizophrenia: a comparative study of clinical features. Dissociation, 3: 127–134, 1990.

24. Frankenburg, F. R., and Zanarini, M. C. Divalproex sodium treatment of women with borderline personality disorder and bipolar II disorder: a double-blind placebo-controlled pilot study. J. Clin. Psychiat., 63:442–446, 2002.

25. Fyer, M. R., Frances, A. J., Sullivan, T., Hurt, S. W., and Clarkin, J. Comorbidity of borderline personality disorder. Arch. Gen. Psychiat., 45:348–352, 1988.

26. Gasperini, M., Battaglia, M., Scherillo, P., Sciuto, G., Diaferia, G., and Bellodi, L. Morbidity risk for mood disorders in the families of borderline patients. J. Affect. Dis., 21:265–272, 1991.

27. Giesen-Bloo, J., van Dyck, R., Spinhoven, P., van Tilburg, W., Dirksen, C., van Asselt, T., Kremers, I., Nadort, M., and Arntz, A. Outpatient psychotherapy for borderline personality disorder: randomized trial of schema-focused therapy vs transference-focused psychotherapy. Arch. Gen. Psychiat., 63:649–658, 2006.

28. Grilo, C. M., Sanislow, C. A., Gunderson, J. G., Pagano, M. E., Yen, S., Zanarini, M. C., Shea, M. T., Skodol, A. E., Stout, R. L., Morey, L. C., and McGlashan, T. H. Two-year stability and change of schizotypal, borderline, avoidant, and obsessive-compulsive personality disorders. J. Consult. Clin. Psychol., 72:767–775, 2004.

29. Grinker, R. R. Neurosis, psychosis, and the borderline states. In *Comprehensive Textbook of Psychiatry*, 2nd edition, Friedman, A. M., Kaplan, H. I., Sadock, B. J. (eds.). Baltimore: Williams & Wilkins, pp. 845–850, 1975.

30. Gross, R., Olfson, M., Gameroff, M., Shea, S., Feder, A., Fuentes, M., Lantigua, R., and Weissman, M. M. Borderline personality disorder in primary care. Arch. Intern. Med., 162:53–60, 2002.

31. Gunderson, J. G., and Ridolfi, M. E. Borderline personality disorder. Suicidality and self-mutilation. Ann. N. Y. Acad. Sci., 932:61–73, 2001.

32. Gunderson, J. G., and Singer, M. T. Defining borderline patients: an overview. Am. J. Psychiat., 132:1–10, 1975.

33. Guze, S. B. Differential diagnosis of the borderline personality syndrome. In *Borderline States in Psychiatry*, Mack, J. E. (ed.). New York: Grune & Stratton, pp. 69–74, 1975.

34. Herpertz, S. C., Dietrich, T. M., Wenning, B., Krings, T., Erberich, S. G., Willmes, K., Thron, A., and Sass, H. Evidence of abnormal amygdala functioning in borderline personality disorder: a functional MRI study. Biol. Psychiat., 50:292–298, 2001.

35. Hudziak, J. J., Boffelli, T. J., Kreisman, J. J., Battaglia, M. M., Stanger, C., Guze, S. B., and Kriesman, J. J. A clinical study of borderline personality disorder: the significance of Briquet's syndrome (hysteria), somatization disorder, antisocial personality disorder, and substance abuse disorders. Am. J. Psychiat., 153:1598–1606, 1996.

36. Johnson, J. G., Cohen, P., Smailes, E. M., Skodol, A. E., Brown, J., and Oldham, J. M. Childhood verbal abuse and risk for personality disorders during adolescence and early adulthood. Compr. Psychiat., 42:16–23, 2001.

37. Johnson, J. G., Smailes, E. M., Cohen, P., Brown, J., and Bernstein, D. P. Associations between four types of childhood neglect and personality disorder symptoms during adolescence and early adulthood: findings of a community-based longitudinal study. J. Personal. Disord., 14:171–187, 2000.

38. Johnson, T. M. Vomiting as a manifestation of borderline personality disorder in primary care. J. Am. Board Fam. Pract., 6:385–394, 1993.

39. Kernberg, O. Borderline personality organization. J. Am. Psychoanal. Assoc., 15:641–685, 1967.

40. Khouri, P. J., Haier, R. J., Rieder, R. O., and Rosenthal, D. A symptom schedule for the diagnosis of borderline schizophrenia: a first report. Br. J. Psychiat., 137:140–147, 1980.

41. Kjelsberg, E., Eikeseth, P. H., and Dahl, A. A. Suicide in borderline patients—predictive factors. Acta Psychiat. Scand., 84:283–287, 1991.

42. Kroll, J. *The Challenge of the Borderline Patient*. New York: W.W. Norton, 1989.

43. Kullgren, G. Factors associated with completed suicide in borderline personality disorder. J. Nerv. Ment. Dis., *176*:40–44, 1988.

44. Larsson, J. O., and Hellzen, M. Patterns of personality disorders in women with chronic eating disorders. Eat. Weight Dis., *9*:200–205, 2004.

45. Lauer, J., Black, D. W., and Keen, P. Multiple personality disorder and borderline personality disorder. Distinct entities or variations on a common theme. Ann. Clin. Psychiat., *5*:129–134, 1993.

46. Leichsenring, F. Quality of depressive experiences in borderline personality disorders: differences between patients with borderline personality disorder and patients with higher levels of personality organization. Bull. Menninger Clin., *68*:9–22, 2004.

47. Lenze, E. L., Miller, A., Munir, Z., Pornoppadol, C., and North, C. S. Psychiatric symptoms endorsed by somatization disorder patients in a psychiatric clinic. Ann. Clin. Psychiat., *11*:73–79, 1999.

48. Lieb, K., Zanarini, M. C., Schmahl, C., Linehan, M. M., and Bohus, M. Borderline personality disorder. Lancet, *364*:453–461, 2004.

49. Linehan, M. M. Dialectical behavior therapy for borderline personality disorder. Theory and method. Bull. Menninger Clin., *51*:261–276, 1987.

50. Linehan, M. M., Armstrong, H. E., Suarez, A., Allmon, D., and Heard, H. L. Cognitive-behavioral treatment of chronically parasuicidal borderline patients. Arch. Gen. Psychiat., *48*:1060–1064, 1991.

51. Linehan, M. M., Tutek, D. A., Heard, H. L., and Armstrong, H. E. Interpersonal outcome of cognitive behavioral treatment for chronically suicidal borderline patients. Am. J. Psychiat., *151*:1771–1776, 1994.

52. Loranger, A. W., and Tulis, E. H. Family history of alcoholism in borderline personality disorder. Arch. Gen. Psychiat., *42*:153–157, 1985.

53. Lyoo, I. K., Han, M. H., and Cho, D. Y. A brain MRI study in subjects with borderline personality disorder. J. Affect. Disord., *50*:235–243, 1998.

54. Matsunaga, H., Kiriike, N., Nagata, T., and Yamagami, S. Personality disorders in patients with eating disorders in Japan. Int. J. Eat. Dis., *23*:399–408, 1998.

55. Matsunaga, H., Kiriike, N., Nagata, T., and Yamagami, S. Personality disorders in patients with eating disorders in Japan. Int. J. Eat. Dis., *23*:399–408, 1998.

56. McQuillan, A., Nicastro, R., Guenot, F., Girard, M., Lissner, C., and Ferrero, F. Intensive dialectical behavior therapy for outpatients with borderline personality disorder who are in crisis. Psychiat. Serv., *56*:193–197, 2005.

57. Millon, T. On the genesis and prevalence of the borderline personality disorder: a social learning thesis. J. Personal. Disord., *1*:354–372, 1987.

58. North, C. S., Hansen, K., Wetzel, R. D., Compton, W., Napier, M., and Spitznagel, E. L. Non-psychotic thought disorder: objective clinical identification of somatization and antisocial personality in language patterns. Compr. Psychiat., *38*:171–178, 1997.

59. North, C. S., Ryall, J. M., Ricci, D. A., and Wetzel, R. D. *Multiple Personalities, Multiple Disorders: Psychiatric Classification and Media Influence*. New York: Oxford, 1993.

60. Nurnberg, H. G., Raskin, M., Levine, P. E., Pollack, S., Siegel, O., and Prince, R. The comorbidity of borderline personality disorder and other DSM-III-R axis II personality disorders. Am. J. Psychiat., 148:1371–1377, 1991.

61. Oldham, J. M. A 44-year-old woman with borderline personality disorder. JAMA, 287:1029–1037, 2002.

62. Ozkan, M., and Altindag, A. Comorbid personality disorders in subjects with panic disorder: do personality disorders increase clinical severity? Compr. Psychiat., 46:20–26, 2005.

63. Paris, J. Memories of abuse in borderline patients: true or false? Harv. Rev. Psychiat., 3:10–17, 1995.

64. Paris, J. Chronic suicidality among patients with borderline personality disorder. Psychiat. Serv., 53:738–742, 2002.

65. Paris, J. The nature of borderline personality disorder: multiple dimensions, multiple symptoms, but one category. J. Personal. Disord., 21:457–473, 2007.

66. Paris, J., Brown, R., and Nowlis, D. Long-term follow-up of borderline patients in a general hospital. Compr. Psychiat., 28:530–535, 1987.

67. Paris, J., and Zweig-Frank, H. A 27-year follow-up of patients with borderline personality disorder. Compr. Psychiat., 42:482–487, 2001.

68. Perry, J. C., and Klerman, G. L. Clinical features of the borderline personality disorder. Am. J. Psychiat., 137:165–173, 1980.

69. Pinto, C., Dhavale, H. S., Nair, S., Patil, B., and Dewan, M. Borderline personality disorder exists in India. J. Nerv. Ment. Dis., 188:386–388, 2000.

70. Pope, H. G., Jr., Jonas, J. M., Hudson, J. I., Cohen, B. M., and Gunderson, J. G. The validity of DSM-III borderline personality disorder. A phenomenologic, family history, treatment response, and long-term follow-up study. Arch. Gen. Psychiat., 40:23–30, 1983.

71. Powell, R. A., and Boer, D. P. Did Freud mislead patients to confabulate memories of abuse? A reply to Gleaves and Hernandez (1999). Psychol. Rep., 95:863–877, 2004.

72. Rinne, T., de Kloet, E. R., Wouters, L., Goekoop, J. G., DeRijk, R. H., and van den Brink, W. Hyperresponsiveness of hypothalamic-pituitary-adrenal axis to combined dexamethasone/corticotropin-releasing hormone challenge in female borderline personality disorder subjects with a history of sustained childhood abuse. Biol. Psychiat., 52:1102–1112, 2002.

73. Riso, L. P., Klein, D. N., Anderson, R. L., and Ouimette, P. C. A family study of outpatients with borderline personality disorder and no history of mood disorder. J. Personal. Disord., 14:208–217, 2000.

74. Robins, E., and Guze, S. B. Establishment of diagnostic validity in psychiatric illness: its application to schizophrenia. Am. J. Psychiat., 126:983–987, 1970.

75. Rosenvinge, J. H., Martinussen, M., and Ostensen, E. The comorbidity of eating disorders and personality disorders: a meta-analytic review of studies published between 1983 and 1998. Eat. Weight Dis., 5:52–61, 2000.

76. Sandell, R., Alfredsson, E., Berg, M., Craford, K., Lagerlof, A., Arkel, I., Cohn, T., Rasch, B., and Rugolska, A. Clinical significance of outcome in long-term follow-up of borderline patients at a day hospital. Acta Psychiat. Scand., 87:405–413, 1993.

77. Sansone, R. A., Wiederman, M. W., and Sansone, L. A. Borderline personality symptomatology, experience of multiple types of trauma, and health care utilization among women in a primary care setting. South. Med. J., 89:1162–1165, 1996.

78. Schmahl, C. G., Vermetten, E., Elzinga, B. M., and Douglas, B. J. Magnetic resonance imaging of hippocampal and amygdala volume in women with childhood abuse and borderline personality disorder. Psychiat. Res., 122:193–198, 2003.

79. Schmideberg, M. The treatment of psychopaths and borderline patients. Am. J. Psychother., 1:45, 1947.

80. Semke, V. I., Polozhii, B. S., Krasik, E. D., Vasil'eva, O. A., Zalevskii, G. V., and Kornetov, N. A. Epidemiology, clinical aspects and prevention of borderline conditions in the regions of Siberia and Far East. Zh. Nevropatol. Psikhiatr. Im S. S. Korsakova, 91:7–11, 1991.

81. Senol, S., Dereboy, C., and Yuksel, N. Borderline disorder in Turkey: a 2- to 4-year follow-up. Soc. Psychiat Psychiat. Epidemiol., 32:109–112, 1997.

82. Shea, M. T., Stout, R., Gunderson, J., Morey, L. C., Grilo, C. M., McGlashan, T., Skodol, A. E., Dolan-Sewell, R., Dyck, I., Zanarini, M. C., and Keller, M. B. Short-term diagnostic stability of schizotypal, borderline, avoidant, and obsessive-compulsive personality disorders. Am. J. Psychiat., 159:2036–2041, 2002.

83. Shearer, S. L. Dissociative phenomena in women with borderline personality disorder. Am. J. Psychiat., 151:1324–1328, 1994.

84. Silverman, J. M., Pinkham, L., Horvath, T. B., Coccaro, E. F., Klar, H., Schear, S., Apter, S., Davidson, M., Mohs, R. C., and Siever, L. J. Affective and impulsive personality disorder traits in the relatives of patients with borderline personality disorder. Am. J. Psychiat., 148:1378–1385, 1991.

85. Skodol, A. E., Gunderson, J. G., McGlashan, T. H., Dyck, I. R., Stout, R. L., Bender, D. S., Grilo, C. M., Shea, M. T., Zanarini, M. C., Morey, L. C., Sanislow, C. A., and Oldham, J. M. Functional impairment in patients with schizotypal, borderline, avoidant, or obsessive-compulsive personality disorder. Am. J. Psychiat., 159:276–283, 2002.

86. Skodol, A. E., Stout, R. L., McGlashan, T. H., Grilo, C. M., Gunderson, J. G., Shea, M. T., Morey, L. C., Zanarini, M. C., Dyck, I. R., and Oldham, J. M. Co-occurrence of mood and personality disorders: a report from the Collaborative Longitudinal Personality Disorders Study (CLPS). Depress. Anxiety, 10:175–182, 1999.

87. Snyder, S., Pitts, W. M., Goodpaster, W. A., Sajadi, C., and Gustin, Q. MMPI profile of DSM-III borderline personality disorder. Am. J. Psychiat., 139:1046–1048, 1982.

88. Soloff, P. H., Cornelius, J., and George, A. The depressed borderline: one disorder or two? Psychopharmacol. Bull., 27:23–30, 1991.

89. Soloff, P. H., George, A., Nathan, R. S., Schulz, P. M., and Perel, J. M. Paradoxical effects of amitriptyline on borderline patients. Am. J. Psychiat., 143:1603–1605, 1986.

90. Soloff, P. H., George, A., Nathan, R. S., Schulz, P. M., Ulrich, R. F., and Perel, J. M. Progress in pharmacotherapy of borderline disorders. A double-blind study of amitriptyline, haloperidol, and placebo. Arch. Gen. Psychiat., 43:691–697, 1986.

91. Soloff, P. H., Lis, J. A., Kelly, T., Cornelius, J., and Ulrich, R. Risk factors for suicidal behavior in borderline personality disorder. Am. J. Psychiat., 151:1316–1323, 1994.

92. Soloff, P. H., and Millward, J. W. Psychiatric disorders in the families of borderline patients. Arch. Gen. Psychiat., 40:37–44, 1983.

93. Spitzer, R. L., Endicott, J., and Gibbon, M. Crossing the border into borderline personality and borderline schizophrenia. The development of criteria. Arch. Gen. Psychiat., 36:17–24, 1979.

94. Stern, A. Psychoanalytic investigation of and therapy in the borderline group of neuroses. Psychoanal. Q., 7:467–489, 1938.

95. Stone, M. H. The borderline syndrome: evolution of the term, genetic aspects, and prognosis. Am. J. Psychother., 31:345–365, 1977.

96. Stone, M. H. Toward a psychobiological theory of borderline personality disorder. Dissociation, 1:2–15, 1988.

97. Swartz, M. S., Blazer, D. G., George, L. K., Winfield, I., Zakris, J., and Dye, E. Identification of borderline personality disorder with the NIMH Diagnostic Interview Schedule. Am. J. Psychiat., 146:200–205, 1989.

98. Tarnopolsky, A., and Berkowitz, M. Borderline personality: a review of recent research. Br. J. Psychiat., 151:724–734, 1987.

99. Tebartz, v. E., Hesslinger, B., Thiel, T., Geiger, E., Haegele, K., Lemieux, L., Lieb, K., Bohus, M., Hennig, J., and Ebert, D. Frontolimbic brain abnormalities in patients with borderline personality disorder: a volumetric magnetic resonance imaging study. Biol. Psychiat., 54:163–171, 2003.

100. Torgersen, S., Kringlen, E., and Cramer, V. The prevalence of personality disorders in a community sample. Arch. Gen. Psychiat., 58:590–596, 2001.

101. Torgersen, S., Lygren, S., Oien, P. A., Skre, I., Onstad, S., Edvardsen, J., Tambs, K., and Kringlen, E. A twin study of personality disorders. Compr. Psychiat., 41:416–425, 2000.

102. Torrens, M., Serrano, D., Astals, M., Perez-Dominguez, G., and Martin-Santos, R. Diagnosing comorbid psychiatric disorders in substance abusers: validity of the Spanish versions of the Psychiatric Research Interview for Substance and Mental Disorders and the Structured Clinical Interview for DSM-IV. Am. J. Psychiat., 161:1231–1237, 2004.

103. van Hanswijck, D. J., Van Furth, E. F., Lacey, J. H., and Waller, G. The prevalence of DSM-IV personality pathology among individuals with bulimia nervosa, binge eating disorder and obesity. Psychol. Med., 33:1311–1317, 2003.

104. Verheul, R., Kranzler, H. R., Poling, J., Tennen, H., Ball, S., and Rounsaville, B. J. Co-occurrence of Axis I and Axis II disorders in substance abusers. Acta Psychiat. Scand., 101:110–118, 2000.

105. Verheul, R., Van Den Bosch, L. M., Koeter, M. W., De Ridder, M. A., Stijnen, T., and van den, B. W. Dialectical behaviour therapy for women with borderline

personality disorder: 12-month, randomised clinical trial in The Netherlands. Br. J. Psychiat., 182:135–140, 2003.

106. Westen, D., Ludolph, P., Misle, B., Ruffins, S., and Block, J. Physical and sexual abuse in adolescent girls with borderline personality disorder. Am. J. Orthopsychiat., 60:55–66, 1990.

107. Wetzel, R. D., Guze, S. B., Cloninger, C. R., Martin, R. L., and Clayton, P. J. Briquet's syndrome (hysteria) is both a somatoform and a "psychoform" illness: a Minnesota Multiphasic Personality Inventory study. Psychosomat. Med., 56:564–569, 1994.

108. Widiger, T. A., and Sanderson, C. J. Personality disorders. In *Psychiatry*, Tasman, A., Kay, J., Lieberman, J. A. (eds.). Philadelphia: Saunders, pp. 1291–1317, 1997.

109. Zanarini, M. C., and Frankenburg, F. R. Olanzapine treatment of female borderline personality disorder patients: a double-blind, placebo-controlled pilot study. J. Clin. Psychiat., 62:849–854, 2001.

110. Zanarini, M. C., and Frankenburg, F. R. The essential nature of borderline psychopathology. J. Personal. Disord., 21:518–535, 2007.

111. Zanarini, M. C., Frankenburg, F. R., Dubo, E. D., Sickel, A. E., Trikha, A., Levin, A., and Reynolds, V. Axis I comorbidity of borderline personality disorder. Am. J. Psychiat., 155:1733–1739, 1998.

112. Zanarini, M. C., Frankenburg, F. R., Dubo, E. D., Sickel, A. E., Trikha, A., Levin, A., and Reynolds, V. Axis II comorbidity of borderline personality disorder. Compr. Psychiat., 39:296–302, 1998.

113. Zanarini, M. C., Frankenburg, F. R., Hennen, J., Reich, D. B., and Silk, K. R. The McLean Study of Adult Development (MSAD): overview and implications of the first six years of prospective follow-up. J. Personal. Disord., 19:505–523, 2005.

114. Zanarini, M. C., Frankenburg, F. R., Hennen, J., and Silk, K. R. The longitudinal course of borderline psychopathology: 6-year prospective follow-up of the phenomenology of borderline personality disorder. Am. J. Psychiat., 160:274–283, 2003.

115. Zanarini, M. C., Frankenburg, F. R., Hennen, J., and Silk, K. R. Mental health service utilization by borderline personality disorder patients and Axis II comparison subjects followed prospectively for 6 years. J. Clin. Psychiat., 65:28–36, 2004.

116. Zanarini, M. C., Frankenburg, F. R., Khera, G. S., and Bleichmar, J. Treatment histories of borderline inpatients. Compr. Psychiat., 42:144–150, 2001.

117. Zanarini, M. C., Frankenburg, F. R., Reich, D. B., Marino, M. F., Lewis, R. E., Williams, A. A., and Khera, G. S. Biparental failure in the childhood experiences of borderline patients. J. Pers. Dis., 14:264–273, 2000.

118. Zanarini, M. C., Frankenburg, F. R., Reich, D. B., Silk, K. R., Hudson, J. I., and McSweeney, L. B. The subsyndromal phenomenology of borderline personality disorder: a 10-year follow-up study. Am. J. Psychiat., 164:929–935, 2007.

119. Zanarini, M. C., Gunderson, J. G., Frankenburg, F. R., and Chauncey, D. L. Discriminating borderline personality disorder from other axis II disorders. Am. J. Psychiat., 147:161–167, 1990.

120. Zanarini, M. C., Ruser, T., Frankenburg, F. R., and Hennen, J. The dissociative experiences of borderline patients. Compr. Psychiat., 41:223–227, 2000.

121. Zanarini, M. C., Yong, L., Frankenburg, F. R., Hennen, J., Reich, D. B., Marino, M. F., and Vujanovic, A. A. Severity of reported childhood sexual abuse and its relationship to severity of borderline psychopathology and psychosocial impairment among borderline inpatients. J. Nerv. Ment. Dis., 190:381–387, 2002.

122. Zhong, J., and Leung, F. Should borderline personality disorder be included in the fourth edition of the Chinese classification of mental disorders? Chin. Med. J. (Engl.), 120:77–82, 2007.

123. Zimmerman, M., and Mattia, J. I. Axis I diagnostic comorbidity and borderline personality disorder. Compr. Psychiat., 40:245–252, 1999.

124. Zimmerman, M., and Mattia, J. I. Differences between clinical and research practices in diagnosing borderline personality disorder. Am. J. Psychiat., 156:1570–1574, 1999.

11

Alcoholism

Alcoholism has been defined by Keller and his associates (71) as the "repetitive intake of alcoholic beverages to a degree that harms the drinker in health or socially or economically, with indication of inability consistently to control the occasion or amount of drinking." A synonym for alcoholism recommended by the World Health Association (40) and American Psychiatric Association (6) (Table 11.1) is *alcohol dependence*.

DSM-IV-TR distinguishes alcohol dependence from alcohol abuse (Table 11.2). The abuse category is for problems resulting from drinking. In addition to these problems, the dependence category includes alcohol-seeking behavior, tolerance to alcohol, and alcohol withdrawal (Table 11.1). Since alcohol dependence can be diagnosed in the absence of tolerance or withdrawal, there is minimal difference between dependence and abuse as defined by *DSM-IV-TR*. Abuse has often been viewed as a milder form of dependence, but the validity of distinguishing between dependence and abuse can be questioned. It is hard to imagine individuals having serious problems from drinking without having some degree of tolerance and at least severe hangovers, which can be viewed as mild forms of withdrawal (because hangovers are relieved by alcohol, as is withdrawal). The term "alcoholism" is still widely used and there are currently no indications that it will be used less in the future. For this reason, the term "alcoholism" is retained in this chapter, referring to both alcohol dependence and alcohol abuse, when the abuse, as defined in Table 11.2, is severe.

TABLE II.I Diagnostic Criteria for Substance Dependence

A maladaptive pattern of substance use, leading to clinically significant impairment or distress, as manifested by three (or more) of the following, occurring at any time in the same 12-month period:

(1) Tolerance, as defined by either of the following:

   (a) A need for markedly increased amounts of the substance to achieve intoxication or desired effect
   (b) Markedly diminished effect with continued use of the same amount of the substance

(2) Withdrawal, as manifested by either of the following:

   (a) The characteristic withdrawal syndrome for the substance (refer to criteria A and B of the criteria sets for withdrawal from the specific substances)
   (b) The same (or a closely related) substance is taken to relieve or avoid withdrawal symptoms

(3) The substance is often taken in larger amounts or over a longer period than was intended.
(4) There is a persistent desire or unsuccessful efforts to cut down or control substance use.
(5) A great deal of time is spent in activities necessary to obtain the substance (e.g., visiting multiple doctors or driving long distances), use the substance (e.g., chain-smoking), or recover from its effects.
(6) Important social, occupational, or recreational activities are given up or reduced because of substance use.
(7) The substance use is continued despite knowledge of having a persistent or recurrent physical or psychological problem that is likely to have been caused or exacerbated by the substance (e.g., current cocaine use despite recognition of cocaine-induced depression, or continued drinking despite recognition that an ulcer was made worse by alcohol consumption).

Note: Criteria for alcohol dependence and abuse are the same as for any substance of abuse (e.g., opiates, cocaine; see Chapter 12).
Adapted from diagnostic criteria in the *DSM-IV-TR* (147).

TABLE II.2 Diagnostic Criteria for Substance Abuse

A. A maladaptive pattern of alcohol use leading to clinically significant impairment or distress, as manifested by one (or more) of the following, occurring within a 12-month period:

   (1) Recurrent substance use resulting in a failure to fulfill major role obligations at work, school, or home (e.g., repeated absences or poor work performance related to substance use; substance-related absences, suspensions, or expulsions from school; neglect of children or household)
   (2) Recurrent substance use in situations in which it is physically hazardous (e.g., driving an automobile or operating a machine when impaired by substance use)
   (3) Recurrent substance-related legal problems (e.g., arrests for substance-related disorderly conduct)
   (4) Continued substance use despite having persistent or recurrent social or interpersonal problems caused or exacerbated by the effects of the substance (e.g., arguments with spouse about consequences of intoxication, physical fights)

B. The symptoms have never met the criteria for Alcohol Dependence.

Adapted from diagnostic criteria in the *DSM-IV-TR* (147).

Historical Background

Six millennia ago at the Sumerian trading post of Godin Tepe in what is now western Iran, people were drinking alcohol. In 1992, chemists analyzed a residue in pottery jars found in the ruins of Godin Tepe and identified it as wine or beer. A scientist said, "I think a lot of serious drinking was going on there." The Sumerians were among the first people to develop a complex, literate society of prospering city-states based on irrigation, agriculture, and widespread trade (52).

Beer-making began almost as soon as (or even before) Mesopotamians domesticated barley to make bread in the early transition to agriculture around 8000 B.C. A longstanding debate in archaeology centers on the question of which came first after the domestication of barley: beer or bread?

There is other evidence that alcohol goes back at least to Paleolithic times. This derives from etymology as well as from studies of Stone Age cultures that survived into the twentieth century. Available to Paleolithic man, presumably, were fermented fruit juice (wine), fermented grain (beer), and fermented honey (mead). Etymological evidence suggests that mead may have been the earliest beverage of choice. The word *mead* derives—by way of *mede* (Middle English) and *meodu* (Anglo-Saxon)—from ancient words of Indo-European stock, such as *methy* (Greek) and *madhu* (Sanskrit). In Sanskrit and Greek, the term means both "honey" and "intoxicating drink." The association of honey rather than grain or fruit with intoxication may indicate its greater antiquity as a source of alcohol (110).

All but three of the numerous Stone Age cultures that survived into modern times have been familiar with alcohol. "The three exceptions," Berton Roueché writes, "are the environmentally underprivileged polar peoples, the ... Australian aborigines, and the ... [people] of Tierra del Fuego" (110). Early European explorers of Africa and the New World invariably discovered that alcohol was important in the local cultures. The Indians of eastern North America, for instance, were using alcohol in the form of fermented birch and sugar maple sap (110).

Alcohol was used medicinally and in religious ceremonies for thousands of years, but it also has a long history of recreational use. Noah, according to the Old Testament, "drank of the wine and was drunken."

Roueché noted that "one of the few surviving relics of the Seventeenth Egyptian Dynasty, which roughly coincided with the reign of Hammurabi, was a hieroglyphic outburst of a female courtier. 'Give me eighteen bowls of wine!' she exclaimed for posterity. 'Behold, I love drunkenness!'" (110). So did other Egyptians of that era. "Drunkenness was apparently not rare," Sigerist remarked, "and seems to have occurred in all layers of society from the farmers to the gods (or ruling class). Banquets frequently ended with the guests, men and women, being sick, and this did not in any way seem shocking" (123).

Descriptions of drunkenness fill the writings of antiquity, but so do pleas for moderation. Dynastic Egypt apparently invented the first temperance tract (110). Moderation was recommended by no less an authority than Genghis Khan: "A soldier must not get drunk oftener than once a week. It would, of course, be better if he did not get drunk at all, but one should not expect the impossible." The Old Testament condemns drunkenness, but not alcohol. "Give strong drink unto him that is ready to perish," the Book of Proverbs proclaims, "and wine unto those that be of heavy hearts. Let him drink, and forget his poverty, and remember his misery no more."

The process of distillation was discovered about 800 A.D. in Arabia. (The word *alcohol* comes from the Arabic *alkuhl*, meaning essence.) For centuries distilled alcohol was used in medicine, but by the seventeenth century it had also become a drug of abuse on a large scale. By the late seventeenth century the annual worldwide production of distilled liquors, chiefly gin, was enormous.

Ancient and classical writers used words that are universally translated as "drunkenness." The people who had it were "drunkards." In the fourteenth century Chaucer used *dronkelewe* to mean addiction to alcohol as a mental illness (26). By the nineteenth century, "inebriety" was the favored descriptor; those who manifested it were not merely inebriated—they were "inebriates." A Swedish public health authority, Magnus Huss, in 1849 coined the term "alcoholism." The word caught on: Danish has *alkoholisme*; Dutch, *alcoholisme*; English, *alcoholism*; Finnish, *alkoholismi*; German, *alkoholismus*; Italian, *alcolismo*; Norwegian, *alkoholisme*; Polish, *alkoholizm*; Portuguese, *alcoolismo*; Russian, *alkogolism*; Serbo-Croatian, *alkoholizam*; Slovene, *alkoholizem*; Spanish, *alcoholismo*; Swedish, *alkoholism* (70).

The "disease concept" of alcoholism originated in the writings of Benjamin Rush and the British physician Thomas Trotter (111), and during the last half of the nineteenth century the notion that alcoholism was a disease became popular with physicians. In the 1830s, Dr. Samuel Woodward, the first superintendent of Worcester State Hospital, Massachusetts, and Dr. Eli Todd of Hartford, Connecticut, suggested establishing special institutions for inebriates. The first was opened in Boston in 1841. In 1904 the Medical Temperance Society changed its name to the American Medical Association for the Study of Inebriety and Narcotics. The *Journal of Inebriety*, established in 1876, was founded on the "fact that inebriety is a neurosis and psychosis." During Prohibition, however, the concept of alcoholism as a disease lost its vogue (67).

With repeal of the Eighteenth Amendment, the disease concept was revived. Pioneering studies performed at the Yale School of Alcohol Studies and the writings of E. M. Jellinek were largely responsible for the popularization of this concept in the twentieth century. In the mid-1960s the U.S. government began supporting alcoholism research on a rather large scale; by the 1980s, the federal government and most state governments were sponsoring alcohol treatment programs, and a large number of proprietary hospitals for alcoholism spanned the continent. Later, for-profit hospitals began to disappear because of the advent of "managed care."

Epidemiology

Alcohol has been the "intoxicant of choice" in Judeo-Christian culture. "To drink is a Christian diversion/Unknown to the Turk and the Persian," wrote Congreve 300 years ago. It was not *totally* unknown to the Turk and the Persian, but it is true that they favored other intoxicants, notably the products of the poppy and hemp plant.

One of the myths of our times is that the "stresses" of modern living have produced a society unusually reliant on alcohol. This is not true. Per capita consumption in the United States was highest in the early 1800s, at an estimated six or seven gallons a year per person (computed in absolute alcohol—200 proof), when whiskey and cider were the favorite beverages (110). One reason was that whiskey is more portable than grain, and cider more portable than apples. Portability was important before trains were developed.

Over the last half century, consumption of alcohol (pure alcohol) by Americans increased to nearly three gallons per person per year in about 1980, with subsequent steady decline to current per capita consumption of a little more than two gallons per year (55, 79). These figures are based on tax data. Untaxed sales, such as those on military installations, are not included, so per capita consumption may be underestimated. Also, because consumption estimates are based on the resident population, when residents of one state cross into another state to purchase lower-priced alcoholic beverages, the result is a higher per capita consumption figure for the state in which sales occur. Washington, DC, and states with high rates of tourism and business travel have higher reported consumption rates because sales to transients are calculated as consumption by the resident population.

International comparisons are difficult at best. Alcohol use patterns have been compared among different countries in a variety of ways. Abstinence appears to be relatively prevalent in Mediterranean countries and uncommon in Denmark. Frequency of alcohol consumption appears to be highest in the European wine-producing countries of Germany and France but also in Denmark, where beer and spirits are preferred over wine. International comparisons of overall consumption are inconsistent, although the United Kingdom and Germany appear to have the highest overall rates of consumption. Ireland, contrary to its popular image, has a lower consumption rate than the United Kingdom. The United States has relatively average alcohol consumption in international comparisons, and Israel has relatively low consumption. Russia (where general under-reporting is well recognized) has no greater than average apparent consumption (95), despite relatively high rates of binge drinking documented among Russian men (17).

Most adults in the United States are light drinkers. About 38% abstain, 43% drink less than three drinks per week, and only 4% consume an average of one ounce or more of alcohol per day (3).

Drinking patterns vary by age and sex. For both men and women, the prevalence of drinking is highest and abstention is lowest in the 25- to 34-year age range (9). Males are two to four times as likely than females to be "heavy" drinkers at all ages (16, 69, 143). For ages 65 years and older, abstainers exceed drinkers in both sexes, and only 10%–12% of men and 2%–3% of women appear to be heavy drinkers (19, 63, 119). "Heavy" drinking, which can be deleterious to the individual's health, is defined by the U.S. government as consuming 14 or more drinks per week for men and 7 or more for women (35, 37, 38, 137).

The level of consumption varies markedly in different segments of the population. In the United States consumption is greatest in the Northeast, lowest in the South. Young males drink more than any other group in the United States (52). The proportion of adolescents who report drinking increases steadily with age, reaching 80%–90% among the oldest school children. By that time, as many girls as boys report "ever" having drunk any alcohol.

Most alcohol is consumed by a small percentage of people: 70% of the drinking population consume only 20% of the total alcohol consumed; 30% of drinkers consume 80% of the alcohol; and 10% consume 50% (95).

Consumption must be distinguished from alcoholism. Is the latter increasing? It could be decreasing (98). In 1795, the distinguished American physician Benjamin Rush estimated that 4,000 Americans died each year from "over-indulgence in ardent spirits." Since the population of the country was about 4 million, this gives a rate of 100 per 100,000. The officially recorded rate of death from alcoholism in the United States today is 2 per 100,000. Granting that Dr. Rush's estimate is suspect, alcoholism in the United States still may be less prevalent today than it was 200 years ago.

There are multiple problems in estimating the prevalence of alcoholism. One is disagreement on the precise definition of alcoholism (58, 96). Second, the conceptualization has evolved over time (80). Third, when household surveys are done, those with alcoholism, more than most people, are not home.

A fourth reason to be skeptical about prevalence estimates is that advocacy is a potent factor in the production of statistics. Government officials spend much of their time trying to wring money out of reluctant legislators and some are caught in the dilemma of, on the one hand, wanting the prevalence of alcoholism to be low to show they are doing a good job and, on the other hand, wanting it to be high to inspire lawmakers to spend more money on the problem. In the late 1960s, for example, the U.S. government announced that 5 million Americans have alcoholism; this number ballooned to 14 million less than three decades later. This increase coincided with increased efforts by the national government to study and treat alcoholism (73).

Nonetheless, keeping all these concerns in mind, there is a need to ascertain with as much accuracy as possible the prevalence of valid disorders. Some would endorse Grant et al. (54) who in 2004 reported that the National Epidemiologic Survey of Alcohol and Related Disorders (NESARC) had found the *DSM-IV* prevalence of alcohol abuse and dependence over a 12-month period to be 4.7% and 3.8%, respectively.

Alcohol problems are correlated with a history of school difficulty (32). High school dropouts and individuals with a record of frequent truancy and delinquency appear to have a particularly high risk of alcoholism.

Individuals in certain occupations are more vulnerable to alcoholism than those doing other types of work. Waiters, bartenders, longshoremen, musicians, authors, and reporters have relatively high cirrhosis rates; accountants, mail carriers, and carpenters have relatively low rates (85).

Clinical Picture

Alcoholism is a behavioral disorder. The specific behavior that causes problems is the consumption of large quantities of alcohol on repeated occasions. The motivation underlying this behavior is often obscure (8). When asked why they drink excessively, individuals with alcoholism occasionally attribute their drinking to a particular mood such as depression or anxiety or to situational problems. They sometimes describe an overpowering "need" to drink, variously described as a craving or compulsion. Just as often, however, the patient with alcoholism is unable to give a plausible explanation of his or her excessive drinking (82).

Like other drug dependencies, alcoholism is accompanied by a preoccupation with obtaining the drug in quantities sufficient to produce intoxication over long periods. It is especially true early in the course of alcoholism that patients may deny this preoccupation or attempt to rationalize their need by assertions that they drink no more than their friends. As part of this denial or rationalization, people who drink to excess tend to spend their time with other heavy drinkers.

An alcoholic patient named David explained (52):

> My need was easy to hide from myself and others (maybe I'm kidding
> myself about the others). I only associated with people who drank. I
> married a woman who drank. There were always reasons to drink.
> I was low, tense, tired, mad, happy. I probably drank as often because
> I was happy as for any other reason. And occasions for drinking—
> when drinking was appropriate, expected—were endless, football
> games, fishing trips, parties, holidays, birthdays, Christmas, or merely
> Saturday night. Drinking became interwoven with everything
> pleasurable—food, sex, social life. When I stopped drinking, these
> things, for a time, lost all interest for me, they were so tied to drinking.

As alcoholism progresses and problems from drinking become more serious, the individual may drink alone, sneak drinks, hide the bottle, and take other measures to conceal the seriousness of their condition. This is almost always accompanied by feelings of guilt and remorse, which in turn may produce more drinking, temporarily relieving the feelings. Remorse may be particularly intense in the morning, when the patient has not had a drink for a number of hours, and this may provoke morning drinking (66):

> For years [David wrote], I drank and had very little hangover, but now
> the hangovers were gruesome. I felt physically bad—headachy,
> nauseous, weak, but the mental part was the hardest. I loathed myself.
> I was waking early and thinking what a mess I was, how I had hurt so
> many others and myself. The words "guilty" and "depression" sound
> superficial in trying to describe how I felt. The loathing was almost
> physical—a dead weight that could be lifted in only one way, and that
> was by having a drink, so I drank, morning after morning. After two or
> three, my hands were steady, I could hold some breakfast down, and
> the guilt was gone, or almost.

Prolonged drinking, even if initiated to relieve guilt and anxiety, commonly produces anxiety and depression (83). The full range of symptoms associated with depression and anxiety disorders—including terminal insomnia, low mood, irritability, and anxiety attacks with chest pain, palpitations, and dyspnea—often appear. Alcohol temporarily relieves these symptoms, resulting in a vicious cycle of drinking-depression-drinking, which may ultimately result in a classical withdrawal syndrome. Often the patient makes a valiant effort to stop drinking and may succeed for a period of several days or weeks, only to fall off the wagon again:

> At some point I was without wife, home, or job. I had nothing to do but drink. The drinking was now steady, days on end. I lost appetite and missed meals (besides money was short). I awoke at night, sweating and shaking, and had a drink. I awoke in the morning vomiting and had a drink. It couldn't last. My ex-wife found me in my apartment shaking and seeing things, and got me in the hospital. I dried out, left, and went back to drinking. I was hospitalized again, and this time stayed dry for 6 months. I was nervous and couldn't sleep, but got some of my confidence back, and found a part-time job. Then my ex-boss offered my job back and I celebrated by having a drink. The next night I had two drinks. In a month I was drinking as much as ever and again unemployed.

Repeated experiences like this easily lead to feelings of despair and hopelessness. By the time patients consult a physician, they have often reached rock bottom. Their situation seems hopeless and, after years of heavy drinking, their problems have become so numerous that they feel nothing can be done about them. At this point, they may be ready to acknowledge their alcoholism but feel powerless to stop drinking. But many do stop—permanently—as will be discussed later.

Alcohol is one of the few psychoactive drugs that produce, on occasion, classical amnesia. Even people who are not alcoholic, when drinking, also experience this amnesia (blackouts), but much less often, as a rule, than do people with alcoholism (25, 68). These episodes of amnesia are particularly distressful to alcoholic individuals because they may fear that they have unknowingly harmed someone or behaved imprudently while intoxicated (52):

> A thirty-nine-year-old salesman awoke in a strange hotel room. He had a mild hangover but otherwise felt normal. His clothes were hanging in the closet: he was clean-shaven. He dressed and went down to the lobby. He learned from the clerk that he was in Las Vegas and that he had checked in two days previously. It had been obvious that he had

been drinking, the clerk said, but he hadn't seemed very drunk. The
date was Saturday the fourteenth. His last recollection was of sitting in
a St. Louis bar on Monday the ninth. He had been drinking all day and
was drunk, but could remember everything perfectly until about
three p.m., when "like a curtain dropping," his memory went blank. It
remained blank for approximately five days. Three years later, those
five days were still a blank. He was so frightened by the experience that
he abstained from alcohol for two years.

Studies of blackouts indicate that the amnesia is anterograde (97). During
a blackout, individuals have relatively intact remote and immediate memory,
but they experience a specific short-term memory deficit in which they are
unable to recall events that happened 5 or 10 minutes before. Because their
other intellectual faculties are well preserved, they can perform complicated
acts and appear normal to the casual observer. For many years it has been
known that alcoholic blackouts represent impaired consolidation of new information rather than repression motivated by a desire to forget events that
happened while drinking (49).

Sometimes, however, a curious thing happens: The drinker recalls things
that happened during a previous drinking period that, when sober, he had
forgotten. For example, people with alcoholism often report hiding money or
alcohol when drinking, forgetting it when sober, and having their memory
return when drinking again (49):

A forty-seven-year-old housewife often wrote letters when she was
drinking. Sometimes she would jot down notes for a letter and start
writing it but not finish it. The next day, sober, she would be unable to
decipher the notes. Then she would start drinking again, and after a
few drinks the meaning of the notes would become clear and she
would resume writing the letter. "It was like picking up the pencil
where I had left off."

Anecdotal reports suggest that benzodiazepine medication combined
with alcohol increases the likelihood of a blackout occurring with smaller
amounts of alcohol than is usually required (93, 120). Benzodiazepines may
also by themselves lead to short-term anterograde memory impairment in a
dose-dependent fashion (15, 84, 99). Benzodiazepines do not typically produce the dense blackouts associated with severe alcoholism. Benzodiazepine-
naïve subjects, however, can have dramatic effects on memory from a single
dose (15).

By the time people with alcohol problems consult a physician, they have often developed medical and social complications from drinking (see section "Complications").

Identifying Alcoholism

Before alcoholism can be treated, it first must be recognized. Physicians are in a particularly good position to identify a drinking problem early through three main approaches: They can take a history, perform a physical examination, and order laboratory tests.

The alcohol inquiry must be designed by the examiner using the physician's own style to elicit the history and eventually the diagnostic criteria. After rapport is developed and the examiner is ready to turn to this section, the clinical approach may be direct ("Tell me about your current and past use of alcohol") or indirect. ("Has alcohol ever interfered with your social, work, interpersonal or legal affairs?") The examiner should avoid a staccato firing of questions, judgmental approach, or aggressive style, all of which will likely inhibit open disclosure by the patient. Over the last 30 years a number of brief screening surveys have been developed for various settings, including the Michigan Alcoholism Screening Test (MAST) (122), CAGE questionnaire (45), Alcohol Use Disorders Identification Test (AUDIT) (114), and TWEAK screening questionnaire (112). While the screening parts of these instruments may be helpful to the clinician in developing a set of questions and even perhaps a style of approach, the reader is reminded that brief surveys neither capture all cases nor diagnose illness. The clinician must take the time to develop rapport and talk with the patient to obtain a specific history of alcohol consumption patterns and sufficient information for diagnostic assessment of problem drinking.

Following are some medical indications of a drinking problem:

1. Arcus senilis—a ringlike opacity of the cornea—occurs commonly with age, causes no visual disturbance, and is considered an innocent condition. The ring forms from fatty material in the blood. Alcohol increases fat in the blood and more patients with alcoholism are reported to have the ring than others their age (13, 46).

2. A red nose (acne rosacea) suggests the owner has a weakness for alcoholic beverages. Often, however, people with red noses are teetotalers or even rabid prohibitionists, and they resent the insinuation.

3. Red palms (palmer erythema) are also suggestive but not diagnostic of alcoholism.

4. Cigarette burns between the index and middle fingers or on the chest and contusions and bruises should raise suspicions of alcoholic stupor.

5. Painless enlargement of the liver may suggest a larger alcohol intake than the liver can process. Severe, constant upper abdominal pain and tenderness radiating to the back indicates pancreatic inflammation, and alcohol sometimes is the cause.

6. Reduced sensation and weakness in the feet and legs may occur from excessive drinking.

7. Laboratory tests provide other clues. The major alcohol biomarkers are gamma-glutamyl transpeptidase (GGT), alanine amino-transferase (ALT), aspartate aminotransferase (AST), mean corpuscular volume (MCV), and carbohydrate-deficient transferring (CDT) (90). Historically, the test used most commonly in clinical practice is GGT. Although more than half of alcoholic patients have increased amounts of this protein, it is nonspecific for alcoholism because it can also be elevated in nonalcoholic liver disease, biliary disease, obesity, and medications. In 2001 a new and more specific test, the carbohydrate-deficient transferrin (CDT) test, was approved by the U.S. Food and Drug Administration (FDA) (10, 90). This biomarker has been widely used in Europe for many years. Few other medical circumstances, such as rare genetic variants, produce false-positive test results (92).

Another approach is to use a wide range of commonly available blood chemistry tests and subject them to quadratic discriminant analysis in a test called the Early Detection of Alcohol Consumption (EDAC) (92). Each value may be in the normal range, but in toto they produce a distinctive "fingerprint" that is highly specific for detecting recent heavy drinking. This test measures heavy alcohol consumption rather than identifying alcoholism. The EDAC is most useful as a screening tool and requires verification with the CDT.

In their search for signs of alcohol abuse, physicians sometimes slip into a moralistic attitude that alienates the patient. For personal reasons, physicians may believe any drinking is wrong, but they still should be aware of relatively recent findings that suggest moderate drinking may actually contribute to longevity (127, 135). Specifically, "beneficial" effects of alcohol may include less likelihood of cardiovascular illness (i.e., myocardial infarction, heart failure, and ischemic stroke thought to be largely conferred through heart-protective effects of increased high-density lipoprotein [HDL] cholesterol) and reduced risk for diabetes mellitus, dementia, and osteo-porosis. The lowest mortality from all causes is associated with consumption of one to two alcoholic beverages per day. Above that level, the risk for medical complications increases dramatically with consumption in what is described as a J-shaped curve (56, 109, 127).

None of this should be interpreted as encouragement of immoderate use of alcohol. The risk for alcohol abuse and dependence preclude recommenda-tions for nondrinkers to initiate alcohol use for potential health benefits. For healthy individuals who demonstrate ability to enjoy alcohol safely, however, recommendation of abstinence is not indicated, although continued moni-toring is (127). In alcoholism, no level of intake is considered beneficial. In addition, moderate drinking may contribute to automobile accidents, high blood pressure, breast cancer, adverse outcomes for patients with hepatitis C, and birth defects associated with drinking during pregnancy (41, 56, 127).

Biological Findings

Current understanding of the biology of alcohol addiction is yet rudimentary. Unlike opioids and nicotine, alcohol has no known receptor in the human brain (43). Alcohol affects a number of neurotransmitter systems in various brain regions that are known to play a role in reward and reinforcement processes considered fundamental to addictions. Administration of alcohol enhances GABA (the brain's main inhibitory neurotransmitter), inhibits glutamate (an excitatory neurotransmitter), and increases dopamine, serotonin, and opioid peptides (21, 43). Research to date suggests that genetic variations in these neurotransmitter systems mediating reward, reinforcement, tolerance, and withdrawal may predispose some individuals to the craving and loss of control that characterize addiction (21, 43).

Natural History

While early studies suggested that the natural history of alcoholism appeared somewhat different in men and women (64, 141), later studies have been less clear. Many of the studies suffer from retrospective nature, short follow-up, select populations, and inconsistent definitions of alcoholism. However, keeping these concerns in mind, there does seem to be—irrespective of gender—either a rapid course from initiation from dependence in several years or a longer course that proceeds over 10 or 15 years.

In men, symptoms of alcoholism do not commonly occur for the first time after age 45 (12, 52). If they do occur, the physician should be alerted to the possibility of primary affective disorder or brain disease. Alcoholism has been studied less extensively in women than in men, but the evidence suggests that the course of the disorder is more variable in women. The onset often occurs later (27, 64) and spontaneous remission apparently is less frequent (36). Women with the disorder are also more likely to have a history of depression (141).

Historically, weight has been given to types or patterns of drinking. The patterns are quite variable, and it is incorrect to associate one particular pattern exclusively with alcoholism. Overall, alcohol dependence is a chronic remitting and relapsing disorder with periods of remission lasting for variable lengths of time.

Alcoholism has a higher "spontaneous" remission rate than is often recognized. The incidence of first admissions to psychiatric hospitals for alcoholism drops markedly in the sixth and seventh decades, as do first arrests for alcohol-related offenses. Although the mortality rate among people with alcoholism is perhaps two to three times that of moderate drinkers, attrition through death is probably insufficient to account for the apparent decrease in problem drinking in middle and late middle life (55, 135).

Based on questionnaire data obtained from alcoholic patients, Jellinek promulgated the view that manifestations of alcoholism follow a natural chronological order, with blackouts being one of the early "prodromal" symptoms of the illness (66). Later studies (25, 49, 97) have challenged this view, and it is now believed that problems from drinking may occur in various sequences and that blackouts have no special significance as a sign of incipient alcoholism. Frequently, after years of heavy problem-free drinking, a person may experience a large number of problems in a brief period. Table 11.3 shows the mean age of onset of alcohol problems in an unselected series of hospitalized alcoholic men.

Historically, Jellinek (67) in 1960 developed an interesting typology subdividing alcoholism along observable drinking patterns. Subsequent research by Edwards and Gross in 1976 (39) moved the field toward establishing a reliable basis for establishing a diagnosis of alcohol dependence syndrome by using criteria. Their "provisional description" of certain observable behaviors (e.g., 1. Narrowing of drinking behaviors, 2. Salience of drink-seeking behavior, 3. Increased tolerance to alcohol, 4. Repeated withdrawal symptoms, 5. Avoidance of withdrawal by further alcohol intake, 6. Awareness of compulsion to drink, and 7. Relapse after abstinence) became the bases for the formalized criteria for alcohol dependence found in *DSM-III-R*, *DSM-IV*, *DSM-IV-TR* (see Table 11.1), and the international diagnostic criteria (*ICD-10*).

TABLE 11.3 Onset of Alcoholic Manifestations among All Subjects (N = 100)

Manifestation	Present (%)	Mean Age at Onset	Percentage of Subjects Reporting Manifestation (by Age at First Occurrence)*										
			<20	20–24	25–29	30–34	35–39	40–44	45–49	50–54	55–59	60–64	65–70
1. Frequent drunken episodes	98	27	18	17	21	18	13	7	3		1	1	
2. Weekend drunken episodes	82	28	11	18	21	32	6	8	2		1		
3. Morning drinking	84	31	2	17	15	25	17	9	11	1	1	1	
4. Benders	76	31	7	14	18	21	13	9	12	5	1		
5. Neglecting meals	86	32	2	11	14	29	15	10	10	6	1		1
6. "Shakes"	88	33	1	11	15	24	17	9	16	3	2		1
7. Job loss from drinking	69	34	3	7	19	19	26	7	9	6	3	1	
8. Separation or divorce from drinking	44	34	3	16	7	23	14	20	14	7			
9. Blackouts	64	35	2	6	16	28	25	8	9	3	3		
10. Joined Alcoholics Anonymous	39	36		8	8	28	20	15	8	10	3		
11. Hospitalization for drinking	100	37	1	3	14	18	20	13	14	9	6		
12. Alcohol withdrawal syndrome	45	38		2	11	11	40	16	7	11	2	1	1

* Figures rounded off to nearest whole number for ease of perusal. Sums may therefore not equal 100%.

Adapted from Goodwin et al. (50).

Complications

Because alcoholism is defined by the problems it creates, symptoms and complications inevitably overlap. For present purposes, we will consider social and medical complications separately.

High rates of marital separation and divorce accompany alcoholism (52). People with alcoholism often have job troubles, including frequent absenteeism and job loss. They also have a high frequency of accidents—in the home, on the job, and while driving automobiles. About 40% of highway fatalities in the United States involve a driver who has been drinking (4). Nearly half of convicted felons are alcoholic (52), and about half of police activities in large cities are associated with alcohol-related offenses. About 10% of pilots killed in private plane crashes had been drinking, according to the Federal Aviation Commission (*New York Times*, April 9, 1995).

Medical complications fall into three categories: *(1)* acute effects of heavy drinking, *(2)* chronic effects of heavy drinking, and *(3)* withdrawal effects. Consumption of very large amounts of alcohol can lead directly to death by depressing the respiratory center in the medulla. Acute hemorrhagic pancreatitis occasionally occurs from a single heavy drinking episode.

Nearly every organ system can be affected, directly or indirectly, by chronic, heavy use of alcohol. The gastrointestinal system is especially vulnerable to damaging effects of alcohol. Chronic gastritis may occur, although chronic *Helicobacter pylori* infection is causal in most alcoholic gastritis rather than the direct effects of alcohol itself. A recent review of related research concluded that the available evidence does not show increased risk of gastric or duodenal ulcer disease in association with acute or chronic alcohol consumption (134).

The most damaging effect of alcohol on the gastrointestinal tract is to the liver. Exactly how alcohol damages the liver is still not clear, despite decades of study. Alcohol induces tissue injury through known pathways involving acetaldehyde production, oxidant injury, and proinflammatory cytokines. The underlying mechanisms in these processes, however, are complex, involving alcohol-induced alteration in cellular pathways of signal transduction, activation of tumor necrosis factor, and generation of free radicals promoting lipid peroxidation, ultimately resulting in oxidant injury in mitochondria (91).

The first stage of alcoholic liver disease is fatty liver, a rapid response to excessive alcohol consumption. While high-fat diets alone cause fatty liver, alcohol produces fatty liver even without dietary fat intake. High-fat diets increase the likelihood of fatty liver and liver disease associated with chronic excessive alcohol intake (77, 81). Although fatty liver is reversible, hepatocytes in this condition are vulnerable to adversity and have reduced survival.

Continued alcohol ingestion leads to a progression of inflammatory responses and fibrosis and ultimately cirrhosis of the liver in some individuals. Although most patients with Laennec cirrhosis in Western countries are excessive drinkers, most people with severe alcoholism do not develop cirrhosis (probably less than 10%). This finding leaves unresolved the question of the direct role of alcohol in producing cirrhosis. It appears that cirrhosis results from the combined effect of alcohol and diet plus other factors, likely including heredity (104).

Because the average alcoholic consumes half of all daily calories from alcohol, insufficient intake of vital nutrients can result in serious malnutrition. Gastrointestinal complications of alcoholism such as pancreatitis can further cause malnutrition through malabsorption. Alcohol also promotes degradation of nutrients such as vitamin A. Although experimental studies have demonstrated that nutritional deficiencies alone may damage the liver, adequate nutrition does not protect the liver against the toxic effects of chronic excessive alcohol consumption (81).

Alcoholism is associated with pathology of the nervous system. It is still debated whether peripheral neuropathy, the most common neurological complication, results from multiple vitamin B deficiencies or direct toxic effects of alcohol (7). It is usually reversible with adequate nutrition. Retrobulbar neuropathy may lead to amblyopia (sometimes called "tobacco-alcohol amblyopia"), which is also usually reversible with vitamin therapy.

Other neurological complications include anterior lobe cerebellar degenerative disease (115) and the Wernicke-Korsakoff syndrome (22). The latter results from thiamine deficiency (52). The acute Wernicke stage consists of ocular disturbances (nystagmus or sixth-nerve palsy), ataxia, and confusion. It usually clears in a few days but may progress to a chronic brain syndrome (Korsakoff psychosis). Short-term memory loss (anterograde amnesia) is the most characteristic feature of Korsakoff psychosis. "Confabulation" (narration of fanciful tales) may also occur. The Wernicke-Korsakoff syndrome is associated with necrotic lesions of the mammillary bodies, thalamus, and other brain stem areas. Thiamine corrects early Wernicke signs rapidly and *may* prevent development of an irreversible Korsakoff dementia. Once the dementia is established, thiamine does not usually help (see also Chapter 13).

Whether excessive use of alcohol produces cortical atrophy has been debated for decades. A confluence of radiological and pathological evidence has reached a consensus that brain shrinkage especially in white matter but also in gray matter occurs with chronic alcoholism. The frontal cortex appears most sensitive to chronic alcohol-induced damage (75, 121, 126, 130). The motor cortex, cerebellum, pons, mammillary bodies, thalamus, and hypothalamus are also affected. Ventricular and cortical sulci are enlarged. Some of these brain matter changes may reverse within a month of abstinence from alcohol, although permanent and irreversible damage may persist, presumably due to neuronal loss (75, 126, 130).

In chronic alcoholism, cognitive impairments are well described in domains of executive functioning (involving judgment, appropriateness of affect, insight, social functioning, motivation, and attention, learning and memory, and abstract problem solving). Longstanding excessive alcohol consumption is particularly disruptive to visuospatial abilities (47) and to functions of gait, balance, and postural stability of the lower extremities (57, 130, 131). Cognitive deficits in chronic alcoholism have long been considered to represent "frontal" brain abnormalities (75), but more recent work has also implicated damage to the pontocerebellar and cerebellothallamocortical systems (57, 131). While the amount of alcohol consumed has not consistently been found to parallel the severity of cognitive deficits in alcoholic patients, lifetime alcohol consumption is related to problems with gait and balance (131). Continued abstinence may permit partial recovery of brain function, but deficits based on neuronal loss may be permanent and irreversible (75, 105, 130).

Other medical complications of alcoholism include cardiomyopathy, thrombocytopenia and anemia, and myopathy. Although excessive alcohol use is clearly associated with increased likelihood of breast cancer, the potential for light to moderate levels of drinking to increase breast cancer risk is still debated (56, 76), and postmenopausal women may have more risk than younger women (127). It has also been reported that alcoholism is associated with increased risk of stroke (88), although light to moderate alcohol consumption could be protective (106).

Teratogenic effects of alcohol have been suspected for centuries, but only in the last few decades has research demonstrated a distinct pattern of birth defects associated with maternal alcoholism during pregnancy. It is called fetal alcohol syndrome. Affected babies are small and exhibit various combinations of developmental delays, craniofacial abnormalities (short palpebral fissures, epicanthal folds, and maxillary hypoplasia), and microcephaly. Associated behavioral and cognitive problems observed in these children are impaired information processing and memory, intellectual deficiencies, hyperactivity, impulsivity, and social and communication skills deficits. Brain abnormalities documented in the hippocampus, corpus callosum, cerebellum (especially anterior vermis), and basal ganglia (especially caudate nucleus) in fetal alcohol syndrome may explain some of the behavioral and cognitive problems (86, 108, 126). Animal studies have now demonstrated specific teratogenic properties of ethyl alcohol in a variety of species, many of the abnormalities being similar to those described in humans (33, 72).

Fetal alcohol syndrome is the leading known cause of mental retardation (44). A comprehensive review of research on the prevalence of fetal alcohol syndrome estimated its occurrence in approximately 0.5 to 2.0 per 1,000 births. The prevalence of all alcohol-related neurodevelopmental disorders is far higher, at least 10 per 1,000 births (87). Far more women drink during pregnancy than have fetal alcohol syndrome babies. Not all children prenatally exposed to heavy alcohol intake develop the full syndrome, many experiencing milder forms of brain abnormalities and associated cognitive and behavioral effects. Moderate drinking during pregnancy in amounts below those known to be associated with fetal alcohol syndrome may also have negative behavioral and neurocognitive consequences; the data on risk for fetal malformations or other gestational problems, however, are inconclusive (56). The amount of alcohol needed to harm a fetus is not established. No threshold has been determined for safe levels of drinking in pregnancy; therefore, general recommendations established by the U.S. Surgeon General in 1981 for abstinence during pregnancy still prevail (56).

Grand mal convulsions ("rum fits") occur occasionally, sometimes as long as 2 or 3 days after drinking stops. As a rule, convulsions in alcoholism do not represent epilepsy; electroencephalograms (EEGs) are normal when the individual is not drinking and convulsions occur only during withdrawal (62).

So-called chronic alcoholic hallucinosis refers to the persistence of hallucinations, usually auditory, for long periods after other abstinence symptoms subside and after the patient has stopped heavy drinking (2). This occurs rarely; after a century of debate concerning the etiology, it has not been resolved whether drinking actually produces the condition.

The term "alcohol withdrawal syndrome" is preferable to "delirium tremens" (DTs). The latter refers to a specific manifestation of the syndrome. The most common withdrawal symptom is tremulousness, which usually occurs only a few hours after cessation of drinking and may even begin while the person is still drinking ("relative abstinence"). Transitory hallucinations also may occur. If so, they usually begin 12 to 24 hours after drinking stops (52). The hallucinations and confusion sometimes associated with this state may precipitate fear and associated behaviors, such as jumping out hospital windows and other forms of disorganized self-harm that represent attempts to escape misperceived terrors. These patients require close monitoring to prevent misadventure.

After a week of heavy drinking and little food, a 30-year-old newspaper reporter tried to drink a morning cup of coffee and found that his hands were shaking so violently he could not get the cup to his mouth.

He managed to pour some whisky into a glass and drank as much as he could. His hands became less shaky but now he was nauseated and began having "dry heaves." He tried repeatedly to drink but could not keep the alcohol down. He felt ill and intensely anxious and decided to call a doctor friend. The doctor recommended hospitalization.

On admission, the patient had a marked resting and exertional tremor of the hands, and his tongue and eyelids were tremulous. He also had feelings of "internal" tremulousness. Lying in the hospital bed, he found the noises outside his window unbearably loud and began seeing "visions" of animals and, on one occasion, a dead relative. He was terrified and called a nurse, who gave him a tranquilizer. He became quieter and his tremor was less pronounced. At all times he realized that the visual phenomena were "imaginary." He always knew where he was and was oriented otherwise. After a few days the tremor disappeared and he no longer hallucinated. He still had trouble sleeping but otherwise felt back to normal and vowed never to drink again. (pp. 41–42) (128)

Alcohol withdrawal syndrome is infrequent and when it does occur is often associated with an intervening medical illness. For a diagnosis of alcohol withdrawal syndrome, gross memory disturbance should be present in addition to other withdrawal symptoms such as agitation and vivid hallucinations. Classically, alcohol withdrawal syndrome begins 2 or 3 days after drinking stops and subsides within 1 to 5 days (2). One must always suspect intercurrent medical illness when delirium occurs during withdrawal. The physician should be particularly alert to hepatic decompensation, pneumonia, subdural hematoma, pancreatitis, and fractures.

Suicide is an important complication of alcoholism. About one-quarter of suicides occur in the context of alcoholism, predominantly among white men over age 35. Apparently alcoholic patients (unlike patients with major depression) are especially likely to commit suicide after loss of a wife, close relative, or other serious interpersonal disruption (31, 133).

Family Studies

Every family study of alcoholism regardless of country of origin has shown much higher rates of alcoholism among the relatives of alcoholic patients than in the general population (43). Having an alcoholic parent, for example, increases a person's risk five-fold. Not everything that runs in families is inherited, however (139). Speaking French, for example, runs in families and

is not inherited. How does one separate nature from nurture in familial illnesses? Both twin and adoption studies have been used to address this question
for many of the conditions described in this book, and this is no less true for
alcoholism. Here, briefly, are the results.

Several twin studies demonstrated significantly greater concordance for
alcoholism in identical twins than in fraternal twins—the more severe the
alcoholism, the greater the difference (43, 103, 136). Early twin studies in
northern Europe, dating to the 1960s to 1980s, described these effects in male
twins, but the situation was not so clear in women. In those days the studies did
not include enough women to provide sufficient statistical power to test for
genetic heritability. Later studies, however, included enough women to demonstrate the same level of genetic heritability in liability for alcoholism as in men—
in the range of 50%–60% (20, 103, 136). Beginning in the early 1970s, results of
several adoption studies in northern Europe and the United States indicated that
alcoholism appears to be inherited through biological fathers, with adoptive
fathers providing no measurable contribution (23, 24, 53, 118). Male biologic
offspring of alcoholic fathers also had elevated rates of childhood conduct disorder compared to offspring of nonalcoholic biological fathers.

Despite overwhelming evidence of genetic liability to risk for alcoholism, it is
easy to overlook reports that alcoholism also occurs in families with no other
alcoholic members. In most studies, about half of hospitalized alcoholic patients
give a family history of alcoholism and about half do not. A number of investigators
have compared the two groups, and two consistent conclusions have emerged.
Alcoholic individuals with familial alcoholism (1) show the first signs of dependence at a younger age than do those without familial alcoholism, and (2) have a
more severe form of dependence with a more rapid, fulminating course (43).

The psychiatric disorders that often accompany alcoholism in individuals
also aggregate in families with alcoholism (especially depressive, anxiety,
somatization, and eating disorders in women and hyperactivity and other
substance use disorders and antisocial personality disorder in men) (43, 100).
There is some evidence to indicate that these comorbid disorders are more
often found in association with nonfamilial alcoholism than in patients who
have alcoholic family members (23, 51). Some studies, however, have suggested
that antisocial personality disorder and childhood conduct disorder and hyperactivity may be specifically associated with the type of alcoholism that runs in
families (61, 101, 133). Cloninger defined two subtypes of alcoholism with
distinct course and relationship to antisocial personality disorder. Type I alcoholism has adult onset and rapid progression to dependence without criminality, and Type II is characterized by male predominance, early onset, and
sociopathy, and is more heritable than Type I (29, 124).

Despite substantial comorbidity (in individuals) and coaggregation (in families) of other psychiatric disorders with alcoholism, available evidence suggests that about 75% of the genetic liability to alcoholism is disease specific (43). Two major studies have demonstrated the familial transmission of opiate, cocaine, and cannabis dependency to be independent of alcohol (14, 89). Nicotine, however, may share its familial transmission of addiction liability with alcohol (43).

Differential Diagnosis

Chronic excessive use of alcohol produces a wide range of psychiatric symptoms that, in various combinations, can mimic other psychiatric disorders. Therefore, while a person is drinking heavily and during the withdrawal period, it is difficult to determine whether he or she suffers from a psychiatric condition other than alcoholism.

Other drug use often accompanies alcoholism. It may be difficult to determine which symptoms are produced by alcohol and which by (crack) cocaine, amphetamines, and so on. Patients who have been drinking heavily and not eating may become hypoglycemic (138), and this condition may produce symptoms resembling those seen in alcohol withdrawal.

A psychiatric condition commonly associated with alcoholism is major depression (18). Women with alcoholism apparently suffer more often from major depression than do their male counterparts (20, 146). The diagnosis of major depression usually can be made by past history or by observing the patient during long periods of abstinence (18). Comorbid major depression is more likely to be the primary diagnosis in women than in men (146); furthermore, family history of major depression and initial onset of the depression before the onset of alcoholism suggest that major depression is the primary disorder (18).

A focused search for an "alcoholic personality" type has been ongoing for nearly a century. Efforts continue (144), but the only personality type found to have some predisposition toward alcoholism has been antisocial personality disorder, with a prevalence of about 15% in alcoholic men and 5% in alcoholic women (60, 107, 116).

Clinical Management

The treatment of alcoholism and the management of alcohol withdrawal symptoms present separate problems. In the absence of serious medical complications, the alcohol withdrawal syndrome is usually transient and self-limited; the patient recovers within several days regardless of treatment (2). Insomnia and irritability may persist for longer periods.

Treatment for withdrawal is symptomatic and prophylactic. Relief of agitation and tremulousness can be achieved with a variety of medications (e.g., including alcohol, paraldehyde, chloral hydrate, clonidine, beta adrenergic antagonists, and carbamazepine), but currently, benzodiazepines (e.g., lorazepam, diazepam, oxazepam, and chlordiazepoxide) are widely considered the drugs of choice for withdrawal. As a class they are considered superior because of efficacy (reduction in withdrawal symptomatology), safety (dosing), possible reduction in seizure risk, and limited side effect profile (particularly compared to the other agents). Several can be administered parenterally to intoxicated patients without apparent significant risk and continued orally during the withdrawal period. Use of phenothiazines should be avoided if possible because these medications lower seizure threshold and are associated with increased mortality, reportedly from hypotension or hepatic encephalopathy.

Some clinicians manage alcohol withdrawal with scheduled benzodiazepines monitored by frequent vital signs checks (every 4 to 6 hours but sometimes up to hourly) and assessment of symptom severity to prompt supplemental medication as needed. Many institutions, however, seem to be moving toward symptom-triggered therapy for alcohol withdrawal. This approach uses the Clinical Institute Withdrawal Assessment for Alcohol revised (CIWA-Ar) (132), a rapidly administered scale, with frequent monitoring (based on the scale), and administration of benzodiazepines as indicated. This approach has been gathering widespread acceptance and has been found to reduce the amount of benzodiazepine needed and to shorten hospitalization (113).

Administration of large doses of vitamins—particularly the B vitamins—is obligatory, given the role of these vitamins in preventing peripheral neuropathy and the Wernicke-Korsakoff syndrome. The B vitamins are water soluble, and there is no apparent danger in administering them in large doses.

Unless the patient is dehydrated because of vomiting or diarrhea, there is no reason to administer fluids parenterally. Contrary to common belief, patients withdrawing from alcohol usually are not dehydrated; actually, they may be overhydrated from consumption of large volumes of fluid (78) and because a resetting of the osmoreceptors in alcohol withdrawal produces an antidiuretic state (42). During the early stages of withdrawal, hyperventilation may cause respiratory alkalosis and this, together with hypomagnesemia, has been reported to produce withdrawal seizures (94). Historically, if the individual had a history of withdrawal seizures, diphenylhydantoin (Dilantin) may have been prescribed, but placebo-controlled trials have now shown the lack of effectiveness of this intervention (62). Fortunately, recent evidence (34) suggests that lorazepam may be helpful in preventing alcohol withdrawal seizures.

Patients who develop delirium should be considered dangerous to themselves and others, and protective measures should be taken. Ordinarily, tranquilizers will calm the patient sufficiently to control agitation, and restraints will not be necessary. Administration of intravenous benzodiazepines in escalating doses may be necessary for severe agitation. Most important, if delirium occurs, further exploration should be conducted to rule out serious medical illness missed in the original examination. When a patient is delirious, as previously noted, an attendant should always be present. It is sometimes helpful to have a friend or relative present.

Uncomplicated outpatient alcohol detoxification has been found to be effective and safe for a significant subset of patients with alcoholism (5, 30, 59, 125, 145). Although the approach varies, nonpharmacologic detoxification is best suited for patients with mild symptoms, only mild to moderate dependence, and no significant withdrawal history. Patients may reside for 3 or 4 days in therapeutic housing that provides support and ensures safety, rest, and proper nutrition. Observation in this setting also allows for medical intervention in case a complication arises.

The treatment of alcoholism should not begin until withdrawal symptoms subside. Treatment has two goals: (1) sobriety and (2) amelioration of psychiatric conditions associated with alcoholism. A small minority of people recovering from alcoholism can eventually drink in moderation, but for several months after a heavy drinking bout, total abstinence is desirable for three reasons. First, it will allow time for assessment of the patient's level of motivation and selection of what may be the optimal approach for achieving the best outcome for the patient. Second, the physician must follow the patient, sober, for a considerable period to potentially diagnose a coexistent psychiatric problem. Third, it is important for the patient to learn that he or she can cope with ordinary life problems without alcohol. Most relapses occur within 6 months of discharge from the hospital; they become less and less frequent after that (102, 142).

For many patients, disulfiram (Antabuse) is helpful in maintaining abstinence. It was the first drug approved by the U.S. Food and Drug Administration (FDA) for the treatment of alcoholism. By inhibiting aldehyde dehydrogenase, this drug leads to an accumulation of acetaldehyde if alcohol is consumed. Acetaldehyde is highly toxic and produces severe anxiety, vomiting, flushing, and headache. Rarely, hypotension may lead to shock and even death (21). In recent years, however, disulfiram has been prescribed in a lower dosage

(250 mg) than was employed previously, and no deaths from its use have been reported for a number of years. The reaction to disulfiram with ingestion of alcohol is sufficiently aversive that most patients who are compliant with it avoid alcohol altogether. In the largest study conducted, those randomized to disulfiram did not have any greater sobriety than those taking placebo; only medication adherence (disulfiram or placebo) predicted sobriety, and only 19% of patients took it consistently (21). The principal disadvantage of disulfiram is therefore not that patients drink while taking the drug but that they stop taking the drug after a brief period. Regardless, discontinuation of disulfiram after several days or weeks of taking it still deters drinking for a 3- to 5-day period because the drug requires that long to be excreted. Thus, it may be useful to give patients disulfiram during office visits at 3- to 4-day intervals early in the treatment program.

In 1995 the FDA approved a second drug, naltrexone (ReVia), for the treatment of alcoholism. A recent meta-analysis of randomized controlled trials with naltrexone found that it significantly reduced the rate of relapse and increased abstinence over 12 weeks (129). The drug's effects are impressive: relapse is prevented in one of every five patients treated with it (142). Although the administration of naltrexone appears beneficial over the short term, evidence for its efficacy in long-term use is less impressive (142).

A third medication was recently approved by the FDA for treatment of alcoholism. Acamprosate (calcium homotaurinate) is thought to modulate the glutaminergic and GABA-ergic systems (142). A systematic review of 15 studies found that this medication in combination with psychosocial treatments reduced relapse rates (68% vs. 80%), not just in the short term but also in the longer term (after 6 months) (21, 142).

In 2001, Project COMBINE, a 4-year study involving 11 academic centers (11), was undertaken to compare the most recently approved pharmacological approaches to alcohol dependence—naltrexone and acamprosate—with combined behavioral interventions (CBI) and placebo. (CBI was defined as flexibly integrated aspects of cognitive-behavioral therapy, 12-step facilitation, motivational interviewing, and support system involvement.) While extended review of the rather complicated findings is beyond the scope of this text, several issues were noteworthy, including (1) Individuals receiving medical management with naltrexone, CBI, or both had the best outcomes; (2) Acamprosate with or without CBI showed no effect; (3) No combination performed better than naltrexone or CBI alone in the presence of medical management; and (4) Placebo pills and meeting with a health care professional had a positive effect above that of CBI during treatment. Only time will tell whether any of these effective interventions will gain widespread acceptance by the field.

Tranquilizers and antidepressants have not been found to be reliably effective in maintaining abstinence or controlled drinking (21, 74, 117).

Historically, various aversive conditioning techniques have been tried and then abandoned: apomorphine and emetine to produce vomiting (140), succinylcholine to produce apnea (28), and electrical stimulation to produce pain (65). Controlled trials required to show that these procedures are effective were never conducted, and ethical questions were raised.

Over the years, a wide variety of psychological approaches have been tried in the treatment of alcoholism. None has proven definitely superior to others (74, 117). Nonetheless, while we do not know how many people with alcohol problems benefit from participation in Alcoholics Anonymous, most clinicians agree that patients with alcoholism should be encouraged to attend their meetings on at least a trial basis. It is now commonly accepted that intensive psychotherapy for alcoholism is not beneficial.

Increasing cost concerns have shifted alcoholism treatment from inpatient to outpatient settings. Residential treatment is reserved for patients with treatment resistance, medical complications, or relapse-conducive home environments. Studies have indicated that most patients benefit as much from brief outpatient services for alcoholism as they do from inpatient care (52, 109). Brief behavioral and educational approaches are simple enough to be conducted in office settings by primary care practitioners. Of note are the results of the MATCH project (1), an 8-year multisite nationwide U.S. clinical study comparing treatment response (defined as decreased alcohol intake) for three dissimilar psychological modalities: *(1)* 12-step facilitation therapy, *(2)* cognitive-behavioral therapy, and *(3)* motivational enhancement therapy. Interestingly, all three modalities demonstrated major improvements in reduction of the frequency of drinking and total amount. Improvements were noted also in depression, alcohol-related problems, and liver functions. The benefits were sustained through 12 months of treatment and at follow-up at 39 months. Detailed discussion of these effective interventions is beyond the scope of this book, but these brief approaches do lend themselves to select populations seen in the primary care physician's office.

In conclusion, while total abstinence is the optimal goal for patients with alcoholism, motivating heavy drinkers to at least reduce their alcohol consumption to nonhazardous levels is a close second outcome. Further, it should be emphasized that relapses are characteristic of alcoholism and that physicians treating this disease should avoid anger or excessive pessimism when such relapses occur. Patients with alcoholism have contact with nonpsychiatric physicians at least as often as they do with psychiatrists, and there is evidence that general practitioners and internists are sometimes more helpful (48). This may be particularly true when the therapeutic approach is warm but authoritarian, with little stress on "insight" or "understanding." Since the cause of alcoholism is unknown, "understanding," in fact, means acceptance of a particular theory. That may provide temporary comfort but probably rarely provides lasting benefit.

REFERENCES

1. Matching alcoholism treatments to client heterogeneity: treatment main effects and matching effects on drinking during treatment. Project MATCH Research Group. J. Stud. Alcohol, 59:631–639, 1998.

2. Alcohol and alcoholism. In Adams and *Victor's Principles of Neurology*, 7th edition, Victor, M., Ropper, A. H. New York: McGraw-Hill, pp. 1004–1015, 2001.

3. Alcohol Consumption, 2000. Atlanta: Centers for Disease Control and Prevention. http://www.infoplease.com/ipa/A0762367. html. Last accessed February 23, 2006.

4. Traffic safety facts 2002: zero tolerance laws. Washington, DC: Traffic Safety Administration, US Department of Transportation. http://www-nrd.nhtsa.dot.gov/pdf/nrd.30/NCSA/TSF 2002/2002old facts.pdf. Last accessed April 4, 2004.

5. Alterman, A. I., Hayashida, M., and O'Brien, C. P. Treatment response and safety of ambulatory medical detoxication. J. Stud. Alcohol, 49:160–166, 1988.

6. American Psychiatric Association. *Diagnostic and Statistical Manual of Mental Disorders*, 4th edition, text revision. Washington, DC: Author, 2000.

7. Ammendola, A., Tata, M. R., Aurilio, C., Ciccone, G., Gemini, D., Ammendola, E., Ugolini, G., and Argenzio, F. Peripheral neuropathy in chronic alcoholism: a retrospective cross-sectional study in 76 subjects. Alcohol Alcohol., 36:271–275, 2001.

8. Anderson, P., Cremona, A., Paton, A., Turner, C., and Wallace, P. The risk of alcohol. Addiction, 88:1493–1508, 1993.

9. Anthony, J. C., and Echeagaray-Wagner, F. Epidemiologic analysis of alcohol and tobacco use. Alcohol Res. Health, 24:201–208, 2000.

10. Anton, R. F., Dominick, C., Bigelow, M., and Westby, C. Comparison of Bio-Rad %CDT TIA and CDTect as laboratory markers of heavy alcohol use and their relationships with gamma-glutamyltransferase. Clinica Chemica Acta, 47:1769–1775, 2001.

11. Anton, R. F., O'Malley, S. S., Ciraulo, D. A., Cisler, R. A., Couper, D., Donovan, D. M., Gastfriend, D. R., Hosking, J. D., Johnson, B. A., LoCastro, J. S., Longabaugh, R., Mason, B. J., Mattson, M. E., Miller, W. R., Pettinati, H. M., Randall, C. L., Swift, R., Weiss, R. D., Williams, L. D., and Zweben, A. Combined pharmacotherapies and behavioral interventions for alcohol dependence: the COMBINE study: a randomized controlled trial. JAMA, 295:2003–2017, 2006.

12. Atkinson, R. M., Tolson, R. L., and Turner, J. A. Late versus early onset problem drinking in older men. Alcohol. Clin. Exp. Res., 14:574–579, 1990.

13. Barchiesi, B. J., Eckel, R. H., and Ellis, P. P. The cornea and disorders of lipid metabolism. Surv. Ophthalmol., 36:1–22, 1991.

14. Bierut, L. J., Dinwiddie, S. H., Begleiter, H., Crowe, R. R., Hesselbrock, V., Nurnberger, J. I., Jr., Porjesz, B., Schuckit, M. A., and Reich, T. Familial

transmission of substance dependence: alcohol, marijuana, cocaine, and habitual smoking: a report from the Collaborative Study on the Genetics of
Alcoholism. Arch. Gen. Psychiat., 55:982–988, 1998.

15. Blin, O., Simon, N., Jouve, E., Habib, M., Gayraud, D., Durand, A., Bruguerolle,
B., and Pisano, P. Pharmacokinetic and pharmacodynamic analysis of sedative
and amnesic effects of lorazepam in healthy volunteers. Clin. Neuropharmacol.,
24:71–81, 2001.

16. Blow, F. C., Barry, K. L., Fuller, B. E., Booth, B. M. Chapter 8. Analysis of the
National Health and Nutrition Examination Survey (NHANES): longitudinal
analysis of drinking over the life span. Rockville, MD: Substance Abuse and
Mental Health Services Administration (SAMHSA), US Department of Health
and Human Services. http://www.oas.samhsa.gov/aging/chap8.htm. Last
accessed February 25, 2006.

17. Bobak, M., McKee, M., Rose, R., and Marmot, M. Alcohol consumption in a
national sample of the Russian population. Addiction, 94:857–866, 1999.

18. Brady, K. T., and Verduin, M. L. Pharmacotherapy of comorbid mood, anxiety,
and substance use disorders. Subst Use Misuse, 40:2021–2028, 2005.

19. Breslow, R. A., Faden, V. B., and Smothers, B. Alcohol consumption by elderly
Americans. J. Stud. Alcohol, 64:884–892, 2003.

20. Brienza, R. S., and Stein, M. D. Alcohol use disorders in primary care: do gender-
specific differences exist? J. Gen. Intern. Med., 17:387–397, 2002.

21. Buonopane, A., and Petrakis, I. L. Pharmacotherapy of alcohol use disorders.
Subst Use Misuse, 40:2001–2008, 2005.

22. Butters, N., and Brandt, J. The continuity hypothesis: the relationship of long-
term alcoholism to the Wernicke-Korsakoff syndrome. Recent Dev. Alcohol,
3:207–226, 1985.

23. Cadoret, R. J., Cain, C. A., and Grove, W. M. Development of alcoholism in
adoptees raised apart from alcoholic biologic relatives. Arch. Gen. Psychiat.,
37:561–563, 1980.

24. Cadoret, R. J., and Gath, A. Inheritance of alcoholism in adoptees. Br. J.
Psychiat., 132:252–258, 1978.

25. Campbell, W. G., and Hodgins, D. C. Alcohol-related blackouts in a medical
practice. Am. J. Drug Alcohol Abuse, 19:369–376, 1993.

26. Chaucer, G. The Canterbury Tales: The Pardoner's Tale. In The Student's
Chaucer, Skeats, W. W. (ed.). New York: Oxford Univ. Press, 1900.

27. Chung, N., Langenbucher, J., McCrady, B., Epstein, E., and Cook, S. Use of
survival analyses to examine onset and staging of DSM-IV alcohol symptoms in
women. Psychol. Addict. Behav., 16:236–242, 2002.

28. Clancy, J., Vanderhoof, E., and Campbell, P. Evaluation of an aversive technique
as a treatment for alcoholism. Q. J. Stud. Alcohol, 28:476–485, 1967.

29. Cloninger, C. R., Sigvardsson, S., Gilligan, S. B., von Knorring, A. L., Reich, T.,
and Bohman, M. Genetic heterogeneity and the classification of alcoholism.
Adv. Alcohol Subst. Abuse, 7:3–16, 1988.

30. Collins, M. N., Burns, T., van den Berk, P. A., and Tubman, G. F. A structured programme for out-patient alcohol detoxification. Br. J. Psychiat., 156:871–874, 1990.

31. Conner, K. R., and Duberstein, P. R. Predisposing and precipitating factors for suicide among alcoholics: empirical review and conceptual integration. Alcohol. Clin. Exp. Res., 28:6S–17S, 2004.

32. Crum, R. M., Ensminger, M. E., Ro, M. J., and McCord, J. The association of educational achievement and school dropout with risk of alcoholism: a twenty-five-year prospective study of inner-city children. J. Stud. Alcohol, 59:318–326, 1998.

33. Cudd, T. A. Animal model systems for the study of alcohol teratology. Exp. Biol. Med. (Maywood), 230:389–393, 2005.

34. D'Onofrio, G., Rathlev, N. K., Ulrich, A. S., Fish, S. S., and Freedland, E. S. Lorazepam for the prevention of recurrent seizures related to alcohol. N. Engl. J. Med., 340:915–919, 1999.

35. Dawson, D. A., Grant, B. F., and Li, T. K. Quantifying the risks associated with exceeding recommended drinking limits. Alcohol. Clin. Exp. Res., 29:902–908, 2005.

36. Dawson, D. A., Grant, B. F., Stinson, F. S., Chou, P. S., Huang, B., and Ruan, W. J. Recovery from DSM-IV alcohol dependence: United States, 2001–2002. Addiction, 100:281–292, 2005.

37. Dawson, D. A., and Room, R. Towards agreement on ways to measure and report drinking patterns and alcohol-related problems in adult general population surveys: the Skarpo conference overview. J. Subst. Abuse, 12:1–21, 2000.

38. Dufour, M. C. If you drink alcoholic beverages do so in moderation: what does this mean? J. Nutr., 131:552S–561S, 2001.

39. Edwards, G., and Gross, M. M. Alcohol dependence: provisional description of a clinical syndrome. Br. Med. J., 1:1058–1061, 1976.

40. Edwards, G., Gross, M. M., Keller, M., Moser, J., and Room, R. Alcohol-Related Disabilities, WHO Offset Publ., no. 32. Geneva: World Health Organization, 1977.

41. Eidelman, R. S., Vignola, P., and Hennekens, C. H. Alcohol consumption and coronary heart disease: a causal and protective factor. Semin. Vasc. Med., 2:253–256, 2002.

42. Emsley, R. A., Potgieter, A., Taljaard, J. J., Coetzee, D., Joubert, G., and Gledhill, R. F. Impaired water excretion and elevated plasma vasopressin in patients with alcohol-withdrawal symptoms. Q. J. Med., 64:671–678, 1987.

43. Enoch, M. A., and Goldman, D. The genetics of alcoholism and alcohol abuse. Curr. Psychiat. Rep., 3:144–151, 2001.

44. Eustace, L. W., Kang, D. H., and Coombs, D. Fetal alcohol syndrome: a growing concern for health care professionals. J. Obstet. Gynecol. Neonatal Nurs., 32:215–221, 2003.

45. Ewing, J. A. Detecting alcoholism. The CAGE questionnaire. JAMA, 252:1905–1907, 1984.

46. Ewing, J. A., and Rouse, B. A. Corneal arcus as a sign of possible alcoholism. Alcohol. Clin. Exp. Res., 4:104–106, 1980.

47. Fama, R., Pfefferbaum, A., and Sullivan, E. V. Perceptual learning in detoxified alcoholic men: contributions from explicit memory, executive function, and age. Alcohol. Clin. Exp. Res., 28:1657–1665, 2004.

48. Ferraro, F. M., Hill, K. G., Kaczmarek, H. J., Coonfield, D. L., and Kiefer, S. W. Naltrexone modifies the palatability of basic tastes and alcohol in outbred male rats. Alcohol, 27:107–114, 2002.

49. Goodwin DW. Blackouts and alcohol induced memory dysfunction. In: Mello, N. K., Mendelson, J. H. (eds.). Recent advances in studies of alcoholism. Publication No. HSM 71-9045. Washington, DC: US Government Printing Office, pp. 508–536, 1971.

50. Goodwin, D. W. Alcohol in suicides and homicides. Q. J. Stud. Alcohol, 34:144–156, 1973.

51. Goodwin, D. W. Commentary: on defining alcoholism and taking stands. J. Clin. Psychiat., 43:394–395, 1982.

52. Goodwin, D. W. *Alcoholism: The Facts*. New York: Oxford Univ. Press, 1995.

53. Goodwin, D. W., and Hill, S. Y. Chronic effects of alcohol and other psychoactive drugs on intellect, learning and memory. In *Chronic Effects of Alcohol and Other Psychoactive Drugs on Cerebral Function*. Toronto: Addiction Research Foundation Press, 1975.

54. Grant, B. F., Dawson, D. A., Stinson, F. S., Chou, S. P., Dufour, M. C., and Pickering, R. P. The 12-month prevalence and trends in DSM-IV alcohol abuse and dependence: United States, 1991–1992 and 2001–2002. Drug Alcohol Depend., 74:223–234, 2004.

55. Greenfield, T. K., and Kerr, W. C. Tracking alcohol consumption over time. Alcohol Res. Health, 27:30–38, 2003.

56. Gunzerath, L., Faden, V., Zakhari, S., and Warren, K. National Institute on Alcohol Abuse and Alcoholism report on moderate drinking. Alcohol. Clin. Exp. Res., 28:829–847, 2004.

57. Harper, C., and Matsumoto, I. Ethanol and brain damage. Curr. Opin. Pharmacol., 5:73–78, 2005.

58. Hasin, D. Classification of alcohol use disorders. Alcohol Res. Health, 27:5–17, 2003.

59. Hayashida, M., Alterman, A. I., McLellan, A. T., O'Brien, C. P., Purtill, J. J., Volpicelli, J. R., Raphaelson, A. H., and Hall, C. P. Comparative effectiveness and costs of inpatient and outpatient detoxification of patients with mild-to-moderate alcohol withdrawal syndrome. N. Engl. J. Med., 320:358–365, 1989.

60. Hesselbrock, M. N. Childhood behavior problems and adult antisocial personality disorder in alcoholism. In *Psychopathology and Addictive Disorders*, Meyer, R. E. (ed.). New York: Guilford Press, pp. 78–94, 1986.

61. Hesselbrock, V. M., Stabenau, J. R., Hesselbrock, M. N., Meyer, R. E., and Babor, T. F. The nature of alcoholism in patients with different family histories for alcoholism. Prog. Neuropsychopharmacol. Biol. Psychiat., 6:607–614, 1982.

62. Hillbom, M., Pieninkeroinen, I., and Leone, M. Seizures in alcohol-dependent patients: epidemiology, pathophysiology and management. CNS Drugs, 17:1013–1030, 2003.

63. Holbert, K. R., and Tueth, M. J. Alcohol abuse and dependence. A clinical update on alcoholism in the older population. Geriatrics, 59:38–40, 2004.

64. Holdcraft, L. C., and Iacono, W. G. Cohort effects on gender differences in alcohol dependence. Addiction, 97:1025–1036, 2002.

65. Hsu, J. J. Electroconditioning therapy of alcoholics. Q. J. Stud. Alcohol, 26:449–459, 1965.

66. Jellinek, E. M. Phases of alcohol addiction. Q. J. Stud. Alcohol, 13:673–684, 1952.

67. Jellinek, E. M. The Disease Concept of Alcoholism. New Haven, CT: College & University Press, 1960.

68. Jennison, K. M., and Johnson, K. A. Drinking-induced blackouts among young adults: results from a national longitudinal study. Int. J. Addict., 29:23–51, 1994.

69. Karlamangla, A., Zhou, K., Reuben, D., Greendale, G., and Moore, A. Longitudinal trajectories of heavy drinking in adults in the United States of America. Addiction, 101:91–99, 2006.

70. Keller, M. On defining alcoholism: with comment on some other relevant words. In Alcohol, Science and Society Revisited. Ann Arbor, MI: University of Michigan Press, 1982.

71. Keller, M., McCormick, M., and Efron, V. A Dictionary of Words about Alcohol, 2nd edition. New Brunswick, NJ: Rutgers University Center of Alcohol Studies, 1982.

72. Kelly, S. J., Day, N., and Streissguth, A. P. Effects of prenatal alcohol exposure on social behavior in humans and other species. Neurotoxicol. Teratol., 22:143–149, 2000.

73. Kessler, R. C., McGonagle, K. A., Zhao, S., Nelson, C. B., Hughes, M., Eshleman, S., Wittchen, H. U., and Kendler, K. S. Lifetime and 12-month prevalence of DSM-III-R psychiatric disorders in the United States. Results from the National Comorbidity Survey. Arch. Gen. Psychiat., 51:8–19, 1994.

74. Kranzler, H. R. Pharmacotherapy of alcoholism: gaps in knowledge and opportunities for research. Alcohol Alcohol., 35:537–547, 2000.

75. Kril, J. J., and Halliday, G. M. Brain shrinkage in alcoholics: a decade on and what have we learned? Prog. Neurobiol., 58:381–387, 1999.

76. Kropp, S., Becher, H., Nieters, A., and Chang-Claude, J. Low-to-moderate alcohol consumption and breast cancer risk by age 50 years among women in Germany. Am. J. Epidemiol., 154:624–634, 2001.

77. Lakshman, M. R. Some novel insights into the pathogenesis of alcoholic steatosis. Alcohol, 34:45–48, 2004.

78. Lambie, D. G. Alcoholic brain damage and neurological symptoms of alcohol withdrawal—manifestations of overhydration. Med. Hypotheses, 16:377–388, 1985.

79. Laskins, N. E., Williams, G. D., Yi, H.-Y., and Smothers, B. A. Surveillance report #66. Apparent per capita ethanol consumption: national, state, and regional trends, 1977–2002, Bethesda, MD: National Institute on Alcohol Abuse and Alcoholism, 2004.

80. Li, T. K., Hewitt, B. G., and Grant, B. F. The Alcohol Dependence Syndrome, 30 years later: a commentary. The 2006 H. David Archibald lecture. Addiction, 102:1522–1530, 2007.

81. Lieber, C. S. Alcoholic fatty liver: its pathogenesis and mechanism of progression to inflammation and fibrosis. Alcohol, 34:9–19, 2004.

82. Ludwig, A. M. On and off the wagon. Reasons for drinking and abstaining by alcoholics. Q. J. Stud. Alcohol, 33:91–96, 1972.

83. Mackenzie, A., Funderburk, F. R., and Allen, R. P. Sleep, anxiety, and depression in abstinent and drinking alcoholics. Subst Use Misuse, 34:347–361, 1999.

84. Maczaj, M. Pharmacological treatment of insomnia. Drugs, 45:44–55, 1993.

85. Mandell, W., Eaton, W. W., Anthony, J. C., and Garrison, R. Alcoholism and occupations: a review and analysis of 104 occupations. Alcohol. Clin. Exp. Res., 16:734–746, 1992.

86. Mattson, S. N., Schoenfeld, A. M., and Riley, E. P. Teratogenic effects of alcohol on brain and behavior. Alcohol Res. Health, 25:185–191, 2001.

87. May, P. A., and Gossage, J. P. Estimating the prevalence of fetal alcohol syndrome. A summary. Alcohol Res. Health, 25:159–167, 2001.

88. Mazzaglia, G., Britton, A. R., Altmann, D. R., and Chenet, L. Exploring the relationship between alcohol consumption and non-fatal or fatal stroke: a systematic review. Addiction, 96:1743–1756, 2001.

89. Merikangas, K. R., Stolar, M., Stevens, D. E., Goulet, J., Preisig, M. A., Fenton, B., Zhang, H., O'Malley, S. S., and Rounsaville, B. J. Familial transmission of substance use disorders. Arch. Gen. Psychiat., 55:973–979, 1998.

90. Miller, P. M., and Anton, R. F. Biochemical alcohol screening in primary health care. Addict. Behav., 29:1427–1437, 2004.

91. Molina, P. E., McClain, C., Valla, D., Guidot, D., Diehl, A. M., Lang, C. H., and Neuman, M. Molecular pathology and clinical aspects of alcohol-induced tissue injury. Alcohol. Clin. Exp. Res., 26:120–128, 2002.

92. Montalto, N. J., and Bean, P. Use of contemporary biomarkers in the detection of chronic alcohol use. Med. Sci. Monit., 9:RA285–RA290, 2003.

93. Morris, H. H., III, and Estes, M. L. Traveler's amnesia. Transient global amnesia secondary to triazolam. JAMA, 258:945–946, 1987.

94. Murck, H., and Steiger, A. Mg2+ reduces ACTH secretion and enhances spindle power without changing delta power during sleep in men—possible therapeutic implications. Psychopharmacol. (Berl)., 137:247–252, 1998.

95. National Institute on Alcohol Abuse and Alcoholism. Drinking in the United States: main findings from the 1992 National Longitudinal Alcohol Epidemiologic Survey (NLAES). In *U.S. Alcohol Epidemiologic Data Reference Manual*, 1st edition. Rockville, MD: Author, 1992.

96. National Institute on Alcohol Abuse and Alcoholism. State trends in alcohol problems 1979–1992. In *U.S. Alcohol Epidemiologic Data Reference Manual, Vol. 5*, 1st edition. Rockville, MD: Author, 1996.

97. Nelson, E. C., Heath, A. C., Bucholz, K. K., Madden, P. A., Fu, Q., Knopik, V., Lynskey, M. T., Lynskey, M. T., Whitfield, J. B., Statham, D. J., and Martin, N. G. Genetic epidemiology of alcohol-induced blackouts. Arch. Gen. Psychiat., 61:257–263, 2004.

98. Nephew, T. M., Williams, G. D., Stinson, F. S., Nguygen, K., and Dufour, M. C. Apparent per capita alcohol consumption: national, state, and regional trends, 1977–1998, Surveillance Report # 55. Rockville, MD: National Institute on Alcohol Abuse and Alcoholism, 2000.

99. Nichols, J. M., and Martin, F. The effect of heavy social drinking on recall and event-related potentials. J. Stud. Alcohol, 57:125–135, 1996.

100. Nurnberger, J. I., Jr., Wiegand, R., Bucholz, K., O'Connor, S., Meyer, E. T., Reich, T., Rice, J., Schuckit, M., King, L., Petti, T., Bierut, L., Hinrichs, A. L., Kuperman, S., Hesselbrock, V., and Porjesz, B. A family study of alcohol dependence: coaggregation of multiple disorders in relatives of alcohol-dependent probands. Arch. Gen. Psychiat., 61:1246–1256, 2004.

101. Penick, E. C., Read, M. R., Crowley, P. A., and Powell, B. J. Differentiation of alcoholics by family history. J. Stud. Alcohol, 39:1944–1948, 1978.

102. Pickens, R. W., Hatsukami, D. K., Spicer, J. W., and Svikis, D. S. Relapse by alcohol abusers. Alcohol. Clin. Exp. Res., 9:244–247, 1985.

103. Prescott, C. A., Caldwell, C. B., Carey, G., Vogler, G. P., Trumbetta, S. L., and Gottesman, I. I. The Washington University Twin Study of alcoholism. Am. J. Med. Genet. B Neuropsychiatr. Genet., 134:48–55, 2005.

104. Ramaiah, S., Rivera, C., and Arteel, G. Early-phase alcoholic liver disease: an update on animal models, pathology, and pathogenesis. Int. J. Toxicol., 23:217–231, 2004.

105. Reed, R. J., Grant, I., and Rourke, S. B. Long-term abstinent alcoholics have normal memory. Alcohol. Clin. Exp. Res., 16:677–683, 1992.

106. Reynolds, K., Lewis, B., Nolen, J. D., Kinney, G. L., Sathya, B., and He, J. Alcohol consumption and risk of stroke: a meta-analysis. JAMA, 289:579–588, 2003.

107. Robins, L. N., Tipp, J., and Przybeck, T. Antisocial personality. In *Psychiatric Disorders in America: The Epidemiologic Catchment Area Study*, Robins, L. N., Regier, D. A. (eds.). New York: The Free Press, 1991.

108. Roebuck, T. M., Mattson, S. N., and Riley, E. P. A review of the neuroanatomical findings in children with fetal alcohol syndrome or prenatal exposure to alcohol. Alcohol. Clin. Exp. Res., 22:339–344, 1998.

109. Room, R., Babor, T., and Rehm, J. Alcohol and public health. Lancet, 365:519–530, 2005.

110. Roueché, B. *Alcohol.* New York: Grove Press, 1962.

111. Rush, B. *An Inquiry into the Effects of Ardent Spirits upon the Human Body and Mind,* 6th edition. New York: Cornelius Davis, 1811.

112. Russell, M. New assessment tools for risk drinking during pregnancy: T-ACE, TWEAK, and others. Alcohol. Health Res. World, 18:55–61, 1994.

113. Saitz, R., Mayo-Smith, M. F., Roberts, M. S., Redmond, H. A., Bernard, D. R., and Calkins, D. R. Individualized treatment for alcohol withdrawal. A randomized double-blind controlled trial. JAMA, 272:519–523, 1994.

114. Saunders, J. B., Aasland, O. G., Babor, T. F., de, l. F., Jr., and Grant, M. Development of the Alcohol Use Disorders Identification Test (AUDIT): WHO Collaborative Project on Early Detection of Persons with Harmful Alcohol Consumption—II. Addiction, 88:791–804, 1993.

115. Scholz, E., Diener, H. C., Dichgans, J., Langohr, H. D., Schied, W., and Schupmann, A. Incidence of peripheral neuropathy and cerebellar ataxia in chronic alcoholics. J. Neurol., 233:212–217, 1986.

116. Schuckit, M. A. The clinical implications of primary diagnostic groups among alcoholics. Arch. Gen. Psychiat., 42:1043–1049, 1985.

117. Schuckit, M. A. Recent developments in the pharmacotherapy of alcohol dependence. J. Consult. Clin. Psychiat., 64:669–676, 1996.

118. Schuckit, M. A., Goodwin, D. A., and Winokur, G. A study of alcoholism in half siblings. Am. J. Psychiat., 128:1132–1136, 1972.

119. Schultz, S. K., Arndt, S., Lutz, G. M., Petersen, A., and Turvey, C. L. Alcohol use among older persons in a rural state. Am. J. Geriat. Psychiat., 10:750–753, 2002.

120. Schwartz, R. H., Milteer, R., and LeBeau, M. A. Drug-facilitated sexual assault ("date rape"). South. Med. J., 93:558–561, 2000.

121. Scroop, R., Sage, M. R., Voyvodic, F., and Kat, E. Radiographic imaging procedures in the diagnosis of the major central neuropathological consequences of alcohol abuse. Australas. Radiol., 46:146–153, 2002.

122. Selzer, M. L. The Michigan alcoholism screening test: the quest for a new diagnostic instrument. Am. J. Psychiat., 127:1653–1658, 1971.

123. Sigerist, H. E. *The History of Medicine.* New York: M.D. Publications, 1960.

124. Sigvardsson, S., Bohman, M., and Cloninger, C. R. Replication of the Stockholm Adoption Study of alcoholism. Confirmatory cross-fostering analysis. Arch. Gen. Psychiat., 53:681–687, 1996.

125. Soyka, M., and Horak, M. Outpatient alcohol detoxification: implementation efficacy and outcome effectiveness of a model project. Eur. Addict. Res., 10:180–187, 2004.

126. Spampinato, M. V., Castillo, M., Rojas, R., Palacios, E., Frascheri, L., and Descartes, F. Magnetic resonance imaging findings in substance abuse: alcohol and alcoholism and syndromes associated with alcohol abuse. Top. Magn. Reson. Imaging, 16:223–230, 2005.

127. Standridge, J. B., Zylstra, R. G., and Adams, S. M. Alcohol consumption: an overview of benefits and risks. South. Med. J., 97:664–672, 2004.

128. Stephens, D. A., Atkinson, M. W., Kay, D. W., Roth, M., and Garside, R. F. Psychiatric morbidity in parents and sibs of schizophrenics and non-schizophrenics. Br. J. Psychiat., 127:97–108, 1975.

129. Streeton, C., and Whelan, G. Naltrexone, a relapse prevention maintenance treatment of alcohol dependence: a meta-analysis of randomized controlled trials. Alcohol Alcohol., 36:544–552, 2001.

130. Sullivan, E. V., and Pfefferbaum, A. Neurocircuitry in alcoholism: a substrate of disruption and repair. Psychopharmacol. (Berl)., 180:583–594, 2005.

131. Sullivan, E. V., Rosenbloom, M. J., and Pfefferbaum, A. Pattern of motor and cognitive deficits in detoxified alcoholic men. Alcohol. Clin. Exp. Res., 24:611–621, 2000.

132. Sullivan, J. T., Sykora, K., Schneiderman, J., Naranjo, C. A., and Sellers, E. M. Assessment of alcohol withdrawal: the revised clinical institute withdrawal assessment for alcohol scale (CIWA-Ar). Br. J. Addict., 84:1353–1357, 1989.

133. Tarter, R. Minimal brain dysfunction as an etiological predisposition in alcoholism. In *Evaluation of the Alcoholic: Implications for Research, Theory and Practice*, Meyer, R., Glueck, J., Babor, T., Jaffe, J., Stanbenau, J. (eds.). Washington, DC: U.S. Department of Health and Human Services, 1971.

134. Teyssen, S., and Singer, M. V. Alcohol-related diseases of the oesophagus and stomach. Best Pract. Res. Clin. Gastroenterol., 17:557–573, 2003.

135. Thun, M. J., Peto, R., Lopez, A. D., Monaco, J. H., Henley, S. J., Heath, C. W., Jr., and Doll, R. Alcohol consumption and mortality among middle-aged and elderly U.S. adults. N. Engl. J. Med., 337:1705–1714, 1997.

136. Tyndale, R. F. Genetics of alcohol and tobacco use in humans. Ann. Med., 35:94–121, 2003.

137. U.S.Department of Health and Human Services and U.S.Department of Agriculture. *Nutrition and Your Health: Dietary Guidelines for Americans*, 5th edition. Washington, DC: USDA, 2000.

138. van de Wiel, A. Diabetes mellitus and alcohol. Diabetes Metab. Res. Rev., 20: 263–267, 2004.

139. Velleman, R., and Orford, J. The adult adjustment of offspring of parents with drinking problems. Br. J. Psychiat., 162:503–516, 1993.

140. Volkow, N. D., Wang, G. J., Hitzemann, R., Fowler, J. S., Overall, J. E., Burr, G., and Wolf, A. P. Recovery of brain glucose metabolism in detoxified alcoholics. Am. J. Psychiat., 151:178–183, 1994.

141. Walter, H., Gutierrez, K., Ramskogler, K., Hertling, I., Dvorak, A., and Lesch, O. M. Gender-specific differences in alcoholism: implications for treatment. Arch. Womens Ment. Health, 6:253–258, 2003.

142. Williams, S. H. Medications for treating alcohol dependence. Am. Fam. Physician, 72:1775–1780, 2005.

143. Wilsnack, R. W., Vogeltanz, N. D., Wilsnack, S. C., Harris, T. R., Ahlstrom, S., Bondy, S., Csemy, L., Ferrence, R., Ferris, J., Fleming, J., Graham, K., Greenfield, T., Guyon, L., Haavio-Mannila, E., Kellner, F., Knibbe, R., Kubicka, L., Loukomskaia, M., Mustonen, H., Nadeau, L., Narusk, A., Neve, R., Rahav, G., Spak, F., Teichman, M., Trocki, K., Webster, I., and Weiss, S. Gender differences in alcohol consumption and adverse drinking consequences: cross-cultural patterns. Addiction, 95:251–265, 2000.

144. Windle, M., and Scheidt, D. M. Alcoholic subtypes: are two sufficient? Addiction, 99:1508–1519, 2004.

145. Wiseman, E. J., Henderson, K. L., and Briggs, M. J. Individualized treatment for outpatients withdrawing from alcohol. J. Clin. Psychiat., 59:289–293, 1998.

146. Zilberman, M. L., Tavares, H., Blume, S. B., and el Guebaly, N. Substance use disorders: sex differences and psychiatric comorbidities. Can. J. Psychiat., 48:5–13, 2003.

147. American Psychiatric Association. *Diagnostic and Statistical Manual of Mental Disorders*, 4th edition, text revision. Washington, DC: Author, 2000.

12

Drug Dependence

Drug dependence refers to the repeated use of a psychoactive drug, causing harm to the user or to others. A multitude of terms have been variously applied to this disorder, and these require definition.

Addiction is used in two senses: physical and psychological. *Physical addiction* refers to a drug-produced condition characterized by tolerance and physical dependence. *Tolerance* refers to an adaptive biological process in which "increasingly larger doses of a drug must be administered to obtain the effect observed with the original dose." *Physical dependence* refers to "the physiological state produced by the repeated administration of the drug which necessitates the continued administration of the drug to prevent the appearance of the stereotyped syndrome, the withdrawal or abstinence syndrome, characteristic for the particular drug" (59).

Psychological addiction (also sometimes referred to as psychological dependence) refers to a "behavioral pattern of compulsive drug use, characterized by overwhelming involvement with the use of a drug, the securing of its supply, and a high tendency to relapse after withdrawal" (59). Physical and psychological addiction may overlap but do not necessarily occur together. For example, a person physically addicted to morphine administered for pain in a hospital may have none of the characteristics of psychological addiction. On the other hand, individuals may be psychologically addicted to drugs with little or no tolerance or physical dependence. Except for the opiates and to a lesser extent the barbiturates, no drugs produce striking degrees of both tolerance and physical dependence and therefore meet the two pharmacological criteria for addiction (3).

Historically, the reader may come across the term *habituation*, which refers to dependence on a drug for an "optimal state of well-being, ranging from a mild desire to a craving or compulsion (a compelling urge) to use the drug" (59).

DSM-IV-TR lists nine symptoms for *substance dependence* (Table 12.1). It also includes a category called *substance abuse* (Table 12.2). Individuals fitting this category do not fulfill the criteria for dependence but repeatedly use drugs despite *(1)* social, occupational, psychological, or physical harm from the substance or *(2)* a risk of drug-related accidents. Examples are persons whose regular use of marijuana aggravates their asthma despite warnings from their physicians, or persons who drive while intoxicated. Alcoholism (alcohol

---

TABLE 12.1 Diagnostic Criteria for Substance Dependence

A maladaptive pattern of substance use, leading to clinically significant impairment or distress, as manifested by three (or more) of the following, occurring at any time in the same 12-month period:

(1) Tolerance, as defined by either of the following:

    (a) A need for markedly increased amounts of the substance to achieve intoxication or desired effect

    (b) Markedly diminished effect with continued use of the same amount of the substance

(2) Withdrawal, as manifested by either of the following:

    (a) The characteristic withdrawal syndrome for the substance (refer to criteria A and B of the criteria sets for withdrawal from the specific substances)

    (b) The same (or a closely related) substance is taken to relieve or avoid withdrawal symptoms.

(3) The substance is often taken in larger amounts or over a longer period than was intended.

(4) There is a persistent desire or unsuccessful efforts to cut down or control substance use.

(5) A great deal of time is spent in activities necessary to obtain the substance (e.g., visiting multiple doctors or driving long distances), use the substance (e.g., chain-smoking), or recover from its effects.

(6) Important social, occupational, or recreational activities are given up or reduced because of substance use.

(7) The substance use is continued despite knowledge of having a persistent or recurrent physical or psychological problem that is likely to have been caused or exacerbated by the substance (e.g., current cocaine use despite recognition of cocaine-induced depression, or continued drinking despite recognition that an ulcer was made worse by alcohol consumption).

Specify if:

WITH PHYSIOLOGICAL DEPENDENCE: evidence of tolerance or withdrawal (i.e., either item 1 or 2 is present)

WITH PHYSIOLOGICAL DEPENDENCE: no evidence of tolerance or withdrawal (i.e., neither item 1 nor 2 is present)

Adapted from diagnostic criteria in the *DSM-IV-TR* (152).

TABLE 12.2 Diagnostic Criteria for Substance Abuse

A. A maladaptive pattern of substance use leading to clinically significant impairment or distress, as manifested by one (or more) of the following, occurring within a 12-month period:

   (1) Recurrent substance use resulting in a failure to fulfill major role obligations at work, school, or home (e.g., repeated absences or poor work performance related to substance use; substance-related absences, suspensions, or expulsions from school; neglect of children or household)

   (2) Recurrent substance use in situations in which it is physically hazardous (e.g., driving an automobile or operating a machine when impaired by substance use)

   (3) Recurrent substance-related legal problems (e.g., arrests for substance-related disorderly conduct)

   (4) Continued substance use despite having persistent or recurrent social or interpersonal problems caused or exacerbated by the effects of the substance (e.g., arguments with spouse about consequences of intoxication, physical fights)

B. The symptoms have never met the criteria for Substance Dependence for this class of substance.

Adapted from diagnostic criteria in the *DSM-IV-TR* (152).

dependence), included in *DSM-IV-TR* as a psychoactive substance use disorder, is discussed in Chapter 11.

While these criteria sets may appear to the trainee somewhat rigid and ill fitting (no real withdrawal syndrome for certain substances, e.g., hallucinogens), the uniform criteria represent a substantial movement forward from previous individualized approaches to the various agents. Further, this rather simplified and streamlined approach facilitates diagnosis, which drives treatment planning for this very significant medical problem that affects so many aspects of society. The reader should be aware that the two categories were created to facilitate diagnosis, but they are not exclusive because a single abuse symptom may be significantly disabling.

Historical Background

> The basic needs of the human race . . . are food, clothing, and shelter.
> To that fundamental trinity most modern authorities would add, as
> equally compelling, security and love. There are, however, many other
> needs whose satisfaction, though somewhat less essential, can seldom
> be comfortably denied. One of these, and perhaps the most insistent, is
> an occasional release from the intolerable clutch of reality. All men
> throughout recorded history have known this tyranny of memory and
> mind, and all have sought . . . some reliable means of briefly loosening
> its grip.
>
> Berton Roueché (115)

Regardless of whether this fully explains the motivation behind the use of intoxicating substances, it is true they have been used by humankind for thousands of years in nearly every part of the world. Except in a few primitive cultures, humans have discovered plants whose juices and powders that on being properly prepared and consumed have caused desirable alterations of consciousness. In ancient times, these substances were widely used in religious ceremonies (as wine is still used in the Catholic mass and peyote by the North American Church), but they also have been used for recreational purposes. As the sciences of medicine and chemistry progressed, the variety of drugs increased and for many years drugs have been diverted from medical use into "illicit" channels as they are today.

The analgesic drugs derived from the opium poppy plant were particularly susceptible to abuse because they produced euphoria as well as analgesia. Drug "epidemics" have occurred periodically in recent centuries. The introduction of opium into England, commercially promoted as part of the Chinese opium trade, led to widespread abuse of the drug in the nineteenth century. With the introduction of the hypodermic needle during the American Civil War period, the use of morphine for nonmedicinal purposes became widespread, and by the turn of the century, large numbers of people were apparently dependent on the drug, taken intravenously or more often as an ingredient of patent medicines (laudanum). (Comprehensive review of these early epidemics is beyond the scope of this book but can be found elsewhere [98]). Heroin, the diethylated form of morphine, was introduced around the turn of the century as a "heroic" solution for the opiate problem (a form of substitution therapy, just as methadone is used today).

Another development of the mid-nineteenth century was the introduction of bromides as sedatives. There was an enormous demand for these compounds and a steady increase in their use. Along with use came misuse, which often resulted in intoxication and psychotic reactions. The bromide problem began to abate in the 1930s as barbiturates and other sedatives became available. The first barbiturate, Veronal, was introduced in 1903, and others appeared in quick succession. The short-acting barbiturates such as pentobarbital and amobarbital became popular in the 1930s and 1940s; their dependence-producing qualities were not immediately recognized (1).

During the late nineteenth century, individuals in the West discovered botanicals used for mind-altering purposes elsewhere, such as cocaine and hashish (the most potent form of cannabis). Cocaine was found to be useful medically (by Freud, among others), and a number of well-known physicians and surgeons became "cocaine addicts."

Ether, also discovered in the nineteenth century, was used recreationally, again often by medical people, as were nitrous oxide and other volatile solvents. Doctors and nurses, presumably because of their access to these drugs and their familiarity with them, were particularly prone to take them, although reliable data regarding drug abuse by physicians at any time in history, including today, are not available. Meperidine, introduced in the 1940s as a "nonaddictive" synthetic narcotic, led to a mild epidemic of abuse among physicians before its addictive potential was appreciated.

In postwar Japan, thousands of young people turned to amphetamines. Drastic measures were required to control the problem, including the establishment of special psychiatric facilities and stringent legal controls.

Further epidemics ensued in the decades to follow. The 1960s witnessed the assimilation of hallucinogens into the American middle-class youth culture of the time. This development originated with Hofmann's discovery in 1953 that lysergic acid diethylamide-25 (LSD) produced perceptual distortions and other aberrant mental phenomena. Once again, physicians were involved in the introduction of the drug for medical use (90). It was first used on the U.S. east and west coasts experimentally because it produced symptoms resembling those seen in psychosis. It was also used therapeutically, usually by psychoanalysts who felt the drug would dissolve "repressions." Because LSD is easy to synthesize, it became widely available and has been used, at least experimentally, by several million people, the majority of them of young age and from the middle or upper-middle class.

As mind-altering drugs became widely publicized in the 1960s, increasing numbers of young people experimented with them. In the early adolescent group, glue sniffing and inhalation of other volatile solvents were apparently widely practiced then, as they have been in recent decades. Individuals in late adolescence and their early 20s, particularly on college campuses in the 1960s and early 1970s, experimented with LSD and other synthetic hallucinogens such as dimethlytryptamine (DMT) as well as other derivatives of the indole and catecholamines that produced psychedelic effects. Beginning in the mid-1970s, the use of LSD and other psychedelics began to decline and has continued to decline since then, although with a slight increase in use in the 1990s (119). Rise in the use of amphetamines in the late 1960s produced a generation of "speed freaks" who injected various amphetamines. Popularity of this class of drugs waned in the 1980s and early 1990s. However, the mid-1990s saw a rise in the use of smoked or injected methamphetamine. "Downers" such as barbiturates and other sedative-hypnotics became popular among young people in the late 1960s. The trend, however, did not appear to continue past the mid-1970s.

Cocaine, the psychoactive component from the coca leaves, first became widely available in the United States in the late nineteenth century (32). It was available in drug stores, grocery stores, and bars and by mail order. Many different preparations included the substance, including wine and Coca-Cola. Problems mounted, and cocaine became Public Enemy Number One with the Harrison Act in 1914 passed to tightly control distribution and sale. Cocaine, sniffed in powdered form, enjoyed resurgence in popularity in the late 1960s and 1970s on college campuses and in suburbia. As in the case of other street drugs, often the "cocaine" people thought they were obtaining was either adulterated or completely absent. During the late 1980s and early 1990s, however, changes in the delivery of available compounds (e.g., "freebase" and "crack" forms) contributed to a significant upsurge in use.

Marijuana became the most widely used illicit drug in America in the 1960s and 1970s because it enhances sensory processes (122), but it also has been found to have psychotomimetic properties (83). Marijuana is the "tobacco" of the hemp plant and has grown wild in America since colonial times or before. Widely condemned in the 1930s as a dangerous drug, marijuana was used recreationally only by small minorities such as jazz musicians and Mexican immigrant workers (15) until the 1960s. Subsequently it has been more widely accepted in Western countries as a benign if not completely innocuous substance. There has been increasing pressure to "decriminalize" the substance if not actually make it legally available. Marijuana and its potent relative, hashish, are still, however, illegal in most countries, many of which are signatories to a U.N. treaty prohibiting its sale. In the mid to late 1970s, daily marijuana use appeared to have peaked at 10% of high school seniors with a fall to 5% in 1984 and to 2% in 1991 (66). However, marijuana abuse/dependence again increased between 1992 and 2002 (26).

Although marijuana and the hallucinogens were being more widely used in the United States in the 1960s, heroin—the fast-acting, potent form of morphine—became a serious medical and legal problem, involving mainly lower-class African-American urban men. By the early 1990s it was estimated that New York City alone had more than 100,000 opiate addicts. Also in the early 1990s there was a change in the demographics with an increase in the opiate use among Hispanic males who were between the ages of 18 and 25 and living in the West (62). Because of the expense of heroin, its use led to widespread criminal activities, including corruption of police authorities. Deaths resulted from overdose, allergic responses, or medical complications following unsterile intravenous injection (bacterial endocarditis, hepatitis B and C, HIV). The heroin "epidemic" was limited somewhat by the high price of the drug and its relative unavailability in noncoastal cities. Resurgence in heroin use during the late 1990s appeared linked to a fall in the price.

Nicotine "addiction" is not discussed at length in this chapter although, according to the U.S. Surgeon General, it is the most addictive substance used by humans. Not too many years ago, half of the adult population in the United States smoked nicotine cigarettes. The figure has now fallen to 25% and will probably drop even further as antismoking sentiment becomes even greater. The idea that nicotine was addictive—as addictive as cocaine or heroin—is a view that became officially "sanctioned" only in the last 20 years (see further below). The government maintains that hundreds of thousands of Americans die every year of nicotine-related illnesses, particularly heart disease and lung cancer. Even secondhand smoke is dangerous, according to the Surgeon General and the Environmental Protection Agency. A brief history of tobacco use therefore seems justified.

In 1492, Columbus recorded in his diary the gift of "strange dry leaves" from a native of San Salvador. Within a few years tobacco had crossed the Atlantic to Europe and became popular for recreational and medical uses. In 1560, Jean Nicot, French ambassador to Portugal, touted tobacco's curative powers. The first commercial tobacco crop was grown in Jamestown in 1612. Within a short time tobacco cultivation spread throughout the colonies. Britain wanted control of tobacco exports, increasing anti-British sentiment. Large plantations sprang up, an impetus for the use of slaves.

In 1881, a cigarette-making machine, capable of making 120,000 cigarettes a day, was invented. Cigarettes became immensely popular; this was met by an enthusiastic antismoking movement, including laws against smoking, which died out in World War I. In 1918, the United States War Department included tobacco in soldiers' rations. By war's end, cigarettes sales had reached 1 billion a year. During World War II and afterward, American cigarettes were accepted as currency around the world.

In 1964, the Surgeon General linked tobacco to cancer, heart disease, and other serious ailments. Warning labels were required on packs. A ban on radio and TV advertising of cigarettes took effect. The 1988 Surgeon General's report concluded the following: (1) cigarettes and other forms of tobacco are addictive; (2) nicotine is the drug in tobacco that causes addiction, and (3) the pharmacologic and behavioral processes that determine addiction are similar to those that determine addiction to drugs such as heroin and cocaine (150). This set the stage for the Food and Drug Administration (FDA) to consider regulation of tobacco in the United States (1994) and still later the World Health Organization (WHO) to consider the international impact and potential control (2005) (150).

Many U.S. workplaces became smoke-free in this political climate. Nonsmokers became increasingly intolerant of cigarette smoke in their environment and many smokers tried to stop but had difficulty. Teenage girls became the last remaining major group of new smokers.

Epidemiology

Epidemiological surveys focusing on prevalence of drug use involve not more than the usual challenges to reliability (e.g., inconsistent population samples, inaccessibility of drug users, self-report data, instrument selection, retrospective design, nondisclosure of criminal activity) expected in prevalence studies but also include issues peculiar to drug studies, especially the rapidly changing patterns of use. Nonetheless, certain broad trends have been identified (131), including the increase in the use of substances in the 1970s with a decrease in the 1980s. Subsequently, there was another upswing in use beginning in 1992 with a peak in 1997 and a leveling off or decline of certain substance use. Of note is a 12-month prevalence study, the National Epidemiologic Survey on Alcohol and Related Condition (NESARC) conducted in 2001–2002 which found only 2% of respondents had a drug use disorder (52).

Nonetheless, many people have been exposed to a wide variety of illicit drugs. More than $1 billion is spent on illicit drugs annually. Another $60 billion is lost every year in drug-related crime, health problems, and lowered productivity. Intravenous drug use is second only to homosexuality as a risk factor for acquired immune deficiency syndrome (AIDS).

The image of drug abusers has changed. Socialites, athletes, and Hollywood celebrities have been arrested in increasing numbers for possession of cocaine. Marijuana has been partially decriminalized in some states: selling it is still a crime, but possession of small amounts is not. Nevertheless, law enforcement devotes substantial resources to combating marijuana use. The popularity of crack—a hazardous derivative of cocaine—in affluent suburbia as well as urban ghettoes seems one of the most serious perils in this very rapidly changing drug scene, whereas use of LSD and the other hallucinogens has declined greatly in use since the 1970s. Particularly problematic has been the recent rise in use of two amphetamines, "meth" (methamphetamine) and "Ecstasy" (3,4-methylenedioxymethamphetamine) along with the widening use of two other "club drugs," ketamine and gamma-hydroxybutyrate (GHB).

Identifying the Drug User

Formal assessment of the patient's substance use is part of every patient's evaluation. While each evaluator develops one's own style of approach to assessment, several major issues need consideration. First, on the whole, a matter-of-fact inquiry embedded in the intake (new out/inpatient, emergency department, consultation setting) is usually most effective. Second, careful attention to the answers provided is necessary to ascertain whether the patient appears to be carefully avoiding disclosure of the whole truth about the patient's substance use. If so, focused follow-up may be necessary and should be preceded by identification of the reasons why it is important that the physician be provided the complete history ("My role here is to fully assess the situation, which is in your best interest. What I need to complete this evaluation is your assistance in providing the full picture.") Should such attempts meet with failure, approaching collateral informants (e.g., spouse, family, friends, workplace informants), within the rules of confidentiality, may yield valuable information. Third, interviewing an intoxicated individual for anything other than the basics may be fruitless or may produce incorrect or misleading information. Fourth, because the examiner will be asking about behaviors that are counter to cultural norms and even perhaps illegal, avoiding a judgmental stance or attitude will facilitate the interview. Finally, inquiry should almost always be made with patients (particularly new patients or those with unknown prior history) into the possibly of pending withdrawal from any agent that may produce significant morbidity (or mortality). Obtaining the history, physical examination and laboratory testing will complete the assessment of these patients. While assessing use of each individual drug for status of abuse versus dependence may prove tedious, establishing the proper diagnosis(es) is the first step toward initiating treatment.

Drug Categories

Opioids

Opioids are derivatives of naturally occurring plant substances (opiates) from which morphine-like effects or opiate-like substances are synthesized or semisynthesized in the laboratory. Opiates include opium, heroin, hydromorphone (Dilaudid), codeine, oxycodone, hydrocodone, and paregoric. Meperidine (Demerol) is a synthetic analgesic structurally dissimilar to morphine but pharmacologically similar. Opium and heroin are only two of these substances that are not available for medical use in the United States.

Historically, opium has been known for millennia to relieve pain and was suggested for surgical use more than 2,000 years ago (38). Oral analgesia was achieved in the 1600s by using tincture of opium, commonly known as laudanum (in various "recipes"). Opium consists of about 10% morphine. Morphine was first isolated in 1805 by Friedrich Sertürner (121) and named after the Greek god of dreams, Morpheus (58). Widespread use in the United States was not seen until the introduction of the intravenous needle, which facilitated analgesia and addiction after the Civil War. As noted previously, heroin was developed as a means of replacement and presumably discontinuation of narcotics dependence/addiction.

Heroin can be snorted (insufflation), smoked, or skin-popped (injected subcutaneously). Most heroin and morphine addicts eventually take opiates intravenously, which produces flushing and a sensation described as similar to orgasm, known as a "rush." Psychomotor activity initially increases, followed by a period of drowsiness and inactivity, a state that has been called "being on the nod" or "nodding out."

In usual therapeutic doses, opioids produce analgesia, drowsiness, and a change in mood described as a sense of well-being. Opioids function to produce constriction of the pupils, constipation, and occasionally nausea and vomiting; they also function as respiratory depressants. Variable potencies of different forms of heroin frequently result in respiratory distress. Many heroin addicts come to the attention of medical authorities after presenting to an emergency department in overdose status.

Obviously, should a somnolent patient present to the emergency department, a drug screen will be undertaken. In outpatient settings the evaluator may notice small, poorly reactive pupils, variability of mentation between visits, needle tracks, lower weight than the ideal, and pain complaints that are out of proportion to the physical exam. The evaluator may then consider ordering a drug screen and may be surprised when the patient volunteers that he has been using a particular narcotic. It is important to ask whether that is the only substance that may be found. Routine drug screens may also be part of the treatment program.

Tolerance develops to most opioid effects, including euphoria. Libido declines; menstruation may cease. Some addicts who are able to obtain an adequate supply of opiates dress properly, maintain nutrition, and discharge social and occupational obligations without gross impairment. Other addicts become socially disabled, because the expense of drugs leads to theft, forgery, prostitution, and the sale of drugs to other users.

The first symptoms of opioid withdrawal usually appear 8–12 hours after the last dose once a habit has been established (Table 12.3). These include lacrimation, rhinorrhea, sweating, and yawning. Thereafter, the addict may fall into a fitful sleep known as "the yen" from which he or she awakens after several hours, restless and miserable. Additional signs and symptoms appear, reaching a peak between 48 and 72 hours after drug discontinuation. These include dilated pupils, anorexia, restlessness, insomnia, irritability, gooseflesh, nausea, vomiting, diarrhea, chills, and abdominal cramps. These manifestations subside gradually. After 7 to 10 days, most signs of withdrawal have disappeared, although the patient may continue to experience insomnia, weakness, and nervousness.

TABLE 12.3 Abstinence Signs in Sequential Appearance After Last Dose of Opiate in Patients with Well-Established Parenteral Habits*

Grades of Abstinence	Signs (Observed in Cool Room, Patient Uncovered or under Only a Sheet)	Hours after Last Dose				
		Morphine	Heroin	Meperidine	Dihydro-Morphinone	Codeine
Grade 0	Craving for drug Anxiety	6	4	2–3	2–3	8
Grade 1	Yawning Perspiration Lacrimation Rhinorrhea Yen sleep	14	8	4–6	4–5	24
Grade 2	Increase in above signs plus: Mydriasis Gooseflesh (piloerection) Tremors (muscle twitches) Hot and cold flashes Aching bones and muscles Anorexia	16	12	8–12	7	48
Grade 3	Increased intensity of above plus: Insomnia Increased blood pressure Increased temperature (1–2) Increased respiratory rate and depth Increased pulse rate Restlessness Nausea	24–36	18–24	16	12	—

continued

TABLE 12.3 (Continued)

Grades of Abstinence	Signs(Observed in Cool Room, Patient Uncovered or under Only a Sheet)	Hours after Last Dose				
		Morphine	Heroin	Meperi-dine	Dihydro-Morphinone	Codeine
Grade 4	Increased intensity of above plus: Febrile facies Position—curled up on hard surface Vomiting Diarrhea Weight loss (5 lb daily) Spontaneous ejaculation or orgasm Hemoconcentration leukocytosis, eosinopenia, increased blood sugar	36–48	24–36	—	16	—

* Not all signs are necessary to diagnose any particular grade. Racemorphan (Dromoran) and levorphanol (Levodromoran), although three times and six times as strong as morphine sulfate, show the same time curve as morphine sulfate. Similarly, paregoric, laudanum, and hydrochlorides of opium alkaloids (Pantopon), depending on their relative content of morphine.

Adapted from Anglin et al. (5).

In addition to acute withdrawal symptoms, opioids may produce a protracted abstinent syndrome lasting several months (22). Body temperature and respiratory rate may be below normal. The patient may have trouble sleeping. More important, the craving for opiates may persist for several months after the last dose. This probably contributes to the high recidivism rate in opiate users. Recidivism has also been attributed to a phenomenon called the "conditioned abstinent syndrome" (22). Detoxified patients who return to the environment in which they used drugs may experience craving for the drug as well as physical manifestations of abstinence because of conditioned stimuli (seeing old friends, familiar places, and so forth).

To ameliorate withdrawal symptoms, oral methadone can be substituted for any opioid. Methadone can then be discontinued gradually over a period of 1 or 2 weeks. (Historically, LAAM, a long-acting form of methadone, was also used, but it has been withdrawn from the European market and no longer marketed in the United States because of cardiac complications.) Naltrexone, an antagonist, has been used with mixed results (69). Clonidine, an alpha-adrenergic agonist given for hypertension, also alleviates the opiate withdrawal syndrome, suggesting that catecholamines are involved in opiate withdrawal.

Clonidine has one advantage over methadone: It allows the patient to become narcotic free (70). The disadvantages of clonidine include sedation, insomnia, and hypotension (6). Most recently, buphrenorphine, a mixed agonist-antagonist opioid has drawn significant attention as a safe and effective detoxification agent in inpatient, outpatient, and primary care settings (4, 21, 63, 75, 84, 85, 101, 103, 105, 137, 141).

The course of opiate addiction varies depending on the population studied. In Vaillant's 12-year follow-up of opiate addicts originally treated at the federal addiction treatment center at Lexington, 98% had returned to the use of opiates within 12 months after release (140). On the other hand, a study of Vietnam veterans who used opium and its products extensively during their tour in Vietnam revealed that less than 10% continued using the drug in the year after their return to the United States (113). This suggests that circumstances of exposure and availability are important factors in maintaining use.

There is some evidence that heroin users who do not die as a result of drugs or criminal activities may spontaneously stop using the drug after their mid-30s. School problems such as delinquency and truancy frequently antedate heroin use (140).

Even in environments where addiction is common, there seems to be a sizable number of occasional or controlled users of heroin; they are sometimes referred to as "chippers." Although well known on the street, they are rarely mentioned in the professional literature, where they are generally assumed to be people in a transition stage leading to either compulsive use or abstinence. In fact, evidence suggests that some people may use heroin occasionally and without signs of addiction for many years (151). In the case of any street drug, however, the purity of the substance must be taken into account. Chippers may be able to control their heroin use because the heroin is of low potency.

Earlier evidence suggested that opiate users had few other diagnosable psychiatric illnesses (except perhaps sociopathy), although many of them take other drugs such as alcohol and benzodiazepines. More recent evidence suggests substance abuse is strongly associated with anxiety, personality, and mood disorders (50, 51, 68, 111, 143).

The mortality from opiate withdrawal is negligible despite the unpleasantness of the withdrawal syndrome. Deaths from medical causes occurring among addicts are mainly due to infection, overdose, and apparent hypersensitivity reactions, possibly from diluents such as quinine. Unsterile injections may produce septicemia, hepatitis B and C, subacute bacterial endocarditis, tetanus, and AIDS. Uncertain dosage is often the cause of death from opiates. The powders sold on the street are highly variable in potency. Accustomed to the normal successive dilutions of the drug as it passes through the distribution channels, addicts may unexpectedly encounter relatively pure heroin and consequently overdose. Opioid overdose may be fatal because of respiratory depression and may require ventilatory assistance in a hospital. Naloxone, an opioid antagonist, will reverse respiratory depression.

No single treatment for opiate addiction has been established as superior to others. More than 40 years ago, methadone maintenance was introduced as a long-term treatment for narcotic users (35). Methadone is given in gradually increasing doses over a period of weeks until a high degree of cross-tolerance to all opiates is established. The euphoric effects of intravenous narcotics are blocked. Some previous drug users have become stabilized as productive citizens with this treatment. Methadone alone apparently is not enough for this outcome in many addicts; a complete program of rehabilitation is necessary.

The original methadone program of Dole and Nyswander (36) was considered impressively successful but has been criticized in that multiple drug users and other presumed poor-prognosis cases were not accepted in the program. The approach also has been challenged because it involves substituting one addiction for another, and it has led to wide dissemination of methadone through illicit channels (100). The consensus at present is that higher doses of methadone are usually required for the program to be effective.

Nevertheless, in many cities, methadone has been given credit for ending the criminal activity of a high percentage of heroin addicts. In a 4-year follow-up of methadone clients, Dole et al. (36) found that the majority were productively employed, living as responsible citizens, and supporting families. Most no longer engaged in criminal activity to support their habit. Naltrexone, an opioid antagonist, appears to be somewhat useful in highly motivated opioid-dependent patients.

Buprenorphine, a relatively new agent with mixed agonist/antagonist properties, has been shown to be helpful in maintaining abstinence and has the added benefits (compared to methadone) of reduced addictive properties, low overdose potential, and fewer withdrawal symptoms (80). Buprenorphine comparison studies with methadone (2, 13, 41, 45, 74, 81, 89, 104, 106, 108, 118, 128, 129, 136) have revealed it to be as effective as methadone. Not surprisingly, reports of buprenorphine abuse (54) arose, but a new preparation was developed that included buprenorphine and noloxone (opiate antagonist). Overall, one very significant advantage of buprenorphine is that the treatment can be provided by qualified physicians in a medical office as opposed to federally approved treatment programs (i.e., methadone clinics).

Various psychosocial treatment models have been put forward for treatment of opiate abuse with less than definitive results (30, 37). Self-help groups made up of former addicts have stimulated enthusiastic responses from some participants, but their efficacy in general remains unknown.

While most of this section has concentrated on heroin dependence, it is important for the reader to be aware of a recent potential change in the longstanding problem of misuse of prescription medications for nonmedical uses. A 2001 survey by Substance Abuse and Mental Health Services Administration (132) found that more than 11 million people had misused a prescription once in their lifetime, which was four times greater than in the 1980s.

Unfortunately, validating this response, at least to some degree, through bad outcomes including emergency department visits (documented by Drug Abuse Warning System [DAWN]) and poison control contacts have been problematic because of retrospective approach, probabilistic analysis (only certain "representative areas" are surveyed), and use of trailing data (1 to 2 years) to identify potential emerging drug trends.

Opioid research has led to exciting findings (5, 6, 11, 16). Injecting opiate compounds labeled with radioactive tracers into rats, investigators discovered that specific opiate receptors, so-called mu (μ) receptors, exist on the surfaces of particular cells in the brain stem and that the attachment of opiates to these cells could be prevented by morphine antagonists. Later, positron emission testing (PET) in humans revealed very high levels of opiate receptors in the areas of the caudate-putamen (43). In 1993 this receptor was cloned (20), allowing further in-depth study. Ultimately, the receptor studies led to the finding that enkephalins are endogenous ligands for the opiate receptor (126).

Sedative-Hypnotics

Sedatives produce calmness; hypnotics produce sleep. Both share similar pharmacological actions, hence the term "sedative-hypnotics." In higher doses, drugs marketed as sedatives also produce sleep. Conversely, hypnotics prescribed in lower doses produce calmness. The most popular class of sedative-hypnotics is the benzodiazepines (discussed in the next section). Benzodiazepines are also called "tranquilizers" or "minor" tranquilizers, in contradistinction to "major" tranquilizers such as the antipsychotic drugs. The term "tranquilizer" originated from the observation that benzodiazepines would "tranquilize" wild animals—make them more tame and manageable—without rendering them unconscious (48). Benzodiazepines are distinguishable from barbiturates and older sedative-hypnotics such as choral hydrate in that animals and people can easily be aroused from benzodiazepine-produced sleep, whereas this is more difficult with the older drugs. This section will confine itself to barbiturates, because encountering one of the older synthetic hypnotics (e.g., glutethimide [Doriden], methyprylon [Noludar], and ethchlorvynol [Placidyl]) is highly unlikely.

In contrast to opioids, barbiturates are usually taken orally. The short- and intermediate-acting barbiturates are most frequently used for nonmedical purposes. In both acute and chronic intoxication as well as the withdrawal syndrome, the clinical picture resembles that produced by alcohol. An intoxicated patient may show lethargy, difficulty in thinking, poor memory, irritability, and self-neglect. Nystagmus, ataxia, and a positive Romberg sign are often present.

Withdrawal symptoms may occur when patients take over 400 mg of barbiturates per day. The patient becomes anxious, restless, and weak during the first 12 to 16 hours after the usual dose has not been supplied. Tremors of the hands are prominent; deep tendon reflexes are hyperactive. During the second or third day, grand mal seizures may occur, sometimes followed by delirium. Deaths have been reported. The syndrome clears in about a week. Long-acting barbiturates such as phenobarbital rarely if ever produce major withdrawal symptoms.

Withdrawal manifestations may be prevented or treated by administering a large dose of a short-acting barbiturate such as secobarbital (800–1,000 mg per 24 hours in divided doses) and then gradually reducing the dose over a period of 7–10 days. If a patient shows evidence of intoxication with the first or second dose (200 mg each), the diagnosis of barbiturate abuse should be questioned in view of the absence of tolerance. Because of cross-tolerance between barbiturates and other sedatives and hypnotics, withdrawal from these drugs may also be accomplished with a short-acting barbiturate.

It is unwise to prescribe barbiturates to depressed patients unless dosage is carefully controlled. Patients may accumulate large amounts of drugs by hoarding. Unintentional death may result from slow absorption rates because large quantities of barbiturates in the stomach diminish gastric and intestinal function (151). Users not getting the desired effect in what seems a long time continue to take tablet after tablet until they are unconscious. In the process, they ingest a lethal dose.

Phenobarbital is useful in detoxifying sedative-hypnotic dependence. The drug is long acting and produces a gradual cessation of withdrawal symptoms: 30 mg of phenobarbital is roughly equivalent to 100 mg of the short-acting barbiturates. Often there is uncertainty about the type and quantity of the sedative-hypnotics the patient has been using. In this event, repeated doses of phenobarbital may be given in smaller amounts to prevent withdrawal (125, 135, 140). The reduced use of the barbiturates as a class makes the possibility of encountering a patient in withdrawal rather uncommon, but knowledge of the potentially serious nature of the withdrawal (and treatment) is exceedingly important.

Benzodiazepines

Benzodiazepines are the most widely prescribed class of medication in the Western world. At least a dozen such drugs are marketed in the United States and perhaps 30 or more are sold throughout the world. Compared to the sedative-hypnotic drugs described earlier, benzodiazepines have the following advantages: (1) they relieve anxiety without necessarily reducing alertness, impairing coordination, or interfering with normal thinking processes; (2) the regularly prescribed doses provide little or no euphoria; (3) they are good muscle relaxants; and (4) they are the safest, most effective drugs for treating alcohol withdrawal and other agitated states produced by many street drugs. Benzodiazepines can be given to intoxicated patients in an emergency room without fear of lethal reactions, although caution should always be exercised.

Benzodiazepines are the most effective drugs available for insomnia. Unlike barbiturates they lose little of their effectiveness over even long periods of usage, and short-acting benzodiazepine hypnotics such as triazolam (Halcion) and temazepam (Restoril) and the alpha-1 and -5 selective agent zolpidem (Ambien) leave few after-effects the next morning. After prolonged use, patients often experience increased insomnia for a few days—possibly a rebound from the previous hypnotic effects—but the difficulty seems to be short lived. Finally, these drugs have one great advantage over the barbiturates and other hypnotics of the past: It is almost impossible to commit suicide by taking an overdose. Very rarely, deaths are reported from overdose, but almost always only when accompanied by other sedative agents or alcohol (48).

Reports of a benzodiazepine withdrawal syndrome have appeared for many years. Although millions of people regularly use these drugs, serious withdrawal symptoms appear to be uncommon (42). The symptoms reported range from panic and hallucinations to disorientation and grand mal seizures. Benzodiazepine users often combine the drug with alcohol or other drugs, and it is usually not clear whether the benzodiazepine alone is responsible for the abstinence syndrome (36). Abstinence syndromes are associated with low doses of benzodiazepines taken over a course of years (23). Nevertheless, in most animal and human studies designed to predict dependence liability, benzodiazepines rank low (79). In one study, subjects were given a choice between 10 mg of diazepam or placebo; they chose the placebo (64). The same subjects preferred a 5-mg dose of dextroamphetamine to placebo. Nevertheless, physicians should be cautious in prescribing the drug for long periods, even in low dosage. Inevitably, some patients will combine them with other substances. Also, abrupt withdrawal of the drugs after relatively high dosages may produce severe anxiety and psychotic symptoms. Alprazolam (Xanax), an effective drug for anxiety, has the particular disadvantage of producing some degree of physical dependence, even when taken in moderate dosage. Withdrawing a patient from alprazolam should be done very slowly, reducing the dosage by as little as 10% per week (92). While discontinuation of the other benzodiazepines used over long periods may be safely accomplished more rapidly, recent recommendations (82) use roughly the same timetable of 10%–12.5% reduction over 1- to 2-week periods. This taper may be adjusted to type of benzodiazepine, diagnosis, personality variables, and support of the patient. Geriatric patients are particularly sensitive to benzodiazepines and should be given smaller doses than younger patients.

While in-depth review of receptor physiology is beyond the scope of this book, it does seem to be a settled issue that GABA (γ-aminobutryic acid) is the major inhibitory neurotransmitter in mammalian brains (148) and its effects are mediated through two receptors—GABA-A and GABA-B. Cloning of parts of the GABA-A receptor in 1991 (86) greatly expanded understanding of its function in relation to benzodiazepines. In particular, the benzodiazepine receptor was found physically linked to the GABA-A receptor and enhancing its responsivity to GABA. Stated more broadly, presence of a benzodiazepine at its receptor causes the GABA-A receptor to be more responsive to synaptic GABA. Activation of the GABA-A receptor facilitates the influx of chloride ions (138), hyperpolarizing the neuron, inhibiting depolarization and therefore transmission. This continues to be an area of intense research focused on "designing" a "benzodiazepine" to reduce anxiety while avoiding sedation, cognitive impairment, and dependence (149).

Marijuana

Cannabis sativa (hemp) contains chemicals called cannabinoids, one of which, Δ-9-tetrahydrocannabinol (THC), is believed to be the most psychoactive constituent of marijuana. The effects of THC depend on dosage, and they range from mild euphoria with small doses to sedation with high doses. Most marijuana originally growing wild in the United States contains insufficient amounts of THC to produce measurable psychological effects. Cannabis imported from Mexico, South America, and India often contains sufficient THC to produce marked euphoria and, depending on the plant preparation used, paranoid delusions and other psychotomimetic effects. Also, THC deteriorates at the rate of 5% per month at room temperature; even imported cannabis eventually loses its potency. However, cannabis in use today tends to have a much higher THC content than that available in the mid-1970s (8, 57).

There are two generally available cannabis preparations: marijuana and hashish. The former consists of a mixture of dried plant products (upper leaves, tops, stems, flowers and seeds). The latter consists of the resins of the plant and is more potent.

Cannabis can be either smoked or eaten. The chemical THC and cannabinoids are lipophilic and rapidly distributed throughout the body, and THC is stored in the adipose tissue and distributed to the body slowly over time. Blood testing can reveal presence of THC more than 30 days after heavy use.

In parts of the world where concentrated cannabis preparations have been used by millions of people for hundreds of years, constant use is said to be associated with serious medical and psychiatric illnesses. Interestingly, early studies conducted in Jamaica, Costa Rica, and Greece—countries where cannabis has been used regularly for many years—failed to reveal any serious pathology associated with the use of the drug (116). However, subsequent evidence accumulated over the past 40 years suggests that regular use of marijuana is associated with the following hazards (19, 67):

1. Bronchial and pulmonary irritation. Marijuana, because of its relatively poor combustibility, has up to 50% more polyaromatic hydrocarbons in its smoke than tobacco does (61, 67). Cigarette for cigarette, the difference between tobacco and marijuana may be even more significant because of the way marijuana typically is smoked—down to a minuscule butt—and because the smoke itself is retained in the lungs for a longer period than tobacco smoke. Multiple studies (14, 133, 134) have found habitual use to be associated with frequent respiratory symptoms, including acute and chronic bronchitis, wheezing, and exertional dyspnea.

2. Marijuana causes tachycardia. Smoking just one marijuana cigarette can significantly reduce exercise tolerance in cardiac patients with anginal syndrome (6). This would militate against marijuana use by persons who have cardiac disorders.

3. THC is a potent immune modulator with significant immunosuppressive effects on various immune cells, including T lymphocytes, macrophages, and natural killer cells (72).

4. Studies consistently show short-term adverse effects of marijuana on cognition and immediate memory (67, 120). These impairments may last for many weeks, months, or years after use (127).

5. Marijuana intoxication impairs reaction time, motor coordination, and visual perception (120). Studies under simulated conditions and in traffic have confirmed that the ability to operate a motor vehicle is adversely affected by marijuana use (67, 73).

Marijuana's association with psychosis and schizophrenia has been the topic of substantial debate. A Swedish study published in late 1987 reported a strong correlation between cannabis use and schizophrenia, defined by *DSM-III* criteria. The study involved a cohort of nearly 50,000 Swedish military conscripts. Those who reported using cannabis on more than 50 occasions were six times more likely subsequently to receive a diagnosis of schizophrenia than were nonusers. The relative risk increased with increased consumption. The study did not demonstrate that cannabis use *caused* schizophrenia; cannabis consumption might, on the contrary, be caused by an emerging schizophrenia. Nevertheless, the association between marijuana use and schizophrenia was significant. Subsequent studies and review (53, 56, 65) have failed to confirm a link between cannabis and psychosis unless there is a preexisting psychotic disorder.

Marijuana does have a certain abuse potential (25, 146, 146). In a follow-up study of 97 regular users, 9% met operational criteria for abuse similar to criteria used in alcohol studies. In other words, marijuana use was associated with a variety of social, psychological, and medical problems in these individuals. Of the abusers, two-thirds had had traffic violations they attributed solely to marijuana intoxication; one-third had engaged in fights, again citing marijuana use as the reason. The latter finding was particularly interesting in view of the widespread observation that marijuana typically has anti-aggressive effects. This, indeed, may be the case in most instances, but "set and setting" notoriously influence the effects of drugs, and it cannot be said that marijuana has exclusively "taming" effects.

Early difficulties isolating the active agent for marijuana were compounded by the fact that many regular users of marijuana also took other drugs. Further, until the 1980s, most marijuana available in the United States contained only small amounts of THC. Intense research located a THC binding site (33) in the rodent brain, and subsequent work (88, 97) revealed two major receptors (CB1 and CB2). Cloning of these receptors (33, 88, 97) allowed discovery of an endogenous lipid agonist in mammals for both CB1 and CB2. Named "ananda-mide" from the Sanskrit word *ananda* (meaning inner bliss and tranquility) (34), this endocannibinoid facilitated pharmacological targeting. Stated differently, marijuana has been used medicinally for thousands of years but with many liabilities (noted above), including addiction. Identification of the receptors may facilitate design of medications that avoid the liabilities and deliver more efficaciously the effects for which marijuana is already touted, including anti-nausea and anti-emetic properties (76), appetite stimulation (91), analgesia (142), anxiolysis (114), anti-spasmodic effects (10), and reduction of intraocular pressure (60).

American attitudes toward marijuana have changed. Experimenters with the drug in the 1960s and 1970s commonly reported mild effects, probably because of the low potency of the drug mainly available at that time. As the THC content of available marijuana increased, there was a corresponding increase in the awareness of risks in using the drug. In 1986, for example, 71% of high school seniors believed that regular marijuana use involved risk, more than double the proportion that believed this in 1978 (96). Unfortunately, as noted earlier, a significant increase in the abuse and dependence of marijuana occurred in the decade from 1991–1992 to 2001–2002 (26).

Phencyclidine

This agent is a member of the ketamine family and was developed as a veterinary anesthetic (Sernylan). Known as "Angel Dust" on the street, phencyclidine was mostly manufactured in home laboratories. Because people present so bizarrely and the drug has been responsible for a number of deaths (99), it is reviewed here briefly. The drug is available in many forms—tablet, powder, leaf, rock crystal—and can be ingested, snorted, smoked, or injected. It is often sold under false guise as THC (tetrahydrocannabinol), LSD, or mescaline. Marijuana and other street drugs were often adulterated with PCP. It has been called the "universal adulterant" (24).

Phencyclidine is a "dissociative" anesthetic. It induces a cataleptic state in which pain is not perceived; the individual's eyes are wide open, but he or she is unconscious and amnestic for the experience. A noteworthy feature of PCP is the behavioral dyscontrol that can produce a variety of bizarre activities or violence that, in turn, results in encounters with police, unusual accidents, strange suicides, impulsive homicides, and lawsuits. The user is often amnestic about these events and may remember only the pleasant, floaty euphoria the drug produces at low doses.

These patients often are admitted to psychiatric hospitals with a diagnosis of acute paranoid or catatonic schizophrenia. Fortunately, the psychosis usually clears. Phenothiazines, the usual drug class of choice for agitated and uncontrollable patients, can cause severe postural hypotension and seizures, and may increase muscle rigidity in patients intoxicated with PCP. Intramuscular benzodiazepines may be a better choice. Talking down a patient intoxicated with PCP may not be as effective as with LSD and other hallucinogens because it may overstimulate the patient (24).

Inhalants

Inhalants represent a significant category of substance abuse that has been understudied for a variety of reasons, including transient use (abused by the young), rareness as a drug of choice, use based on availability (or lack of availability of more desirable substances), poorly understood chemistry (not originally developed as a medication), and difficulty conducting studies (other than surveys). Nonetheless, inhalant abuse has been found to be second only to marijuana abuse in 12–17 year olds in the 1990s (39, 130). Between 1994 and 2000 the number of new inhalant users increased more than 50%, from 618,000 to 970,000 (132). Because of the potential for serious complications (18), including liver damage, cardiac arrhythmias, brain damage, and death (17), some knowledge of the available agents is desirable. Inquiry into inhalant use should be part of intake evaluations on children, adolescents, and young adults.

Inhalants are often divided into three types: nitrous oxide, nitrites, and volatile solvents. Nitrous oxide or "laughing gas" has many industrial and medical uses. When used as an anesthetic, some perceive it as precipitating euphoria. Certain individuals report a dissociative experience with numbness, tingling, dizziness, warmth, stiffness, and auditory hallucinations (9). Nitrites consist of amyl, butyl, and isobutyl nitrite, which are available in room odorizers and over-the-counter preparations. Primary uses include euphoria and enhancing the sexual response. Volatile substances comprise the largest group, encompassing gasoline (with or without lead), solvents (correction fluid, paint thinner, nail polish remover, fuel [butane], lighter fluid), cleaning agents (spot remover, degreaser, dry cleaning, spark plug cleaner), adhesives (rubber cement, airplane glue, and PVC cement), and aerosols (spray paint, hair spray, deodorants, room freshener, analgesic spray, asthma sprays) (17). While many of the active ingredients are well known, such as toluene, butane, hexane, trichloroethylene, fluorocarbons, and acetone, the precise pathophysiology of most has not been identified. The usual primary effect of all of these agents is euphoria.

Amphetamines

This group of stimulants includes d-amphetamine (Dexedrine), dl-amphetamine (Benzedrine—withdrawn from the market), methamphetamine (Desoxyn, Methedrine), and dextromethamphetamine ("ice"). Their effects include elevated mood, increased energy and alertness, decreased appetite, and slight improvement in task performance. Amphetamines may be taken orally, smoked, or injected intravenously.

Drug-induced psychosis is common among individuals taking large doses of amphetamines (over 50 mg per day). Such psychosis may resemble paranoid schizophrenia with persecutory delusions occurring despite a clear sensorium. Hallucinations are common. Usually the psychosis subsides 1 or 2 weeks after drug use stops. When an apparent amphetamine psychosis persists, a hidden source of drugs or the diagnosis of schizophrenia should be considered.

No specific amphetamine withdrawal syndrome has been described; however, users complain of fatigue and depression after discontinuing the drug, and these have been temporally associated with a decrease in the excretion of 3-methoxy-4-hydroxphenylglycol (MHPG), a metabolite of norepinephrine (107). Tolerance may be striking. "Speed freaks" sometimes take as much as 1 or 2 g per day (the usual therapeutic dose is 5–30 mg per day).

Since their introduction in the early 1930s, amphetamines have been prescribed by physicians for a variety of conditions, including depression, obesity, and narcolepsy. Beginning in the 1960s, increasing amounts of amphetamine entered illegal distribution channels and became available on the street. Amphetamine use declined in the 1980s, partly because of physicians' reluctance to prescribe the drug, and partly because of the growing popularity of cocaine.

Concern about the increased use of amphetamines and other stimulants led to a marked curtailment of their production and availability. Cocaine, considered by many in the 1970s to be a relatively benign drug, substantially replaced amphetamines as a street drug. The trade-off—for society and for individuals—did not work (47). First, experience since the 1980s indicates that cocaine (particularly "crack") may be more dependence producing and dangerous than the amphetamines. Second, the previous beneficial uses of amphetamines for medical purposes were virtually denied. In some countries, amphetamines were removed from the market. Yet the evidence was strong that these and similar drugs are useful for treating patients with narcolepsy, attention-deficit disorders, and depression. Supporting this point in a general way is the 1987 report by the National Institute on Drug Abuse, which concluded that nonmedical use of prescription drugs as an individual's only form of drug abuse was relatively rare, although this may be changing as noted previously.

Drug epidemics tend to wax and wane, and this has also been true of amphetamine abuse. With the introduction of "ice" in Hawaii in the early 1990s, reason for concern about amphetamines has reemerged. Ice, also known as "crystal" or "rock," and chemically named dextromethamphetamine, is a designer drug that can be smoked and thus will deliver methamphetamine to the brain even faster than when injected. (Designer drugs have been defined as substances created by the manipulation of molecular structure to avoid prosecution for the manufacture of a scheduled drug that nonetheless retains psychoactive properties.) Ice has a long duration of action—up to eighteen hours. It stimulates the brain to a greater degree than regular methamphetamine but stimulates the heart, blood vessels, and lungs less. Its effects can be devastating, sometimes leading to a severe psychosis and intense depression as the drug wears off. Users often become paranoid. Acute hypertensive crisis and violence are possible. Haloperidol can usually control the psychotic symptoms, and antidepressants can usually control the withdrawal effects. One "advantage" of ice is that it eliminates the use of needles—reducing the risk of AIDS. A disadvantage is that the drug affects the user's judgment regarding safe sexual practices—increasing the risk of AIDS.

The Midwest and Western states saw a significant upsurge in the use of methamphetamine in the late 1990s and into the next decade (110). Efforts to stem the production of this easily synthesized and inexpensive-to-produce (in bulk) substance consisted of attempting to control legally the availability of the precursors. Once restrictions on precursors were in place in most states, suppliers began to provide the substance from outside the country. Impact of this regional epidemic has been substantial. In particular, leaving aside the direct effect on the individual's mental status and physical well-being, the burden on families, social networks, criminal justice, education, workplace environment, and mental health services has been extraordinary (29, 94, 110).

"Ecstasy," or 3, 4-methylenedioxymethamphetamine (MDMA), was patented by Dr. E. Merck in 1914 as an appetite suppressant (93). Rediscovered in the 1970s, it was touted as an adjunct to therapy (123) and its use expanded. While it was legally available at one time, evidence eventually came to light that it was neurotoxic and therefore required categorization as a Schedule I substance. Unfortunately, notoriety probably increased demand. Surveys in the early 2000s suggested increased use (12, 131). It is also clear that use of this substance is associated with significant morbidity and mortality (55, 117), including cerebrovascular accident, liver failure, hyponatremia (and cerebral edema), serotonin syndrome, and exertional hyperpyrexia leading to rhabdomyolysis along with multi-organ failure.

Cocaine

The United States has experienced two major epidemics of cocaine abuse. The first occurred in the last decades of the nineteenth century when physicians, in particular, became addicted to the drug (thinking, as did Freud at first, that it was relatively benign and nonaddictive). The second epidemic began in the mid-1970s and has continued ever since (although abating somewhat in the 1990s). Cocaine remains a major drug of abuse throughout the United States.

In the early 1980s, increasing numbers of white, employed, middle-class people in their late 20s and 30s who had never before sought psychological help sought treatment for cocaine dependence. A cocaine hot line in Washington, DC, received more than 14,000 calls daily (47, 144, 144). Many of the callers were college graduates, professionals, and business executives. Half had incomes over $25,000 per year and cocaine habits costing $600 a week. Dependence on the drug was intense. Nearly all callers said they could not turn the drug down when it was available. Most said cocaine had become more important to them than food or sex. They had physical complaints: headaches, sinus infections, and sexual malfunctioning. Some had seizures or became paranoid.

The demographics of the epidemic changed as the country moved into the second half of the 1980s. Use among women, minority groups, lower-income groups, and adolescents increased. Cocaine problems infiltrated the small towns of the Midwest. Once called the champagne of drugs, cocaine became less expensive, freebasing (smoking cocaine) became popular, and cheap freebase, known as "crack," invaded the slums as well as suburbia. By the mid-1980s, cocaine was universally considered a dangerous drug (109). With recognition of its danger, cocaine use plateaued and then began falling in the early 1990s. Interestingly, by 1996 the number of occasional users (less than 12 days per year) had decreased to 2.5 million as opposed to 7 million in 1985 (31).

Cocaine resembles amphetamines in many ways, but whereas amphetamines are synthetic drugs, cocaine is of botanical origin, originating from shrubs grown in the Andes. Its effects last for a shorter period than those of amphetamines. Like amphetamines, cocaine is a powerful stimulant of the nervous system, producing euphoria, increasing alertness, suppressing fatigue and boredom (102). Cocaine intoxication is usually recognized by anxiety, agitation, suspiciousness extending to paranoia, tremor, mydriasis, tachycardia, diaphoresis, hypertension, and hyperpyrexia. After regular, heavy use of the drug, a withdrawal syndrome may occur, in which formication (a sensation of bugs crawling under the skin) is frequent, together with depression and lassitude (144).

Heavy use of cocaine may produce a schizophreniform psychosis resembling paranoid schizophrenia. Occasional users sometimes report a profound dysphoria, persisting for several days after they have used the drug. Cocaine may have a deleterious effect on the health of pregnant women and on fetal development. Used during pregnancy, it may cause irregularities of placental blood flow, abruptio placentae, and premature labor. Reported effects on fetal development include low birth weight, malformations of the urogenital system, cerebral infarction and seizures, and sudden death syndrome.

Until the late 1980s the cocaine most often used and most widely available on the street was cocaine hypochloride, a powdered form that was ingested by snorting (49). However, in the mid-1970s some Americans adopted a method similar to the South American practice of smoking cocoa paste (base)—a potent extract from cocoa leaves. Users can "free" street cocaine from its salts and cutting agents by a chemical process—potentially hazardous because it involves heating flammable solvents. The purified cocaine base that remains, mainly cocaine alkaloid, is highly potent when smoked. It increases heart rate and blood pressure (145); produces tremors, anorexia, insomnia; sometimes causes hallucinations (124), paranoia, and depression; and even results in occasional cardiac arrest (87) and lung damage (28). Nevertheless, according to a 1985 National Household Survey, 20% of cocaine users were using freebase despite its known dangers. The rate of administration—intranasal, smoking, or intravenous—is relevant to the dependence potential of the drug (49). The inhaled form of the freebase—crack, relatively inexpensive and enormously popular in the urban ghetto—is considered by many authorities the most dangerous of all forms of cocaine. It has accounted for a number of deaths among celebrities, and it is associated with drug-related crime and murder. Because crack is inhaled and enters the brain rapidly, it is highly addictive. There was little evidence in the mid- to late-1990s that its use was subsiding in urban settings. About 25% of users prefer the IV route—the route still most associated with dependence.

Neuroleptics may be used to treat the symptoms of amphetamine and cocaine psychoses. Antidepressants may be used to treat associated depressive symptoms (7, 44, 44). Intravenous diazepam can be used to control seizures. Multiple medications have been tried and continue to be tried, but no single agent (27) has consistently demonstrated positive results in treating cocaine dependence. Neither has any psychosocial treatment approach yielded convincing replicated evidence of an efficacious approach to this disorder.

Hallucinogens

Perceptual distortions are the primary effect of hallucinogenic drugs, which include LSD, mescaline, psilocybin, and a family of compounds chemically resembling either LSD or the amphetamines (e.g., DMT, STP [2,5-dimethoxy-4-methylamphetamine], and MDMA [3, 4-methylenedioxymethamphetamine]—"Ecstasy"). Our discussion will focus on LSD because it has been the most widely used and studied hallucinogen. The use of LSD peaked in the 1970s and was in steady decline until the drug had a slight increase in popularity in the mid-1990s.

Together with perceptual distortions, including illusions and hallucinations, LSD "trips" produce altered time sense, disturbed judgment, and sometimes confusion and disorientation (95). Some LSD trips are unpleasant. Users of LSD may be brought to emergency rooms for bad trips characterized by panic and sometimes persecutory delusions. There are reports of prolonged or flashback effects (a resurgence of the drug effect days, weeks, months, or even years subsequent to the end of a trip). Although flashbacks have not been studied systematically, they are reported so commonly that some authorities believe individuals do experience them. A number of deaths have been attributed to LSD, primarily from suicide or homicide, although a causal connection remains unclear (92).

Repeated use of LSD results in marked tolerance. No withdrawal syndrome has been reported. The drug usually produces euphoria, but dysphoria may occur. No deaths have been reported from LSD overdose.

Treatment for acute adverse reactions to LSD consists of reassurance and, if this fails, tranquilizers. Diazepam appears to be as effective as phenothiazines and is somewhat safer because it is less likely to produce hypotension.

Hallucinogens have complicated the problem of diagnosing psychiatric disorders among young drug users. Prolonged psychotic episodes are probably more often attributable to schizophrenia or other psychiatric illness than to LSD toxicity. To determine whether a patient has a psychiatric illness that is not associated with drug abuse, the patient must be drug free for a lengthy period.

Tobacco

For the last 50 years tobacco, and more precisely nicotine, has been the focus of intense scientific research, scientific argument, public health proclamations, regulation, public debate, and extensive litigation. It appears highly unlikely that until the conclusions by the 1988 Surgeon General's report noted earlier (and more precisely, "... pharmacologic and behavioral processes that determine tobacco addiction are similar to those that determine addiction to drugs such as heroin and cocaine") are scientifically proven *and* accepted by society, the issue of addiction to this substance will not be resolved. Further discussion of addiction and related issues are beyond the scope of this book, but the reader should be aware of various pathways and interventions to cessation after nicotine dependence is established.

First, epidemiologic studies have demonstrated that the majority of successful attempts at quitting smoking occur without medical or pharmacological assistance (46, 139). Advising patients to quit has contributed to doubling the quit rates (112). Generally, addressing motivational issues and using motivational techniques with education regarding associated risks can be helpful. Second, a number of other nonpharmacologic interventions have been found to be efficacious, including self-help materials, proactive telephone counseling, group counseling, individual counseling, intra-treatment social support, and extra-treatment social support (40, 77). Third, acupuncture, mesotherapy, hypnosis, and auriculotherapy have not been found to have positive outcomes on smoking cessation (40, 78). Fourth, pharmacologic interventions include nicotine replacement therapy (various forms), bupropion, and varenicline. These treatments have been found to be effective in controlled clinical trials with behavioral support when "nicotine dependence" was moderate to severe (40, 71, 78, 147). No one agent was found superior, and choice by the clinician would rest on patient preference and medical profile.

REFERENCES

1. Dependence on barbiturates and other sedative drugs. JAMA, *193*:107–111, 1965.
2. Ahmadi, J. Methadone versus buprenorphine maintenance for the treatment of heroin-dependent outpatients. J. Subst. Abuse Treat., *24*:217–220, 2003.
3. Altman, I., Kroeger, H. H., Clark, D. A., Johnson, A. C., and Sheps, C. G. Dependence on barbiturates and other sedative drugs. JAMA, *193*:673–677, 1965.
4. Amass, L., Bickel, W. K., Higgins, S. T., and Hughes, J. R. A preliminary investigation of outcome following gradual or rapid buprenorphine detoxification. J. Addict. Dis., *13*:33–45, 1994.
5. Anglin, M. D., Brecht, M. L., Woodward, J. A., and Bonett, D. G. An empirical study of maturing out: conditional factors. Int. J. Addict., *21*:233–246, 1986.
6. Ansubel, D. P. Methadone maintenance treatment: the other side of the coin. Int. J. Addict., *18*:851–862, 1983.
7. Arndt, I., Dorozynsky, L., Woody, G., McLellan, A. T., and O'Brien, C. P. Desipramine treatment of cocaine abuse in methadone-maintained patients, National Institute on Drug Abuse Research Monograph 95. In *Problems of Drug Dependence*, Harris, L. (ed.). Rockville, MD: NIDAR, 1990.

8. Ashton, C. H. Pharmacology and effects of cannabis: a brief review. Br. J. Psychiat., 178:101–106, 2001.

9. Atkinson, R. M., and Green, J. D. Personality, prior drug use, and introspective experience during nitrous oxide intoxication. Int. J. Addict., 18:717–738, 1983.

10. Baker, D., Pryce, G., Croxford, J. L., Brown, P., Pertwee, R. G., Huffman, J. W., and Layward, L. Cannabinoids control spasticity and tremor in a multiple sclerosis model. Nature, 404:84–87, 2000.

11. Ball, J. C., Lange, W. R., Myers, C. P., and Friedman, S. R. Reducing the risk of AIDS through methadone maintenance treatment. J. Health. Soc. Behav., 29:214–226, 1988.

12. Banken, J. A. Drug abuse trends among youth in the United States. Ann. N. Y. Acad. Sci., 1025:465–471, 2004.

13. Bickel, W. K., Stitzer, M. L., Bigelow, G. E., Liebson, I. A., Jasinski, D. R., and Johnson, R. E. A clinical trial of buprenorphine: comparison with methadone in the detoxification of heroin addicts. Clin. Pharmacol. Ther., 43:72–78, 1988.

14. Bloom, J. W., Kaltenborn, W. T., Paoletti, P., Camilli, A., and Lebowitz, M. D. Respiratory effects of non-tobacco cigarettes. Br. Med. J. (Clin. Res. Ed.), 295:1516–1518, 1987.

15. Bloomquist, E. R. *Marijuana.* Toronto: Glencoe Press, 1968.

16. Bouckoms, A. J., Masand, P., Murray, G. B., Cassem, E. H., Stern, T. A., and Tesar, G. E. Chronic nonmalignant pain treated with long-term oral narcotic analgesics. Ann. Clin. Psychiat., 4:185–192, 1992.

17. Bowen, S. E., Daniel, J., and Balster, R. L. Deaths associated with inhalant abuse in Virginia from 1987 to 1996. Drug Alcohol Depend., 53:239–245, 1999.

18. Brouette, T., and Anton, R. Clinical review of inhalants. Am. J. Addict., 10:79–94, 2001.

19. Busto, U., Sellers, E. M., Naranjo, C. A., Cappell, H., Sanchez-Craig, M., and Sykora, K. Withdrawal reaction after long-term therapeutic use of benzodiazepines. N. Engl. J. Med., 315:854–859, 1986.

20. Chen, Y., Mestek, A., Liu, J., Hurley, J. A., and Yu, L. Molecular cloning and functional expression of a mu-opioid receptor from rat brain. Mol. Pharmacol., 44:8–12, 1993.

21. Cheskin, L. J., Fudala, P. J., and Johnson, R. E. A controlled comparison of buprenorphine and clonidine for acute detoxification from opioids. Drug Alcohol Depend., 36:115–121, 1994.

22. Childress, A. R., McLellan, A. T., and O'Brien, C. P. Abstinent opiate abusers exhibit conditioned craving, conditioned withdrawal and reductions in both through extinction. Br. J. Addict., 81:655–660, 1986.

23. Closser, M. H., and Brower, K. J. Treatment of alprazolam withdrawal with chlordiazepoxide substitution and taper. J. Subst. Abuse Treat., 11:319–323, 1994.

24. Cohen, S. Angel dust. JAMA, 238:515–516, 1977.

25. Committee to study the health-related effects of cannabis and its derivatives of the National Academy of Sciences and the Institute of Medicine. Marijuana and Health. Washington, DC: National Academy Press, 1992.

26. Compton, W. M., Grant, B. F., Colliver, J. D., Glantz, M. D., and Stinson, F. S. Prevalence of marijuana use disorders in the United States: 1991–1992 and 2001–2002. JAMA, 291:2114–2121, 2004.

27. Cornish, J. W., and O'Brien, C. P. Crack cocaine abuse: an epidemic with many public health consequences. Annu. Rev. Publ. Health, 17:259–273, 1996.

28. Cregler, L. L., and Mark, H. Medical complications of cocaine abuse. N. Engl. J. Med., 315:1495–1500, 1986.

29. Cretzmeyer, M., Sarrazin, M. V., Huber, D. L., Block, R. I., and Hall, J. A. Treatment of methamphetamine abuse: research findings and clinical directions. J. Subst. Abuse Treat., 24:267–277, 2003.

30. Crits-Christoph, P., and Siqueland, L. Psychosocial treatment for drug abuse. Selected review and recommendations for national health care. Arch. Gen. Psychiat., 53:749–756, 1996.

31. Crits-Christoph, P., Siqueland, L., Blaine, J., Frank, A., Luborsky, L., Onken, L. S., Muenz, L. R., Thase, M. E., Weiss, R. D., Gastfriend, D. R., Woody, G. E., Barber, J. P., Butler, S. F., Daley, D., Salloum, I., Bishop, S., Najavits, L. M., Lis, J., Mercer, D., Griffin, M. L., Moras, K., and Beck, A. T. Psychosocial treatments for cocaine dependence: National Institute on Drug Abuse Collaborative Cocaine Treatment Study. Arch. Gen. Psychiat., 56:493–502, 1999.

32. Das, G. Cocaine abuse in North America: a milestone in history. J. Clin. Pharmacol., 33:296–310, 1993.

33. Devane, W. A., Dysarz, F. A., III, Johnson, M. R., Melvin, L. S., and Howlett, A. C. Determination and characterization of a cannabinoid receptor in rat brain. Mol. Pharmacol., 34:605–613, 1988.

34. Devane, W. A., Hanus, L., Breuer, A., Pertwee, R. G., Stevenson, L. A., Griffin, G., Gibson, D., Mandelbaum, A., Etinger, A., and Mechoulam, R. Isolation and structure of a brain constituent that binds to the cannabinoid receptor. Science, 258:1946–1949, 1992.

35. Dole, V. Research on methadone maintenance treatment. Proceedings of the 2nd National Conference on Methadone Maintenance, New York: National Association for the Prevention of Addiction to Narcotics (NAPAN), pp. 359–370, 1969.

36. Dole, V. P., Nyswander, M. E., and Warner, A. Successful treatment of 750 criminal addicts. JAMA, 206:2708–2711, 1968.

37. Dutra, L., Stathopoulou, G., Basden, S. L., Leyro, T. M., Powers, M. B., and Otto, M. W. A meta-analytic review of psychosocial interventions for substance use disorders. Am. J. Psychiat., 165:179–187, 2008.

38. Dwarakananth, S. C. Use of opium and cannabis in traditional systems of medicine in India. Bull. Narcotics, 17:15–19, 1965.

39. Edwards, R., Oetting, E. Inhalant use in the United States. National Institute on Drug Abuse Research Monograph Series, 148: 8–28. Rockville, MD: National Institute on Drug Abuse, 1995.

40. Fiore, M., Bailey, W., Cohen, S., Dorfman, S. F., Goldstein, M. G., Gritz, E. R., Heyman, R. B., Holbrook, J., Jaen, C. R., Kottke, T. E., Lando, H. A., Mecklenburg, R. E., Mullen, P. D., Nett, L. M., Robinson, L., Stilzer, M. L., Tommasello, A. C., Villejo, L.,

and Vewers, M.E. Treating tobacco use and dependence. Clinical practice guideline. Rockville, MD: US Department of Health and Human Services, Public Health Service, 2000.

41. Fischer, G., Gombas, W., Eder, H., Jagsch, R., Peternell, A., Stuhlinger, G., Pezawas, L., Aschauer, H. N., and Kasper, S. Buprenorphine versus methadone maintenance for the treatment of opioid dependence. Addiction, 94:1337–1347, 1999.

42. Fleischhacker, W. W., Barnas, C., and Hackenberg, B. Epidemiology of benzo-diazepine dependence. Acta Psychiat. Scand., 74:80–85, 1986.

43. Frost, J. J., Wagner, H. N., Jr., Dannals, R. F., Ravert, H. T., Links, J. M., Wilson, A. A., Burns, H. D., Wong, D. F., McPherson, R. W., Rosenbaum, A. E., Kuhar, M. J., and Solomon, S. H. Imaging opiate receptors in the human brain by positron tomography. J. Comput. Assist. Tomogr., 9:231–236, 1985.

44. Gawin, F. H. New uses of antidepressants in cocaine abuse. Psychosomat., 27:24–29, 1986.

45. Gerra, G., Borella, F., Zaimovic, A., Moi, G., Bussandri, M., Bubici, C., and Bertacca, S. Buprenorphine versus methadone for opioid dependence: predictor variables for treatment outcome. Drug Alcohol Depend., 75:37–45, 2004.

46. Giovino, G. A. Epidemiology of tobacco use in the United States. Oncogene, 21:7326–7340, 2002.

47. Gold, M. S., Galanter, M., and Stimmel, B., eds. In *Cocaine: Pharmacology, Addiction and Therapy.* New York: Haworth Press, 1987.

48. Goodwin, D. W. *Anxiety.* New York: Ballantine Books, 1986.

49. Gossop, M., Griffiths, P., Powis, B., and Strang, J. Cocaine: patterns of use, route of administration, and severity of dependence. Br. J. Psychiat., 164:660–664, 1994.

50. Grant, B. F. Comorbidity between DSM-IV drug use disorders and major depression: results of a national survey of adults. J. Subst. Abuse, 7:481–497, 1995.

51. Grant, B. F., Hasin, D. S., Stinson, F. S., Dawson, D. A., Patricia, C. S., June, R. W., and Huang, B. Co-occurrence of 12-month mood and anxiety disorders and personality disorders in the US: results from the national epidemiologic survey on alcohol and related conditions. J. Psychiat. Res., 39:1–9, 2005.

52. Grant, B. F., Stinson, F. S., Dawson, D. A., Chou, S. P., Dufour, M. C., Compton, W., Pickering, R. P., and Kaplan, K. Prevalence and co-occurrence of substance use disorders and independent mood and anxiety disorders: results from the National Epidemiologic Survey on Alcohol and Related Conditions. Arch. Gen. Psychiat., 61:807–816, 2004.

53. Gruber, A., and Pope, H. Cannabis psychotic disorder: does it exist? Am. J. Addict., 3:72–83, 1994.

54. Hakansson, A., Medvedeo, A., Andersson, M., and Berglund, M. Buprenorphine misuse among heroin and amphetamine users in Malmo, Sweden: purpose of misuse and route of administration. Eur. Addict. Res., 13:207–215, 2007.

55. Hall, A. P., and Henry, J. A. Acute toxic effects of "Ecstasy" (MDMA) and related compounds: overview of pathophysiology and clinical management. Br. J. Anaesth., 96:678–685, 2006.

56. Hall, W., and Degenhardt, L. Cannabis use and psychosis: a review of clinical and epidemiological evidence. Aust. N. Z. J. Psychiat., *34*:26–34, 2000.

57. Hall, W., and Solowij, N. Adverse effects of cannabis. Lancet, *352*:1611–1616, 1998.

58. Hamilton, G. R., and Baskett, T. F. In the arms of Morpheus: the development of morphine for postoperative pain relief. Can. J. Anaesth., *47*:367–374, 2000.

59. Hardman, J. G., Lindbird, L. E., and Goodman, G. A. (eds.). *Goodman & Gilman's The Pharmacological Basis of Therapeutics*, 10th edition. New York: McGraw-Hill, 2001.

60. Hepler, R. S., and Frank, I. R. Marihuana smoking and intraocular pressure. JAMA, *217*:1392, 1971.

61. Hoffman, D., Brunnermann, K. D., Gori, G. B., Wynder, G. B. Carcinogenicity of marihuana smoke. In *Recent Advances of Phytochemistry*, Runeckles, V. C. (ed.). New York: Plenum, 1975.

62. Hughes, P. H., and Rieche, O. Heroin epidemics revisited. Epidemiol. Rev., *17*:66–73, 1995.

63. Janiri, L., Mannelli, P., Persico, A. M., Serretti, A., and Tempesta, E. Opiate detoxification of methadone maintenance patients using lefetamine, clonidine and buprenorphine. Drug Alcohol Depend., *36*:139–145, 1994.

64. Johanson, C. E., and Uhlenhuth, E. H. Drug preferences in humans. Fed. Proc., *41*:228–233, 1982.

65. Johns, A. Psychiatric effects of cannabis. Br. J. Psychiat., *178*:116–122, 2001.

66. Johnston, L. D., O'Malley, P. M., and Bachman, J. C. *Monitoring the Future National Survey Results on Drug Use 1975–2001. Vol I: Secondary School Students*, NIH Publ. No. 01-5106. Bethesda, MD: National Institute on Drug Abuse, 2002.

67. Kalant, H. Adverse effects of cannabis on health: an update of the literature since 1996. Prog. Neuropsychopharmacol. Biol. Psychiat., *28*:849–863, 2004.

68. Kessler, R. C., Aguilar-Gaxiola, S., Andrade, L., Bijl, R., Borges, G., Caraveo-Anduaga, J. J., Dewitt, D. J., Kolody, B., Merikangas, K. R., Molnar, B. E., Vega, W. A., Walters, E. D., Wittchen, H.-U., and Ustun, T. B. Mental substance comorbidities in the ICPE surveys. Psychiat. Fenn., *32*:62–79, 2001.

69. Kleber, H. D. Ultrarapid opiate detoxification. Addiction, *93*:1629–1633, 1998.

70. Kleber, H. D., Topazian, J., Gaspari, J., Riordan, C. D., and Kosten, T. Clonidine and naltrexone in the outpatient treatment of heroin withdrawal. Am. J. Drug Alc. Abuse, *13*:1–17, 1987.

71. Kleber, H. D., Weiss, R. D., Anton, R. F., Jr., George, T. P., Greenfield, S. F., Kosten, T. R., O'Brien, C. P., Rounsaville, B. J., Strain, E. C., Ziedonis, D. M., Hennessy, G., Connery, H. S., McIntyre, J. S., Charles, S. C., Anzia, D. J., Cook, I. A., Finnerty, M. T., Johnson, B. R., Nininger, J. E., Summergrad, P., Woods, S. M., Yager, J., Pyles, R., Cross, C. D., Peele, R., Shemo, J. P., Lurie, L., Walker, R. D., Barnovitz, M. A., Gray, S. H., Saxena, S., Tonnu, T., Kunkle, R., Albert, A. B., Fochtmann, L. J., Hart, C., and Regier, D. Treatment of patients with substance use disorders, 2nd edition. American Psychiatric Association. Am. J. Psychiat., *164*:5–123, 2007.

72. Klein, T. W., Friedman, H., and Specter, S. Marijuana, immunity and infection. J. Neuroimmunol., *83*:102–115, 1998.

73. Klonoff, H. Marihuana and driving in real-life situations. Science, *186*:317–324, 1974.

74. Kosten, T. R., Schottenfeld, R., Ziedonis, D., and Falcioni, J. Buprenorphine versus methadone maintenance for opioid dependence. J. Nerv. Ment. Dis., *181*:358–364, 1993.

75. Kutz, I., and Reznik, V. Rapid heroin detoxification using a single high dose of buprenorphine. J. Psychoactive Drugs, *33*:191–193, 2001.

76. Kwiatkowska, M., Parker, L. A., Burton, P., and Mechoulam, R. A comparative analysis of the potential of cannabinoids and ondansetron to suppress cisplatin-induced emesis in the Suncus murinus (house musk shrew). Psychopharmacol. (Berl)., *174*:254–259, 2004.

77. Lancaster, T., Stead, L., Silagy, C., and Sowden, A. Effectiveness of interventions to help people stop smoking: findings from the Cochrane Library. Br. Med. J., *321*:355–358, 2000.

78. Le Foll, B., Melihan-Cheinin, P., Rostoker, G., and Lagrue, G. Smoking cessation guidelines: evidence-based recommendations of the French Health Products Safety Agency. Eur. Psychiat., *20*:431–441, 2005.

79. Leighton, D. C., Harding, J. S., Macklin, D. B., Macmillan, A. M., and Leighton, A. H. *The Character of Danger: Psychiatric Systems in Selected Communities.* New York: Basic Books, 1963.

80. Ling, W., Charuvastra, C., Collins, J. F., Batki, S., Brown, L. S., Jr., Kintaudi, P., Wesson, D. R., McNicholas, L., Tusel, D. J., Malkerneker, U., Renner, J. A., Jr., Santos, E., Casadonte, P., Fye, C., Stine, S., Wang, R. I., and Segal, D. Buprenorphine maintenance treatment of opiate dependence: a multicenter, randomized clinical trial. Addiction, *93*:475–486, 1998.

81. Ling, W., Wesson, D. R., Charuvastra, C., and Klett, C. J. A controlled trial comparing buprenorphine and methadone maintenance in opioid dependence. Arch. Gen. Psychiat., *53*:401–407, 1996.

82. Lingford-Hughes, A. R., Welch, S., and Nutt, D. J. Evidence-based guidelines for the pharmacological management of substance misuse, addiction and comorbidity: recommendations from the British Association for Psychopharmacology. J. Psychopharmacol., *18*:293–335, 2004.

83. Linszen, D., and van Amelsvoort, T. Cannabis and psychosis: an update on course and biological plausible mechanisms. Curr. Opin. Psychiat., *20*:116–120, 2007.

84. Lintzeris, N., Bammer, G., Rushworth, L., Jolley, D. J., and Whelan, G. Buprenorphine dosing regime for inpatient heroin withdrawal: a symptom-triggered dose titration study. Drug Alcohol Depend., *70*:287–294, 2003.

85. Lintzeris, N., Bell, J., Bammer, G., Jolley, D. J., and Rushworth, L. A randomized controlled trial of buprenorphine in the management of short-term ambulatory heroin withdrawal. Addiction, *97*:1395–1404, 2002.

86. Luddens, H., and Wisden, W. Function and pharmacology of multiple GABAA receptor subunits. Trends Pharmacol. Sci., *12*:49–51, 1991.

87. Mathias, D. W. Cocaine-associated myocardial ischemia. Am. J. Med., *81*:675–678, 1986.

88. Matsuda, L. A., Lolait, S. J., Brownstein, M. J., Young, A. C., and Bonner, T. I. Structure of a cannabinoid receptor and functional expression of the cloned cDNA. Nature, 346:561–564, 1990.

89. Mattick, R. P., Ali, R., White, J. M., O'Brien, S., Wolk, S., and Danz, C. Buprenorphine versus methadone maintenance therapy: a randomized double-blind trial with 405 opioid-dependent patients. Addiction, 98:441–452, 2003.

90. McGlothlin, W. H., and Arnold, D. O. LSD revisited. A 10 year follow-up of medical LSD use. Arch. Gen. Psychiat., 24:35–49, 1971.

91. Mechoulam, R., and Hanu, L. The cannabinoids: an overview. Therapeutic implications in vomiting and nausea after cancer chemotherapy, in appetite promotion, in multiple sclerosis and in neuroprotection. Pain Res. Manag., 6:67–73, 2001.

92. Mellman, T. A., and Uhde, T. W. Withdrawal syndrome with gradual tapering of alprazolam. Am. J. Psychiat., 143:1464–1466, 1986.

93. Merck, E. Verfahren zur darstellng von alkyloxyaryl-dialyloxyaryl und alkylene-dioxy-arylaminopropanen bzw deren am stickstoffmonalkylieten derivaten. German Patient # 273, 350. Berlin, Germany, 1914.

94. Meredith, C. W., Jaffe, C., Ang-Lee, K., and Saxon, A. J. Implications of chronic methamphetamine use: a literature review. Harv. Rev. Psychiat., 13:141–154, 2005.

95. Meyer, R. E. Adverse reactions to hallucinogenic drugs. Washington, DC: U.S. GPO, NIMH, 1967.

96. Millman, R. B., and Sbriglio, R. Patterns of use and psychopathology in chronic marijuana users. Psychiat. Clin. N. Am., 9:533–545, 1986.

97. Munro, S., Thomas, K. L., and Abu-Shaar, M. Molecular characterization of a peripheral receptor for cannabinoids. Nature, 365:61–65, 1993.

98. Musto, D. F. *The American Disease: Origins of Narcotic Control*, 3rd edition. New York: Oxford University Press, 1999.

99. Newman, R. G. Frustrations among professionals working in drug treatment programs. Br. J. Addict., 82:115–117, 1987.

100. Newman, R. G. Methadone treatment: defining and evaluating success. N. Engl. J. Med., 317:447–450, 1987.

101. Nigam, A. K., Srivastava, R. P., Saxena, S., Chavan, B. S., and Sundaram, K. R. Naloxone-induced withdrawal in patients with buprenorphine dependence. Addiction, 89:317–320, 1994.

102. Noble, E. P., Blum, K., Khalsa, M. E., Ritchie, T., Montgomery, A., Wood, R. C., Fitch, R. J., Ozkaragoz, T., Sheridan, P. J., Anglin, M. D., Paredes, A., Treiman, L. J., and Sparkes, R. S. Allelic association of the D2 dopamine receptor gene with cocaine dependence. Drug Alcohol Depend, 33:271–285, 1993.

103. O'Connor, P. G., Carroll, K. M., Shi, J. M., Schottenfeld, R. S., Kosten, T. R., and Rounsaville, B. J. Three methods of opioid detoxification in a primary care setting. A randomized trial. Ann. Intern. Med., 127:526–530, 1997.

104. Oliveto, A. H., Feingold, A., Schottenfeld, R., Jatlow, P., and Kosten, T. R. Desipramine in opioid-dependent cocaine abusers maintained on buprenorphine vs methadone. Arch. Gen. Psychiat., 56:812–820, 1999.

105. Palmstierna, T. Effects of a high-dose fast tapering buprenorphine detoxification program on symptom relief and treatment retention. J. Psychoactive Drugs, 36:273–277, 2004.

106. Pani, P. P., Maremmani, I., Pirastu, R., Tagliamonte, A., and Gessa, G. L. Buprenorphine: a controlled clinical trial in the treatment of opioid dependence. Drug Alcohol Depend., 60:39–50, 2000.

107. Paul, S. M., Hulihan-Giblin, B., and Skolnick, P. (+)-Amphetamine binding to rat hypothalamus: relation to anorexic potency of phenylethylamines. Science, 218:487–489, 1982.

108. Petitjean, S., Stohler, R., Deglon, J. J., Livoti, S., Waldvogel, D., Uehlinger, C., and Ladewig, D. Double-blind randomized trial of buprenorphine and methadone in opiate dependence. Drug Alcohol Depend., 62:97 104, 2001.

109. Position statement on psychoactive substance use and dependence: up-date on marijuana and cocaine. Am. J. Psychiat., 144:5, 1987.

110. Rawson, R. A., Anglin, M. D., and Ling, W. Will the methamphetamine problem go away? J. Addict. Dis., 21:5–19, 2002.

111. Regier, D. A., Farmer, M. E., Rae, D. S., Locke, B. Z., Keith, S. J., Judd, L. L., and Goodwin, F. K. Comorbidity of mental-disorders with alcohol and other drug abuse. Results from the Epidemiologic Catchment Area (ECA) study. JAMA, 264:2511–2518, 1990.

112. Rigotti, N. A. Clinical practice. Treatment of tobacco use and dependence. N. Engl. J. Med., 346:506–512, 2002.

113. Robins, L. N. Follow-Up of Vietnam Drug Users. Washington, DC: National Institute of Drug Abuse, Special Action Office, 1973.

114. Rodriguez, D. F., Carrera, M. R., Navarro, M., Koob, G. F., and Weiss, F. Activation of corticotropin-releasing factor in the limbic system during cannabinoid withdrawal. Science, 276:2050–2054, 1997.

115. Roueché, B. Alcohol. New York: Grove Press, 1962.

116. Rubin, V., and Comitas, L. Ganja in Jamaica. The Hague and Paris: Mouton, 1975.

117. Schifano, F. A bitter pill. Overview of ecstasy (MDMA, MDA) related fatalities. Psychopharmacol. (Berl)., 173:242–248, 2004.

118. Schottenfeld, R. S., Pakes, J. R., Oliveto, A., Ziedonis, D., and Kosten, T. R. Buprenorphine vs methadone maintenance treatment for concurrent opioid dependence and cocaine abuse. Arch. Gen. Psychiat., 54:713–720, 1997.

119. Schwartz, R. H. LSD. Its rise, fall, and renewed popularity among high school students. Pediat. Clin. N. Am., 42:403–413, 1995.

120. Secretary of HEW. Marihuana and Health. 8th Annual Report to the U.S. Congress from the Secretary of HEW. Washington, DC: U.S. GPO, 1980.

121. Sertürner, F. W. Trommsdorff's Journal der Pharmazie fur Aerzte, Apotheker und Chemisten, 14:47–93, 1806.

122. Sharma, T. D. Clinical observations of patients who used tetrahydrocannabinol (THC) intravenously. Beh. Neuropsychiat., 4:17–19, 1972.

123. Shulgin, A. T., and Nichols, D. E. Characterization of three new psychomimetics. In *The Pharmacology of Hallucinogens*, Stillman, R., Willette, R. (eds.). New York: Pergamon Press, pp. 74–83, 1978.

124. Siegel, R. K. Cocaine hallucinations. Am. J. Psychiat., 135:309–314, 1978.

125. Smith, D. E., and Wesson, D. R. A new method for treatment of barbiturate dependence. JAMA, 213:294–295, 1970.

126. Snyder, S. H., and Pasternak, G. W. Historical review: opioid receptors. Trends Pharmacol. Sci., 24:198–205, 2003.

127. Solowij, N. *Cannabis and Cognitive Functioning*. New York: Cambridge University Press, 1998.

128. Strain, E. C., Stitzer, M. L., Liebson, I. A., and Bigelow, G. E. Buprenorphine versus methadone in the treatment of opioid-dependent cocaine users. Psychopharmacol. (Berl)., 116:401–406, 1994.

129. Strain, E. C., Stitzer, M. L., Liebson, I. A., and Bigelow, G. E. Comparison of buprenorphine and methadone in the treatment of opioid dependence. Am. J. Psychiat., 151:1025–1030, 1994.

130. Substance Abuse and Mental Health Services Administration. *Preliminary Estimates from the 1995 National Household Survey on Drug Abuse, Advance Report 18*. Rockville, MD: U.S. Department of Health and Human Services, 1996.

131. Substance Abuse and Mental Health Services Administration. *Results from the 2002 National Survey on Drug Use and Health: National Findings*. NHSDA Series H-22, DHHS Publication SMA 03-3836. Rockville, MD: Substance Abuse and Mental Health Services Administration, Office of Applied Studies, 2003.

132. Substance Abuse and Mental Health Services Administration. *Results from the 2001 National Household Survey on Drug Abuse: Volume 1. Summary of National Findings*. Office of Applied Studies, NHSDA Series H-17 ed. (BKD461, SMA 02-3758). Washington, DC: U.S. Government Printing Office, 2008.

133. Tashkin, D. P., Coulson, A. H., Clark, V. A., Simmons, M., Bourque, L. B., Duann, S., Spivey, G. H., and Gong, H. Respiratory symptoms and lung function in habitual heavy smokers of marijuana alone, smokers of marijuana and tobacco, smokers of tobacco alone, and nonsmokers. Am. Rev. Respir. Dis., 135:209–216, 1987.

134. Taylor, D. R., Poulton, R., Moffitt, T. E., Ramankutty, P., and Sears, M. R. The respiratory effects of cannabis dependence in young adults. Addiction, 95:1669–1677, 2000.

135. Treatment of acute drug abuse reactions. Med. Lett. Drug Ther., 29:83–86, 1987.

136. Uehlinger, C., Deglon, J., Livoti, S., Petitjean, S., Waldvogel, D., and Ladewig, D. Comparison of buprenorphine and methadone in the treatment of opioid dependence. Swiss multicentre study. Eur. Addict. Res., 4 Suppl 1:13–18, 1998.

137. Umbricht, A., Montoya, I. D., Hoover, D. R., Demuth, K. L., Chiang, C. T., and Preston, K. L. Naltrexone shortened opioid detoxification with buprenorphine. Drug Alcohol Depend., 56:181–190, 1999.

138. Unwin, N. Structure and action of the nicotinic acetylcholine receptor explored by electron microscopy. FEBS Lett., *555*:91–95, 2003.

139. US Centers for Disease Control and Prevention, *Reducing tobacco use: a report of the Surgeon General*. Atlanta: US Department of Health and Human Services, US Centers for Disease Control and Prevention, National Center for Chronic Disease Prevention and Health Promotion, Office on Smoking and Health, 2000.

140. Vaillant, G. E. A 12-year follow-up of New York narcotic addicts. Arch. Gen. Psychiat., *15*:599–609, 1966.

141. Vignau, J. Preliminary assessment of a 10-day rapid detoxification programme using high dosage buprenorphine. Eur. Addict. Res., *4 Suppl 1*:29–31, 1998.

142. Walker, J. M., and Huang, S. M. Cannabinoid analgesia. Pharmacol. Ther., *95*:127–135, 2002.

143. Warner, L. A., Kessler, R. C., Hughes, M., Anthony, J. C., and Nelson, C. B. Prevalence and correlates of drug use and dependence in the United States. Results from the National Comorbidity Survey. Arch. Gen. Psychiat., *52*:219–229, 1995.

144. Washton, A. M., and Gold, M. S. *Cocaine: A Clinician's Handbook*. New York: Guilford Press, 1987.

145. Weinstein, S. P., Gottheil, E., Smith, R. H., and Migrala, K. A. Cocaine users seen in medical practice. Am. J. Drug Alcohol Abuse, *12*:341–354, 1986.

146. Weller, R. A., and Halikas, J. A. Objective criteria for the diagnosis of marihuana abuse. J. Nerv. Ment. Dis., *168*:98–103, 1980.

147. West, R., McNeill, A., and Raw, M. Smoking cessation guidelines for health professionals: an update. Health Education Authority. Thorax, *55*:987–999, 2000.

148. Whiting, P. GABA. In *Encyclopedia of Molecular Biology*, Creighton, T. E. (ed.). Hoboken, NJ: Wiley Interscience, pp. 1957–1959, 1999.

149. Whiting, P. J. GABA-A receptors: a viable target for novel anxiolytics? Curr. Opin. Pharmacol., *6*:24–29, 2006.

150. World Health Organization. WHO Framework Convention on Tobacco Control. Geneva, Switzerland: WHO Document Production Services, 2005.

151. Zinberg, N. E., and Jacobson, R. C. The natural history of "chipping." Am. J. Psychiat., *133*:37–40, 1976.

152. American Psychiatric Association. *Diagnostic and Statistical Manual of Mental Disorders*, 4th edition, text revision. Washington, DC: Author, 2000.

13

Delirium and Dementia (Acute and Chronic Brain Syndromes)

Delirium, amnestic disorders, and dementia are often referred to as organic brain syndromes, or simply brain syndromes. The clinical diagnosis is based primarily on the mental status examination and usually is applied to patients with recognizable medical and neurological disorders affecting brain structure and/or function. In *DSM-IV-TR*, these conditions are described as "Delirium, Dementia, and Amnestic and Other Cognitive Disorders." The older, very broad term, "brain syndrome," can still be found in the literature, and "acute brain syndrome" and "chronic brain syndrome" are still utilized by many outside psychiatry. They are used in this introduction for historical accuracy and as points of reference. In psychiatry, an acute brain syndrome is known as a delirium, and it is usually brief and presumably reversible. Delirium is associated with excitement and agitation, and it is also frequently associated with hallucinations and delusions. Amnestic disorders are uncommon and are characterized by a disturbance of memory. Chronic brain syndrome, or dementia, is frequently progressive and chances of recovery are often limited.

The diagnosis depends on finding impairment of consciousness/inattention, orientation, memory, and other intellectual or cognitive functions. Additional psychiatric symptoms may occur, including delusions, hallucinations, depression, obsessions, and personality change. Judgment is impaired. Patients may or may not be aware of experiencing the disorder.

Historical Background

It is not known with any certainty when the clinical picture of brain syndrome was first recognized as distinct from other psychiatric disorders. On this subject, extensive interesting material is presented in an annotated anthology of selected medical texts (49).

One of the earliest descriptions in English was provided in 1615 by a clergyman, Thomas Adams, in his treatise *Mystical Bedlam, the World of Mad-Men* (3). He referred to "some mad, that can rightly judge of the things they see, as touching imagination and phantasie: but for cogitation and reason, they swarve from naturale judgment." In 1694 William Salmon (78) described in detail a case of dementia and noted that the patient was "not mad, or distracted like a man in Bedlam [but] decayed in his Intellectuals."

In 1761 Giovanni Battista Morgagni, the great Italian pioneer in morphologic pathology, who first systematically correlated clinical features and course with postmortem findings, described certain areas of "hardness" in the brains of former mental patients (63). He emphasized, however, that the correlation between clinical picture and anatomical findings was not consistent. Morgagni's work set the stage for Antoine Laurant Jesse Bayle who, in 1822, published the first systematic clinicopathologic study of paresis. In this study the clinical symptoms, including progressive dementia, were correlated with changes in brain parenchyma and meninges (9). Bayle's findings were confirmed in 1826 by Louis Florentin Calmeil (21).

Another milestone in the understanding of brain syndrome was Korsakoff's investigation of the disorder that bears his name (90). His observations, reported between 1887 and 1891, correlated to a particular form of dementia manifested by extreme amnesia with lesions of the brain stem.

Years of accumulation of case reports and clinical experience indicated that inattention to surroundings, disorientation, and memory impairment were the hallmarks of a clinical syndrome seen frequently in the presence of intoxications, systemic infections, or demonstrable brain damage. Early systematic investigations were infrequent. However, modern necropsy studies have consistently found that brain syndromes, particularly the chronic forms, are associated with organic brain pathology.

Epidemiology

There have been a number of relatively narrow epidemiologic studies of delirium. It occurs commonly in the presence of pneumonia, systemic infections, AIDS, congestive heart failure, high fever, fluid and electrolyte imbalance, burns, dialysis, transplant, stroke, postoperative state (particularly cardiac and hip), post-injury state, advanced age, and intoxication/withdrawal with alcohol or other drugs. Reports of prevalence in hospitalized general medical patients range from 10% to 30% and in the hospitalized elderly from 10% to 40% (57). Up to 51% of postoperative patients (88) and 80% of terminal patients near death (61) develop delirium. While several new instruments have been developed to aid assessment, concerns about ascertainment, definition of delirium, wide range of estimates, and generalizability abound. One issue endorsed by almost all experts is the concern that prevalence numbers significantly underestimate the problem.

The prevalence of the amnestic syndrome known as Wernicke-Korsakoff syndrome has been estimated through postmortem studies at between 0.8% and 2.8% (12, 44). The upper range estimate is based on an epidemic of cases in Australia in the 1970s and 1980s.

Early epidemiologic studies of dementia had serious flaws related to a number of factors, such as extrapolation from hospitalization rates (59). It is now known that dementia of the Alzheimer type (DAT) and vascular disease of the brain are two of the most common and perhaps best understood of the illnesses manifesting as dementia. Other causes of dementia, including Parkinson disease with dementia, dementia with Lewy bodies, and the fronto-temporal dementias (2, 14, 48) are described, but are much less well understood. The prevalence of DAT and vascular disease increases with age. Recent estimates of the incidence and prevalence of DAT find the illness to be rare in individuals under the age of 50, but approximately 1% of people between the ages of 60 and 64 demonstrate symptoms of the illness. Subsequently, the prevalence of the illness is thought to double every 5 years, and one-third of people over the age of 85 manifest symptoms of DAT (17).

Clinical Picture

Delirium is nearly always associated with medical, surgical, or neurological disorders, or with drug intoxications/withdrawal. This association is so consistent that an unexplained delirium should alert the physician to the likelihood that such a disorder exists or is developing. A patient with pneumonia, for example, will sometimes present with a delirium hours before the other clinical findings appear.

A delirium may vary clinically, but two features are of special diagnostic importance: disorder of consciousness (i.e., reduced awareness of the environment) and change in cognition (i.e., impairment of recent memory and/or orientation). Without at least one of these, the diagnosis can only be suspected.

Patients may complain that they do not understand where they are and that they cannot find the bathroom; or they may bitterly insist that no one has fed them, even though the remains of the last meal are on the tray next to their bed. Other common clinical features include a depressed or fearful mood; apathy; irritability; impaired judgment; suspiciousness; delusions; hallucinations; and combative, uncooperative, or frightened behavior.

Examples of clinical features of delirium are a labile, shifting affect with sudden crying spells; an argumentative, demanding manner ("I've called and called and no one pays any attention to me"); visual hallucinations of frightening or threatening faces ("They're grinning at me all the time, . . .they know something bad will happen"); unreasonable pressure for changes in room, personnel, or food; and inappropriate efforts to get dressed and leave the hospital or to "escape" other patients who "want to hurt me."

The combination of impairment of consciousness/inattention, disorientation, impaired memory, suspiciousness, hallucinations, and combative or frightened behavior constitutes delirium. This is the most dramatic, clinically severe form of delirium. It may develop rapidly without any preceding manifestations or gradually in a patient who has been quietly confused and apathetic for many hours or days. Sometimes it may complicate a chronic state of dementia. The diagnostic criteria for delirium, according to *DSM-IV-TR*, are presented in Table 13.1.

TABLE 13.1 Diagnostic Criteria for Delirium due to . . . [*Indicate the General Medical Condition*]

A. Disturbance of consciousness (i.e., reduced clarity of awareness of the environment) with reduced ability to focus, sustain, or shift attention

B. A change in cognition (such as memory deficit, disorientation, language disturbance) or the development of a perceptual disturbance that is not better accounted for by a preexisting, established, or evolving dementia

C. The disturbance develops over a short period of time (usually hours to days) and tends to fluctuate during the course of the day.

D. There is evidence from the history, physical examination, or laboratory findings that the disturbance is caused by the direct physiological consequences of a general medical condition.

Adapted from diagnostic criteria in the *DSM-IV-TR* (94).

A delirium may fluctuate strikingly from day to day and even from hour to hour. Some patients show a diurnal pattern with the most obvious and severe manifestations at night. They may appear normal in the morning except for haziness about the night before and yet be frankly disoriented, confused, and hallucinating at night. In some cases, the patient's mental status must be checked repeatedly to elicit disorientation or recent memory difficulty.

Disorientation may relate to time, place, or person. The first is the most common, the last the least common. Minor errors by patients who have been sick or hospitalized for some time should not receive undue emphasis. But persistent inability to recall the month or year correctly, especially if the correct answers have been offered recently, recurrent failure to identify where the patient is, or repeated inability to recall recent events correctly, is diagnostic. Because the manifestations are often more definite at night, the first indication of delirium may be recorded in the nurse's notes. A report of the patient mistaking the nurse for someone else—such as a neighbor or relative ("What is my sister doing here?") or experiencing hallucinations—is sometimes ignored until the patient is frankly disoriented and combative.

Delirium seen in a general hospital usually indicates that the patient is seriously ill physically. Available evidence suggests that when the condition interferes with nursing care or treatment or when it disturbs other patients, the prognosis is poorer than is the case for patients with similar medical illnesses matched for age, sex, and race who do not have delirium (23, 35). Wernicke-Korsakoff syndrome (amnestic disorder) is associated with a long history of alcohol use along with the thiamine deficiency that results in a delirium (Wernicke encephalopathy). It can also be caused by malnourishment related to other illnesses, including marasmus, gastric cancer, and HIV (52). Patients presenting with the delirium may clear or they may develop Korsakoff syndrome, a permanent memory impairment. Patients with the memory impairment cannot recall (anterograde) newly learned information (e.g., nurse's name, ward number, etc.) or remember (retrograde) information after the Wernicke encephalopathy began (e.g., how they got to the hospital, who came with them, etc.). Individuals with the severe memory disturbance have significant functional disturbance of everyday living characterized by not being able to meet their basic needs.

Diagnostic criteria for dementia, according to *DSM-IV-TR*, are presented in Table 13.2. Many patients with dementia may present with depressive symptoms (54) or somatic complaints such as headache, abdominal pain, and constipation. Others are brought to physicians by relatives because of temper outbursts, socially embarrassing behavior, or suspiciousness. The cognitive and memory impairment may become evident only as the patient's history is elicited.

TABLE 13.2 Diagnostic Criteria for Dementia due to Other General Medical
             Conditions

A. The development of multiple cognitive deficits manifested by both:

    (1) Memory impairment (impaired ability to learn new information or to recall previously
        learned information)

    (2) One (or more) of the following cognitive disturbances:

        (a) Aphasia (language disturbance)

        (b) Apraxia (impaired ability to carry out motor activities despite intact motor function)

        (c) Agnosia (failure to recognize or identify objects despite intact sensory function)

        (d) Disturbance in executive functioning (i.e., planning, organizing, sequencing,
            abstracting)

B. The cognitive deficits in criteria A1 and A2 each cause significant impairment in social or
   occupational functioning and represent a significant decline from a previous level of
   functioning.

C. There is evidence from the history, physical examination, or laboratory findings that the
   disturbance is the direct physiological consequence of one of the general medical conditions
   listed below:

   Dementia due to HIV disease

   Dementia due to head trauma

   Dementia due to Parkinson's disease

   Dementia due to Huntington's disease

   Dementia due to Creutzfeld-Jacob disease

   Dementia due to other general medical conditions not listed above, for example, normal-
   pressure hydrocephalus, hypothyroidism, brain tumor, or vitamin B-12 deficiency.

D. The deficits do not occur exclusively during the course of a delirium.

Adapted from diagnostic criteria in the *DSM-IV-TR* (94).

Patients with depression may complain of poor memory, and some studies
have revealed impairment of short-term memory in many. The memory difficulty improves with remission of the depression (83). Sometimes, however, it is
important to distinguish between complaints of memory difficulty (pseudodementia) and actual impairment of memory. Some have argued that the term
"pseudodementia" can be misleading because depression may also include
significant cognitive impairment as part of the clinical picture, especially in
older patients.

It has therefore been suggested that a more appropriate name for this
condition might be *cognitive impairment of depression*. In some middle-aged and
older patients suffering from depression, the complaint of memory impairment
is disproportionately greater than the degree of memory impairment noted on
systematic testing, and the perceived memory difficulty subsides as the

depression improves (22, 50, 62, 92). Clearly the relationship between depression and cognitive impairment may sometimes be puzzling. It is important to recognize that some patients with depression, especially older ones, may present with enough cognitive difficulty to raise differential diagnostic problems. In such cases, physicians should be cautious about making a firm diagnosis and be prepared to change their diagnosis as the clinical picture unfolds.

In dementia, the patient's insight may vary greatly. Sometimes, especially earlier in the illness, the patient may volunteer that, "I keep losing things. I don't know where I left them. I occasionally can't remember the directions when I drive home." Often, however, and especially as the illness progresses, the patient may deny any memory difficulty and insist that he was preoccupied or distracted by worries or interruptions. Inability to follow directions and confusion about what others intend may lead to irritability and anger: "Nobody tries to explain things to me. Nobody cares about how I feel—I'll show them." Frustration at being unable to accomplish specific tasks, including specific cognitive tests, frequently leads to suspicion and resistance: "That's a silly thing to do. I could do it if I really wanted to, but I don't see a good reason for it. You're trying to trip me up and fool me." Inattention to cleanliness and grooming, deterioration in table manners, the use of abusive and foul language, social withdrawal and a generally inconsiderate manner, sudden and seemingly unprovoked outbursts of anger, and even physical violence present increasingly heavy burdens to the family as the disorder worsens; they may necessitate institutionalization.

The most important point about dementia is that in some cases the underlying illness is treatable (46). These cases should be recognized as early as possible because recovery may be related to the duration of the dementia. Drug intoxication (10, 69, 81, 87, 89), liver failure (79), hypothyroidism (34, 82), pernicious anemia (84), paresis (40), subdural hematomas, benign brain tumors (5), and normal-pressure hydrocephalus (55, 70) are infrequent but recognizable causes of dementia, though debate continues about the diagnosis and validity of the last entity (4). Recurrent hypoglycemia because of insulin treatment of diabetes, pancreatic islet-cell tumors, or the too-rapid alimentary absorption of glucose in patients who have undergone subtotal gastric resection may also lead to severe dementia (6, 7, 20). All these disorders may be correctable. Chronic alcohol abuse has been associated with a memory impairment (58, 60, 75) that is distinct from the Wernicke-Korsakoff syndrome and, if recognized early, often can be reversed by abstention from further drinking; however, debate continues about the validity of an alcohol-induced dementia separate from Wernicke encephalopathy or hepatic encephalopathy (86). Dementia caused by aluminum intoxication from the water used in such great quantities during chronic renal dialysis is now avoided through modern water purification techniques in use since 1980 (1, 71).

Most cases of dementia are the result of intrinsic brain disease (Table 13.3) or arteriosclerotic changes in the blood vessels supplying the brain (Table 13.4). The term "vascular dementia" (Table 13.4) is preferred over the older term "arteriosclerotic dementia," reflecting the recognition that the dementia results from loss of brain tissue. Other causes of dementia include a variety of previously mentioned presenile brain degenerations (mostly untreatable), central nervous system (CNS) disease (some treatable), systemic disease (mostly treatable), and medications/substances (some correctable) (Table 13.5). Of particular interest is a relatively new "form" of dementia associated with the CNS involving the acquired immune deficiency syndrome (AIDS). Indeed, dementia may be an early or even the first clinical manifestation of human immunodeficiency virus (HIV) infection (41). Finally, dementia may arise from more than one etiology and sometimes from multiple etiologies, making it difficult for clinicians to address the source of the problem (Table 13.6).

TABLE 13.3 Diagnostic Criteria for Dementia of the Alzheimer Type

---

A. The development of multiple cognitive deficits manifested by both:

    (1) Memory impairment (impaired ability to learn new information or to recall previously learned information)
    (2) One (or more) of the following cognitive disturbances:
        (a) Aphasia (language disturbance)
        (b) Apraxia (impaired ability to carry out motor activities despite intact motor function)
        (c) Agnosia (failure to recognize or identify objects despite intact sensory function)
        (d) Disturbance in executive functioning (i.e., planning, organizing, sequencing, abstracting)

B. The cognitive deficits in Criteria A1 and A2 each cause significant impairment in social or occupational functioning and represent a significant decline from a previous level of functioning.
C. The course is characterized by gradual onset and continuing cognitive decline.
D. The cognitive deficits in Criteria A1 and A2 are not due to any of the following:

    (1) Other central nervous system conditions that cause progressive deficits in memory and cognition (e.g., cerebrovascular disease, Parkinson disease, Huntington disease, subdural hematoma, normal-pressure hydrocephalus, brain tumor)
    (2) Systemic conditions that are known to cause dementia (e.g., hypothyroidism, vitamin B12 or folic acid deficiency, niacin deficiency, hypercalcemia, neurosyphilis, HIV infection)
    (3) Substance-induced conditions

E. The deficits do not occur exclusively during the course of a delirium.
F. The disturbance is not better accounted for by another Axis I disorder (e.g., major depressive disorder, schizophrenia).

Adapted from diagnostic criteria in the *DSM-IV-TR* (94).

TABLE 13.4 Diagnostic Criteria for Vascular Dementia

A. The development of multiple cognitive deficits manifested by both:

   (1) Memory impairment (impaired ability to learn new information or to recall previously learned information)

   (2) One (or more) of the following cognitive disturbances:

      (a) Aphasia (language disturbance)

      (b) Apraxia (impaired ability to carry out motor activities despite intact motor function)

      (c) Agnosia (failure to recognize or identify objects despite intact sensory function)

      (d) Disturbance in executive functioning (i.e., planning, organizing, sequencing, abstracting)

B. The cognitive deficits in Criteria A1 and A2 each cause significant impairment in social or occupational functioning and represent a significant decline from a previous level of functioning.

C. Focal neurological signs and symptoms (e.g., exaggeration of deep tendon reflexes, extensor plantar response, pseudobulbar palsy, gait abnormalities, weakness of an extremity) or laboratory evidence indicative of cerebrovascular disease (e.g., multiple infarctions involving cortex and underlying white matter) that are judged to be etiologically related to the disturbance

D. The deficits do not occur exclusively during the course of a delirium

Adapted from diagnostic criteria in the *DSM-IV-TR* (94).

TABLE 13.5 Causes of Dementia

Primary CNS degenerative disorders (not including DAT/vascular dementia)

   1. Frontotemporal dementias (including Pick disease)

   2. Dementia with Lewy bodies

   3. Parkinson disease with dementia

   4. Huntington disease

CNS disease

   1. Brain injury (concussion/damage)

   2. Neoplasms

   3. Vascular disease

   4. Normal pressure hydrocephalus

   5. Viral/bacterial infections

   6. Subdural hematoma

   7. Chronic seizures

Systemic disease

   1. Nutritional deficits (niacin, B-12)

   2. Hepatic disease

   3. Renal disease

   4. Wilson disease

   5. Endocrine (hypothyroidism, hypoparathyroidism)

   6. Multiple sclerosis

   7. Chronic metabolic dysregulation (hypocalcemia, hypoglycemia)

   8. Autoimmune disease

   9. Immune system disease

  10. Cardiovascular disease

Medication(s)/substance(s)

   1. Alcohol dementia

Adapted from diagnostic criteria in the *Diagnostic and Statistical Manual of Mental Disorders*, fourth edition text revision. Washington, DC: American Psychiatric Association, 2000.

TABLE 13.6 Diagnostic Criteria for Dementia due to Multiple Etiologies

A. The development of multiple cognitive deficits manifested by both:

   (1) Memory impairment (impaired ability to learn new information or to recall previously learned information)
   (2) One (or more) of the following cognitive disturbances:
       (a) Aphasia (language disturbance)
       (b) Apraxia (impaired ability to carry out motor activities despite intact motor function)
       (c) Agnosia (failure to recognize or identify objects despite intact sensory function)
       (d) Disturbance in executive functioning (i.e., planning, organizing, sequencing, abstracting)

B. The cognitive deficits in Criteria A1 and A2 each cause significant impairment in social or occupational functioning and represent a significant decline from a previous level of functioning.
C. There is evidence from the history, physical examination, or laboratory findings that the disturbance has more than one etiology (e.g., head trauma plus chronic alcohol use, dementia of the Alzheimer type with the subsequent development of vascular dementia).
D. The deficits do not occur exclusively during the course of a delirium.

Adapted from diagnostic criteria in the *DSM-IV-TR* (94).

Natural History

As noted, delirium may occur in the course of various medical illnesses. Often it is impossible to determine the most crucial factor in a patient with simultaneous heart failure, infection, fever, and dehydration who is also receiving a variety of medications. Generally, the delirium subsides as the underlying abnormalities are corrected. Sometimes, when patients have been very sick and have had a prolonged delirium, many days pass after medical abnormalities are controlled before the mental picture clears. Acute delirium resulting from drug intoxication or drug withdrawal (e.g., alcohol, barbiturates, or benzodiazepines) nearly always subsides within a few days after discontinuing the drug.

Wernicke-Korsakoff syndrome develops after many years of heavy alcohol use and poor nutrition. Patients usually present in a marked delirious state without other classic signs of delirium tremens (autonomic instability and tremulousness). Patients may demonstrate ataxia. As the confusion clears, significant anterograde and retrograde amnesia become prominent. Interestingly, remote memory and intellectual function is spared. The deficit can be permanent (52), although in one series of patients, 20% did resolve (77).

Dementia usually develops insidiously. The early manifestations may be subtle, and only in retrospect does their significance become evident. Fatigability, moodiness, distractibility, depression, irritability, and carelessness may be present long before memory difficulty, intellectual deterioration, and disorientation can be clearly and easily detected. Depending on the underlying brain disease, the dementia may either stabilize for long periods or progress to total incapacity and death (13, 59, 76, 91). Both delirium and dementia appear to be associated with an excess mortality (11).

Biological Findings

Delirium is a perturbation in the function of the brain caused by extrinsic factors. Certain vulnerabilities to this alteration, including age, illness, brain disease, or medication(s), may all play a part in this disorder. Genetic factors are not considered to play an active role.

Wernicke-Korsakoff syndrome is widely accepted to be produced also by an extrinsic factor, namely thiamine deficiency. Because other causes of thiamine deficiency produce the same type of disorder, genetic factors are not considered to actively contribute to the illness. The generally agreed-upon pathological lesions are located bilaterally in the temporal lobes and involve the associated hippocampus and mammillary body (44).

For many years a distinction was made between Alzheimer disease (DAT), a presenile dementia, and senile brain disease or dementia, despite the fact that the anatomical findings (senile plaques, neurofibrillary tangles, and granulo-vacuolar degenerative changes) in the two groups of patients are similar. (See also the section "Family Studies.") In current practice, the two conditions are viewed as identical (76, 91). Recent work indicates that dementia of the Alzheimer type, whether presenile or senile, is associated with a variety of pathological and biochemical changes involving many brain areas and systems (53). Evidence suggests that the neurofibrillary tangles characteristic of Alzheimer disease originate from neurotubules and that plaques arise from amyloid deposits (27, 42, 53). The production, processing, and deposition of amyloid appear to be at the core of this puzzle and are the focus of tremendous interest.

The role of impaired cholinergic function in DAT is unclear, but there is evidence suggesting that age-related memory disturbances in animals and humans may also be associated with cholinergic dysfunction (8, 28, 68, 93). Whether the problem in Alzheimer patients is simply a more rapid progression of age-related changes or whether it involves certain more specific factors is not yet clear.

Vascular dementia is generally thought to result from cerebrovascular disease or trauma. The course is usually associated with the underlying cause and may be rapid, stepwise progressive, or plateau without advance. The association between large strokes and detectable changes in cognition is understandable, but the precise correspondence of slow loss of neurons to progression of formal dementia is less clear.

Computerized tomography (CT), magnetic resonance imaging (MRI), and positron emission testing (PET) may contribute valuable information for the diagnosis of dementia, but it is important to appreciate that the correlation between cognitive impairment and the radiological findings is sometimes poor. It is likely, however, that refinements in all techniques will improve such correlations in the future.

Complications

Faulty judgment in important decisions, inability to care for oneself, accidents, aggression, and suicide are the principal complications of delirium and dementia. One of the more difficult decisions physicians must make concerns patients with delirium/dementia whose behavior raises questions about their mental capacity. At some point in the course of many chronic brain illnesses, the patients' confusion, forgetfulness, temper outbursts, and questionable financial dealings will lead relatives and friends to question whether they are still competent to handle their affairs and care for themselves properly. Losing or giving away large sums of money, writing bad checks, extreme carelessness of dress, unprecedented sexual behavior (e.g., displaying genitals or molesting children), wandering away from home, getting lost, and unpredictable temper displays may require legal action to protect patients from their own acts and permit extended placement in a safe environment. In some cases of delirium it is not possible to tell whether the patient jumped from a window with the intention of committing suicide or fell because of confusion and fear.

Dementia complicated by secondary depression is one of the psychiatric disorders associated with suicide risk, though it accounts for only a small portion of suicides (72). The role of dementia—especially that of Alzheimer disease—as an important risk factor for serious falls has also been recognized (64).

Family Studies

Investigations of the familial prevalence of dementia have primarily focused on the most frequent form of dementia, namely Alzheimer dementia (DAT). Substantial numbers of family (15, 16) and linkage (37, 38) studies over the last 20 years have shown that less than 5% of DAT cases occur with early onset (prior to age 65), follow an autosomal dominate pattern of transmission, and are linked to three chromosomes (1, 14, and 21) (37, 43). Each gene was located by studying multiple generations of families with early DAT and identifying the mutations (Chromosome 1—Presenilin-2, Chromosome 14—Presenilin-1, and Chromosome 21—Amyloid precursor protein) (39, 45, 47, 56, 80), which alter the production of proteins responsible for DAT. Careful elucidation of these mechanisms also led to the finding that late-onset DAT is associated with Apolipoprotein E (APOE) (65) and chromosome 19 (66). Of note, family studies revealed smaller aggregates and no clear Mendelian inheritance. APOE is not a mutation but is considered a susceptibility gene, meaning that it is neither necessary nor sufficient to cause DAT. However, presence of the APOE-4 allele increases the risk of the disorder. Calculations of the risk of DAT in a multitude of studies have revealed that one APOE-4 allele increases chances three-fold to five-fold and two APOE-4 alleles renders an eight-fold risk (24, 67). While APOE is the most significant known genetic risk, it does not explain all the genetic risk (67). Much work remains to fully understand the genetic (and environmental) contribution(s) to this disorder.

Differential Diagnosis

Other psychiatric conditions may be mimicked by delirium/dementia: patients' anxiety attacks may suggest a primary anxiety disorder; low mood and apathy, an affective disorder; hallucinations and delusions, schizophrenia. The crucial question in each case is whether the patient exhibits definite inattention, disorientation, or memory impairment. These mental status abnormalities, when clearly present, are pathognomonic of a brain syndrome; they are not manifestations of an uncomplicated, so-called functional disorder. If a patient with another psychiatric illness develops inattention, disorientation, or memory impairment, one should suspect that something else has developed: a drug reaction or medical or neurologic illness.

When a patient is unable or unwilling to cooperate in the mental status examination, a delirium may be suspected. If there has been a sudden change in behavior, speech, or manner, and if the behavioral change develops in a clinical situation that frequently predisposes to a delirium, the diagnosis should be considered. A definitive diagnosis must await evidence of inattention, disorientation, or memory impairment; these will usually become apparent as the patient is observed carefully.

Clinical Management

Correction of the underlying medical or neurological condition, whenever possible, is the principal aim of therapy for patients with delirium/dementia. At the same time, certain measures often help in the management of the brain syndrome itself. Good nursing care is very important. A calm, sympathetic, reassuring approach can turn a frightened, combative patient into a quiet, cooperative one. A patient with a delirium often misinterprets stimuli and has unpredictable emotional responses. It is important, therefore, to provide a familiar, stable, unambiguous environment for such patients. Repeated simple explanations and frequent reassurance from familiar nurses, attendants, or relatives may be helpful. Patients do better with constant light; shadows or the dark easily frightens them.

Only the smallest effective doses of drugs acting on the CNS should be used because patients with delirium are frequently sensitive to these agents. Delirium is, in fact, often precipitated by sedatives or hypnotics and may subside when such drugs are discontinued. No CNS active medicine is entirely safe. Careful attention to dosage and mental status is most important.

Some patients need to be kept from harming themselves. Usually a relative, friend, or nurse who is able to be with the patient constantly—talking to him, explaining things, reassuring him—can calm him enough to permit appropriate care without restraints on a general hospital service. When this does not work or is not possible, rather than risk having a confused and frightened patient fall out of bed or jump out a window, physical restraint or transfer to the psychiatric service may be necessary.

If a psychiatric unit is not available or if the patient's medical condition and treatment require bed rest, a body restraint may be necessary. Obviously, a restrained patient should be watched carefully, and the previously described measures should be continued with the hope of calming him quickly, making any period of restraint brief.

The specific treatment for Wernicke-Korsakoff is initially parental thiamine followed by oral. Abstinence from further use of alcohol and good nutrition are the goals (52). A significant number of these individuals require careful monitoring in the home or institution.

Organized groups (e.g., Alzheimer's Association and others) for relatives of patients with dementia patients can be very helpful in providing emotional support and practical suggestions for handling the wide range of problems that dementia presents to families (36). Too often the impact on family members is overwhelming, and this must be considered by the physician so that appropriate steps can be taken to reduce the burden, at least intermittently (31–33).

It should be noted that a number of new medications are being developed to treat Alzheimer dementia (27). Potent, centrally active, reversible acetylcholinesterase inhibitors—tacrine, donepezil, rivastigmine, and galantamine—have been reported to have efficacy in clinical trials (18, 19, 29, 51, 74) and are standard therapy (30), but are not without risks. All have been associated with improvements in global functioning and cognition (25, 73, 85). The result of these improvements has been a reduction in impaired behavior, stabilization (albeit temporary) of daily living activities, delay of placement in the nursing home setting, and decreased caregiver burden (26).

REFERENCES

1. Dialysis dementia in Europe. Report from the Registration Committee of the European Dialysis and Transplant Association. Lancet, 2:190–192, 1980.
2. Cummings, J. L. (ed.). *The Neuropsychiatry of Alzheimer's Disease and Related Dementias.* London: Martin Duntiz, 2003.
3. Adams, T. *Mystical Bedlam, the World of Mad-Men.* London: George Purslowe for Clement Knight, 1615.
4. Anderson, M. Normal pressure hydrocephalus. Br. Med. J., *293*:837–838, 1986.
5. Avery, T. L. Seven cases of frontal tumour with psychiatric presentation. Br. J. Psychiat., *119*:19–23, 1971.
6. Bale, R. N. Brain damage in diabetes mellitus. Br. J. Psychiat., *122*:337–341, 1973.
7. Banerji, N. K., and Hurwitz, L. J. Nervous system manifestations after gastric surgery. Acta Neurol. Scand., *47*:485–513, 1971.
8. Bartus, R. T., Dean III, R. L., Beer, B., and Lippa, A. S. The cholinergic hypothesis of geriatric memory dysfunction. Science, *217*:408–414, 1982.
9. Bayle, A. L. J. *Reserches sur l'arachnitis chronique.* Paris: Gabon, 1822.
10. Bergman, H., Borg, S., and Holm, L. Neuropsychological impairment and exclusive abuse of sedatives or hypnotics. Am. J. Psychiat., *137*:215–217, 1980.
11. Black, D. W., Warrack, G., and Winokur, G. The Iowa record-linkage study. I. Excess mortality among patients with organic mental disorders. Arch. Gen. Psychiat., *42*:78–81, 1985.
12. Blansjaar, B. A., Horjus, M. C., and Nijhuis, H. G. Prevalence of the Korsakoff syndrome in The Hague, The Netherlands. Acta Psychiat. Scand., *75*:604–607, 1987.
13. Blessed, G., and Wilson, I. D. The contemporary natural history of mental disorder in old age. Br. J. Psychiat., *141*:59–67, 1982.
14. Bolla, L. R., Filley, C. M., and Palmer, R. M. Dementia DDx. Office diagnosis of the four major types of dementia. Geriatrics, *55*:34–46, 2000.
15. Breitner, J. C., Folstein, M. F., and Murphy, E. A. Familial aggregation in Alzheimer dementia—I. A model for the age-dependent expression of an autosomal dominant gene. J. Psychiat. Res., *20*:31–43, 1986.
16. Breitner, J. C., Murphy, E. A., and Folstein, M. F. Familial aggregation in Alzheimer dementia—II. Clinical genetic implications of age-dependent onset. J. Psychiat. Res., *20*:45–55, 1986.

17. Brookmeyer, R., Gray, S., and Kawas, C. Projections of Alzheimer's disease in the United States and the public health impact of delaying disease onset. Am. J. Publ. Health, 88:1337–1342, 1998.

18. Bullock, R. New drugs for Alzheimer's disease and other dementias. Br. J. Psychiat., 180:135–139, 2002.

19. Bullock, R. Galantamine: use in Alzheimer's disease and related disorders. Expert Rev. Neurother., 4:153–163, 2004.

20. Burton, R. A., and Raskin, N. H. Alimentary (post gastrectomy) hypoglycemia. Arch. Neurol., 23:14–17, 1970.

21. Calmiel, L. F. De la paralysie considérée chez les aliénés, Paris: 1826.

22. Cavenar, J. O., Maltbie, A. A., and Austin, L. Depression simulating organic brain disease. Am. J. Psychiat., 136:521–523, 1979.

23. Cole, M. G., and Primeau, F. J. Prognosis of delirium in elderly hospital patients. Can. Med. Ass. J., 141:41–46, 1991.

24. Corder, E. H., Saunders, A. M., Strittmatter, W. J., Schmechel, D. E., Gaskell, P. C., Small, G. W., Roses, A. D., Haines, J. L., and Pericak-Vance, M. A. Gene dose of apolipoprotein E type 4 allele and the risk of Alzheimer's disease in late onset families. Science, 261:921–923, 1993.

25. Corey-Bloom, J., Anand, R., and Veach, J. A randomized trial evaluating the efficacy and safety of ENA 713 (rivastigmine tartrate), a new acetylcholinesterase inhibitor, in patients with mild to moderately severe Alzheimer's disease. Int. J. Geriat. Psychopharm., 1:55–65, 1998.

26. Cummings, J. L. Cholinesterase inhibitors: A new class of psychotropic compounds. Am. J. Psychiat., 157:4–15, 2000.

27. Dahl, D., Selkoe, D. J., Pero, R. T., and Bignami, A. Immunostaining of neurofibrillary tangles in Alzheimer's senile dementia with a neurofilament antiserum. J. Neurosci., 2:113–119, 1982.

28. Davis, K. L., Mohs, R. C., and Tinklenberg, J. R. Enhancement of memory by physostigmine (letter to the editor). N. Engl. J. Med., 301:946, 1979.

29. Davis, K. L., Thal, L. J., Gamzu, E. R., Davis, C. S., Woolson, R., Gracon, S. I., Drachman, D. A., Schneider, L. S., Whitehouse, P. J., Hoover, T. M., and et al. A double-blind, placebo-controlled multicenter study of tacrine for Alzheimer's disease. The Tacrine Collaborative Study Group. N. Engl. J. Med., 327:1253–1259, 1992.

30. Doody, R. S., Stevens, J. C., Beck, C., Dubinsky, R. M., Kaye, J. A., Gwyther, L., Mohs, R. C., Thal, L. J., Whitehouse, P. J., DeKosky, S. T., and Cummings, J. L. Practice parameter: management of dementia (an evidence-based review). Report of the Quality Standards Subcommittee of the American Academy of Neurology. Neurology, 56:1154–1166, 2001.

31. Eagles, J. M., Beattie, J. A., Blackwood, G. W., Restall, D. B., and Ashcroft, G. W. The mental health of elderly couples: I. The effects of a cognitively impaired spouse. Br. J. Psychiat., 150:299–303, 1987.

32. Eagles, J. M., Craig, A., Rawlinson, F., Restall, D. B., Beattie, J. A., and Besson, J. A. The psychological well-being of supporters of the demented elderly. Br. J. Psychiat., 150:293–298, 1987.

33. Eagles, J. M., Walker, L. G., Blackwood, G. W., Beattie, J. A., and Restall, D. B. The mental health of elderly couples: II. Concordance for psychiatric morbidity in spouses. Br. J. Psychiat., 150:303–308, 1987.

34. Easson, W. Myxedema with psychosis. Arch. Gen. Psychiat., 14:277–283, 1966.

35. Francis, J., Martin, D., and Kapoor, W. N. A prospective study of delirium in hospitalized elderly. JAMA, 263:1097–1101, 1990.

36. Fuller, J., Ward, E., Evans, A., Massam, K., and Gardner, A. Dementia: supportive groups for relatives. Br. Med. J., 1:1684–1685, 1979.

37. George-Hyslop, P. H. Molecular genetics of Alzheimer's disease. Biol. Psychiat., 47:183–199, 2000.

38. George-Hyslop, P. H., Myers, R. H., Haines, J. L., Farrer, L. A., Tanzi, R. E., Abe, K., James, M. F., Conneally, P. M., Polinsky, R. J., and Gusella, J. F. Familial Alzheimer's disease: progress and problems. Neurobiol. Aging, 10:417–425, 1989.

39. George-Hyslop, P. H., Tanzi, R. E., Polinsky, R. J., Haines, J. L., Nee, L., Watkins, P. C., Myers, R. H., Feldman, R. G., Pollen, D., and Drachman, D. The genetic defect causing familial Alzheimer's disease maps on chromosome 21. Science, 235:885–890, 1987.

40. Gjestland, T. The Oslo study of untreated syphilis; an epidemiologic investigation of the natural course of the syphilitic infection based upon a re-study of the Boeck-Bruusgaard material. Acta Derm. Venereol., 35:3–368, 1955.

41. Grant, I., and Martin, A. Neuropsychology of HIV Infection. New York: Oxford University Press, 1994.

42. Grundke-Iqbal, I., Johnson, A. B., Wisniewski, H. M., Terry, R. D., and Iqbal, K. Evidence that Alzheimer neurofibrillary tangles originate from neurotubules. Lancet, 1:578–580, 1979.

43. Hardy, J. Amyloid, the presenilins and Alzheimer's disease. Trends Neurosci., 20:154–159, 1997.

44. Harper, C., Rodriguez, M., Gold, J., and Perdices, M. The Wernicke-Korsakoff syndrome in Sydney—a prospective necropsy study. Med. J. Aust., 149:718, 720, 1988.

45. Harrison, P. Alzheimer's disease and chromosome 14. Different gene, same process? Br. J. Psychiat., 163:2–5, 1993.

46. Hendrie, H. C., Unverzagt, F. W., and Austrom, M. G. The dementing disorders. Psychiat. Q., 68:261–279, 1997.

47. Heston, L. L., Orr, H. T., Rich, S. S., and White, J. A. Linkage of an Alzheimer disease susceptibility locus to markers on human chromosome 21. Am. J. Med. Genet., 40:449–453, 1991.

48. Holmes, C., Cairns, N., Lantos, P., and Mann, A. Validity of current clinical criteria for Alzheimer's disease, vascular dementia and dementia with Lewy bodies. Br. J. Psychiat., 174:45–50, 1999.

49. Hunter, R., and Macalpine, I. Three Hundred Years of Psychiatry. 1535–1860, London: Oxford University Press, 1963.

50. Kahn, R. L., Zarit, S. H., Hilbert, N. M., and Niederehe, G. Memory complaint and impairment in the aged. The effect of depression and altered brain function. Arch. Gen. Psychiat., 32:1569–1573, 1975.

51. Knapp, M. J., Knopman, D. S., Solomon, P. R., Pendlebury, W. W., Davis, C. S., and Gracon, S. I. A 30-week randomized controlled trial of high-dose tacrine in patients with Alzheimer's disease. JAMA, 271:985–991, 1994.

52. Kopelman, M. D. The Korsakoff syndrome. Br. J. Psychiat., 166:154–173, 1995.

53. Kosik, K. S. Alzheimer's disease: a cell biological perspective. Science, 256:780–783, 1992.

54. Lazarus, L. W., Newton, H., Cohler, B., Lesser, J., and Schweon, C. Frequency and presentation of depressive symptoms in patients with primary degenerative dementia. Am. J. Psychiat., 144:41–45, 1987.

55. Leading article. Communicating hydrocephalus. Lancet, 2:1011–1012, 1977.

56. Levy-Lahad, E., Wasco, W., Poorkaj, P., Romano, D. M., Oshima, J., Pettingell, W. H., Yu, C. E., Jondro, P. D., Schmidt, S. D., Wang, K., Crowley, A.C., Fu, Y.-H., Guenette, S. Y., Galas, D., Nemens, E., Wijsman, E.W., Bird, T. D., Schellenberg, G. D., and Tanzi, R. E. Candidate gene for the chromosome 1 familial Alzheimer's disease locus. Science, 269:973–977, 1995.

57. Lipowski, Z. J. Delirium (acute confusional states). JAMA, 258:1789–1792, 1987.

58. Lishman, W. A. Cerebral disorder in alcoholism. Syndromes of impairment. Brain, 104:1–20, 1981.

59. Liston, E. H. The clinical phenomenology of presenile dementia. A critical review of the literature. J. Nerv. Ment. Dis., 167:329–336, 1979.

60. Martin, P. R., McCool, B. A., and Singleton, C. K. Genetic sensitivity to thiamine deficiency and development of alcoholic organic brain disease. Alcohol. Clin. Exp. Res., 17:31–37, 1993.

61. Massie, M. J., Holland, J., and Glass, E. Delirium in terminally ill cancer patients. Am. J. Psychiat., 140:1048–1050, 1983.

62. McAllister, R. W., and Price, T. R. Severe depressive pseudodementia with and without dementia. Am. J. Psychiat., 139:626–629, 1982.

63. Morgagni, G. B. *The Seats and Causes of Diseases Investigated by Anatomy*, Alexander, B., trans. edition. London: Millar et al., 1769.

64. Morris, J. C., Rubin, E. H., Morris, E. J., and Mandel, S. A. Senile dementia of the Alzheimer's type: an important risk factor for serious falls. J. Gerontol., 42:412–417, 1987.

65. Myers, R. H., Schaefer, E. J., Wilson, P. W., D'Agostino, R., Ordovas, J. M., Espino, A., Au, R., White, R. F., Knoefel, J. E., Cobb, J. L., McNulty, K. A., Beiser, A., and Wolf, P. A. Apolipoprotein E epsilon4 association with dementia in a population-based study: the Framingham study. Neurology, 46:673–677, 1996.

66. Pericak-Vance, M. A., Bebout, J. L., Gaskell, P. C., Jr., Yamaoka, L. H., Hung, W. Y., Alberts, M. J., Walker, A. P., Bartlett, R. J., Haynes, C. A., Welsh, K. A., Heyman, E.A., Clark, C. M., Roses, A. D. Linkage studies in familial Alzheimer disease: evidence for chromosome 19 linkage. Am. J. Hum. Genet., 48:1034–1050, 1991.

67. Plassman, B. L., and Breitner, J. C. The genetics of dementia in late life. Psychiat. Clin. N. Am., 20:59–76, 1997.

68. Potamianos, G., and Kellett, J. M. Anti-cholinergic drugs and memory: the effects of benzhexol on memory in a group of geriatric patients. Br. J. Psychiat., 140:470–472, 1982.

69. Preskorn, S. H., and Simpson, S. Tricyclic-antidepressant-induced delirium and plasma drug concentration. Am. J. Psychiat., *139*:822–823, 1982.

70. Rice, E., and Gendelman, S. Psychiatric aspects of normal pressure hydrocephalus. JAMA, *223*:409–412, 1973.

71. Rob, P. M., Niederstadt, C., and Reusche, E. Dementia in patients undergoing long-term dialysis: aetiology, differential diagnoses, epidemiology and management. CNS Drugs, *15*:691–699, 2001.

72. Robins, E., Murphy, G. E., Wilkinson, R. H., Jr., Gassner, S., and Kayes, J. Some clinical considerations in the prevention of suicide based on a study of 134 successful suicides. Am. J. Publ. Health, *49*:888–899, 1959.

73. Rogers, S. L., Farlow, M. R., Doody, R. S., Mohs, R., and Friedhoff, L. T. A 24-week, double-blind, placebo-controlled trial of donepezil in patients with Alzheimer's disease. Donepezil Study Group. Neurology, *50*:136–145, 1998.

74. Rogers, S. L., Friedhoff, L. T., and the Donepezil Study Group. The efficacy and safety of donepezil in patients with Alzheimer's disease: results of a US multicentre, randomized, double-blind, placebo-controlled trial. Dementia, *7*:293–303, 1996.

75. Ron, M. A. Brain damage in chronic alcoholism: a neuropathological, neuroradiological and psychological review. Psychol. Med., *7*:103–112, 1977.

76. Ron, M. A., Toone, B. K., Garralda, M. E., and Lishman, W. A. Diagnostic accuracy in presenile dementia. Br. J. Psychiat., *134*:161–168, 1979.

77. Ropper, A. H., and Brown, R. H. *Adams and Victor's Principles of Neurology*, 8th edition. New York: McGraw-Hill, 2005.

78. Salmon, W. *Iatrica: Sen Praxis Medendi. The Practice of Curing Disease*, 3rd edition. London: Rolls, 1964.

79. Schafer, D. F., and Jones, E. A. Hepatic encephalopathy and the gamma aminobutyric-acid neurotransmitter system. Lancet, *1*:18–20, 1982.

80. Schellenberg, G. D., Bird, T. D., Wijsman, E. M., Orr, H. T., Anderson, L., Nemens, E., White, J. A., Bonnycastle, L., Weber, J. L., Alonso, M. E., Potter, H., Heston, L. L., and Martin, G. M. Genetic linkage evidence for a familial Alzheimer's disease locus on chromosome 14. Science, *258*:668–671, 1992.

81. Schentag, J. J., Cerra, F. B., Calleri, G., DeGlopper, E., Rose, J. Q., and Bernhard, H. Pharmacokinetic and clinical studies in patients with cimetidine-associated mental confusion. Lancet, *1*:177–181, 1979.

82. Smith, C. K., Barish, J., Correa, J., and Williams, R. H. Psychiatric disturbance in endocrinologic disease. Psychosomat. Med., *34*:69–86, 1972.

83. Sternberg, D. E., and Jarvik, M. E. Memory functions in depression. Arch. Gen. Psychiat., *33*:219–224, 1976.

84. Strachan, R., and Henderson, J. Psychiatric syndromes due to avitaminosis B12 with normal blood and marrow. Q. J. Med., *34*:303–317, 1965.

85. Tariot, P. N., Solomon, P. R., Morris, J. C., Kershaw, P., Lilienfeld, S., and Ding, C. A 5-month, randomized, placebo-controlled trial of galantamine in AD. The Galantamine USA-10 Study Group. Neurology, *54*:2269–2276, 2000.

86. Thomas, P. K. Brain atrophy and alcoholism. Br. Med. J., 292:787, 1986.

87. Trimble, M. R., and Reynolds, E. H. Anticonvulsant drugs and mental symptoms: a review. Psychol. Med., 6:169–178, 1976.

88. Tune, L. E. Postoperative delirium. Int. Psychogeriatr., 3:325–332, 1991.

89. Tune, L. E., Damlouji, H. F., Holland, A., Gardner, T. J., Folstein, M. F., and Coyle, J. T. Association of postoperative delirium with raised serum levels of anticholinergic drugs. Lancet, 2:651–653, 1981.

90. Victor, M., Adams, R. D., and Collins, G. H. *The Wernicke-Korsakoff Syndrome.* Philadelphia: F.A. Davis, 1971.

91. Wells, C. E. Chronic brain disease: an overview. Am. J. Psychiat., 135:1–12, 1978.

92. Wells, C. E. Pseudodementia. Am. J. Psychiat., 136:895–900, 1979.

93. Whitehouse, P. J. The cholinergic deficit in Alzheimer's disease. J. Clin. Psychiat., 59 *Suppl* 13:19–22, 1998.

94. American Psychiatric Association. *Diagnostic and Statistical Manual of Mental Disorders*, 4th edition, text revision. Washington, DC: Author, 2000.

14

The Psychiatric Evaluation

Such is man that if he has the name for something, it ceases
to be a riddle.

—Isaac Bashevis Singer

The purpose of a psychiatric evaluation is to examine psychological function and to diagnose a psychiatric disorder(s) if present. To elicit enough information about the disorder(s) to make a diagnosis, one must know the signs, symptoms, course, and complications. This is the primary reason this chapter concludes the book.

Eliciting clinical information is an art. It can be only partially learned in a formal manner. Establishing rapport and trust between the doctor and patient facilitates accurate history gathering, communicates empathy, and allows logical arrival at reasoned conclusions regarding clinical status and diagnosis(es). This ability is essential, and it cannot be learned from textbooks. Below we offer advice on interviewing, provide a logical framework for organizing observations, and suggest how case histories should be presented. We begin with just a few words about terminology and time.

The *mental status* examination is the part of the physical examination that deals with the patient's thoughts, feelings, and behavior at a particular point in time. This term is often used as a synonym for a *psychiatric examination*, but *mental status* refers to one part of the psychiatric examination: the current thoughts, feelings, and behavior of the patient. *Psychiatric evaluation* includes the past history (medical, social, family, records, collateral information) of the patient as well. The distinction between the two terms is somewhat artificial. Similar to *liver status* or *cardiac status*, what exists now is inseparable from what came before; a certain amount of historical background is unavoidable in describing the current mental status of a patient. Nonetheless, the term "mental status" is used when the *primary* focus of the questioning is on current functioning.

Internists, family practitioners, and other nonpsychiatrists generally have little time to conduct a physical examination: often no more than 15 or 20 minutes. If the examination is "complete," it will include some attention to the mental status of the patient. This may be limited to a few minutes. While managed care may put extra time pressure on the clinician, the expenditure of at least a few moments will broaden the perspective about the patient (whether the answers are positive or negative) and may save substantial time during the course of treatment. For example, learning that an obviously depressed individual also has a history of one or more manic episodes will not only change the diagnosis from major depression to bipolar affective disorder but also the treatment that may have otherwise switched the patient from a depressive episode into a manic phase.

Later we will provide some screening questions that will help nonpsychiatrists quickly ascertain whether the mental state of the patient is abnormal. For now, we will assume the mental status examination is being conducted by a psychiatrist, a student, or a resident in psychiatry who has the luxury of being able to spend a fair amount of time with the patient, observing him or her and asking questions.

Advice on Interviewing

Following are four rules for conducting a psychiatric evaluation:

1. *Start open ended.* After exchanging friendly greetings with the patient and attempting to set a relaxed tone, the interviewer should ask an open-ended question such as, "What is the problem that brings you here?" "What can I do for you?" Unless the patient is uncooperative or incapable of free expression (perhaps because of physical disability), let the patient tell his or her story with little or no interruption during the first 5 to 15 minutes.

   The patient is often anxious early in the interview and this tension may indeed stimulate the information flow. A patient with a *formal thought disorder* (where the thoughts do not connect coherently) will reveal this quickly. Much of the information needed for the diagnosis is often provided in the first few minutes if the patient proceeds without interruption. Early steering of the interview through certain question lines may result in missing important material.

On the other hand, for a particularly tense patient, more structure at the beginning of the interview may lead to easier communication. The interviewer can ask specific questions that are emotionally neutral. Questions about the patient's background, including where the patient grew up and attended school, marital status, employment history, and other physicians seen, can provide a comfortable transition into asking about a presenting problem.

2. *Ask specific questions later.* One purpose of the mental status examination is to make a diagnosis, if possible. This requires specific questions if merely to rule out remote possibilities. For example, patients often avoid volunteering information about hallucinations. "Do you hear voices or see things that others do not hear or see?" or some variation on this query is often necessary to determine whether the patient is psychotic. "Do you feel in danger?" may elicit persecutory delusions. "Do you have a special mission in life?" may bring out grandiose delusions. "What are your plans after leaving the hospital?" may bring out unrealistic thinking, raising questions about judgment.

Even with the advantage of a long interview, the psychiatric examiner must ask specific questions bearing on a reasonable differential diagnosis. There is usually no point, for example, in going through a complete review of systems if the patient experiences excellent health and presents with symptoms of a psychiatric condition in which physical symptoms do not usually play a role.

Details about positive early life experiences rarely bear on the problem of making a differential diagnosis in adults. School and social history are often important, but not always, particularly in dealing with elderly people.

3. *Establish the chronology of the illness.* Kraepelin (3) noted that the course of a psychiatric illness is as important as the symptoms. Sydenham (5) said that "true" illnesses should have common symptoms and a common course. Few, if any, pathognomonic symptoms exist in psychiatry. We agree with Kraepelin that establishing the course of an illness is as important as recognizing current symptoms.

When did the symptoms begin? Was the patient ever free of psychiatric symptoms? When? Age of onset is an important clue to diagnosis as many conditions typically begin at particular times in life.

Has the illness been continual, always present with fluctuations, or episodic in the sense that symptoms sometimes go away entirely? How rapid was the onset? (Psychotic illnesses with abrupt onsets generally have a better prognosis than those with a gradual onset.) Have professional interventions (medications, psychotherapy) altered the course of illness? In general, has the patient tended to improve or get worse?

"Diagnosis is prognosis" is an old saying in medicine, and knowledge of the course of illness as well as the symptoms forms the basis for determining prognosis.

4. *Be friendly, sympathetic, respectful.* Establish good eye contact and listen attentively. Encourage the patient to tell his or her history through noninterfering encouragement (e.g., smiling, nodding, reflecting the patient's expressed feelings). Adult patients should be called "Mr." or "Mrs." or "Ms.," at least until the clinician knows them well. Clinicians should never insult patients. They should never make fun of them. This may seem obvious, but there are subtle ways of betraying disrespect.

Be sensitive to the emotional state of the patient. If certain questioning makes the patient angry, anxious, depressed, or tearful, this may offer an opportunity to enhance the patient's ability to communicate, though sometimes a return to more neutral ground is indicated so that the patient is not overwhelmed by emotion.

A word about the uncooperative patient: to say, "I can't help you unless you help me" sometime works, but usually it does not. Asking specific questions such as "What led to your coming here?" or "Whose idea was it that you come here?" may help lower resistance. Sometimes the interview must be postponed until another time when the patient may be more helpful. Anger toward the uncooperative patient is never appropriate.

Psychiatry, probably more than any other specialty, benefits greatly from informants—friends and family who will tell what the patient will not (or cannot). Although caution should be exercised in judging the merit of such information, it can be very helpful in making a diagnosis. One should also remember to obtain permission from the patient before seeking outside or collateral information.

The Decision Tree

Except for open-ended questions at the beginning and specific questions toward the end, history taking should flow easily and casually, as in a conversation.

Initially, patients should be permitted to talk about what they want to talk about, but eventually they should be gently guided back into channels that provide information the examiner requires for a diagnosis. From the moment a patient walks into the examination room, however, the examiner's mental "computer" starts making relevant observations. How is the patient dressed and groomed? Does the patient have a normal gait and range of motion? Is the patient hostile or friendly? How old does the patient appear to be?

Based on early impressions, the interviewer starts constructing the differential diagnosis. Over the course of the interview, the examiner's choices about *probable* diagnoses will determine which areas to emphasize and which to skip over lightly or omit entirely. The examiner's mind, indeed, functions as a computer. By the end of the interview—if it is successful—the choices will have narrowed to one or a few.

Table 14.1 shows a highly simplified branching process for approaching the diagnosis of psychiatric disorders. The first important decision concerns psychosis. Is the patient psychotic or nonpsychotic? Psychosis can be both broadly and narrowly defined. Broadly defined, it refers to the gravity or seriousness of the condition; a suicidal patient might be called psychotic because suicide is serious. Narrowly defined, as here, psychosis means the presence of persistent hallucinations and/or delusions and/or disordered thoughts.

As shown in Table 14.1, the diagnostic possibilities for a nonpsychotic person would include the anxiety disorders (there are twelve in *DSM-IV-TR*) (1), mood disorder, chemical dependence, antisocial personality, other personality disorder, eating disorders, and somatization disorder. Thus, in some conditions such as mood disorders and drug dependence, the patient may or may not be psychotic.

A psychotic individual may suffer from schizophrenia, a mood disorder, or drug intoxication. Hallucinogens, amphetamines, and phencyclidine (PCP) are

TABLE 14.1 Major Branches in Diagnosis Making

Nonpsychotic	Psychotic		Impaired Memory	
Anxiety disorders	Schizophrenia	Acute	Chronic	
Panic	Acute	(Delirium)		
Obsessional	Chronic			
Phobic	Affective disorders		Dementia	Retardation
Somatization disorder	Depression			
Antisocial personality	Mania			
Other personality disorder	Both			
Chemical dependence	Chemical			
Affective disorders	dependence			

commonly associated with psychosis. Please see earlier chapters for fuller discussion of the various diagnoses and their many presentations.

The second early decision concerns memory. If the memory is abnormal, one moves toward the right of the center line in Table 14.1. Memory problems can usually be sorted into acute or chronic conditions. The nomenclature and presentations were reviewed in detail in Chapter 13. Several issues warrant review. First, poor intellectual functioning is associated with, and often indistinguishable from, bad memory. Impaired memory *produces* impaired intellectual functioning. Intelligence encompasses more than memory, but even those skills not normally associated with memory (e.g., reasoning ability) often suffer when memory is impaired. Second, patients with major depression sometimes have difficulty with memory, and this is called "pseudodementia." Their memory improves as their depression improves. Finally, patients with gross memory impairment (as distinguished from absentmindedness, normal forgetting, or "not paying attention") may display any psychiatric symptom associated with disorders on the left side of Table 14.1. While symptoms of disorders on the left side of Tables 14.1 may temporally correspond to or antedate onset of memory impairment, identification of a new organic impairment is *of paramount importance*. Diagnosis of a new onset of an organic disorder is one of the most important things a psychiatrist can do because it initiates a search for the *cause* of the disorder that may be *treatable*. Physicians are uniquely qualified among mental health professionals to identify the organic disease. Trained in anatomy, physiology, and biochemistry, and aided by modern imaging and laboratory techniques, physicians can evaluate the entire range of sources of organic disorders, including brain tumors, endocrine disorders, metabolic illness, and infections.

In most hospitals, about one-fifth of the patients who clearly have psychiatric abnormalities do not meet criteria for the categories in Table 14.1. The suitable label for these people is *undiagnosed*. One advantage of this term is that physicians who deal with the patient in the future will not be biased by having a poorly grounded diagnosis in the chart. Another advantage is the sense of modesty it correctly implies. In particular, there is no diagnostic test to conclusively establish a psychiatric diagnosis other than delirium and dementia.

Unfortunately, many insurance companies *require* a diagnosis. One can include the most likely diagnosis or diagnoses prefaced by the term "rule out." Many insurance companies will accept this practice. Alternatively, use of the diagnostic category, Not Otherwise Specified (NOS) (e.g., anxiety disorder, Not Otherwise Specified) may suffice and be clinically useful because it conveys the core symptom(s) without overstating certitude.

Outside of hospitals, many patients who consult psychiatrists do not have a diagnosable illness. They even lack symptoms of sufficient severity to justify being called "undiagnosed." One label for these more or less normal people who see psychiatrists is "problem of living," which suggests, if nothing else, that no conventional diagnosis seems to fit them.

The Mental Status Format

The purpose of the mental status format is to help the interviewer organize and communicate his or her observations about a patient. Minor deviations occur in the format from expert to expert, but some framework for observations is necessary to facilitate thinking and communication. The format presented here is commonly used and includes the following categories:

Appearance and behavior
Form and content of thought
Affect and mood
Memory and intellectual functioning
Insight and judgment

Appearance and Behavior

The patient's appearance is often relevant to the diagnosis. Patients with schizophrenia, for example, may sometimes appear poorly groomed or even dirty. Patients with major depression can be negligent about their dress and grooming. Patients with mania may wear odd or unusual clothing. Sunglasses worn indoors may suggest paranoia; a puffy face and red palms are suggestive, but not diagnostic, of alcohol abuse/dependence.

A physical appearance older than the patient's stated age may suggest depression or long-term substance abuse. If this is the case, a more youthful appearance may be restored as the patient recovers.

The patient's attitude toward the interviewer may be significant. Patients who are paranoid are often suspicious, guarded, or hostile. Patients with somatization disorder sometimes try to flatter interviewers by comparing them favorably with previous doctors; they are often dramatic, friendly—sometimes seductive. During manic episodes, patients may crack jokes and occasionally are quite funny—when they are not irritable or obnoxious. Sociopathic patients may seem like con men—and sometimes are.

The patient may be agitated—unable to sit still, moving constantly. Others are retarded, slumping in their seats, slow in movement and speech. Talking may seem an effort. Disturbance of motor function may have several causes. Neuroleptic medications may produce a restlessness called "akathisia," in which the patient cannot sit still and feels compelled to walk. Neuroleptics also may produce Parkinson-type symptoms, including tremor and an expressionless face. Pacing and handwringing may be expressions of depression; joviality and volubility may portray mania.

Neuroleptics are given so commonly that it is often impossible to determine whether abnormal movements are drug induced or are catatonic symptoms. In fact, similar involuntary movements were observed in schizophrenia years ago before medications were introduced. It is said that catatonic symptoms (cataplexy, stupor, hyperkinesiae) are disappearing, but what previously was called catatonic may now be interpreted as drug induced without knowing whether medications are responsible.

Schizophrenia also may involve psychomotor disturbances such as mannerisms, posturing, stereotypical movements, and negativism (doing the opposite of what is requested). Also seen is *echopraxia*, in which movements of another person are imitated, and *catalepsy*, in which awkward positions are maintained for long periods without apparent discomfort. Some patients say nothing. Called "mutism," this behavior may be seen in schizophrenia, depression, delirium/dementia, and drug intoxication.

Form and Content of Thought

Form refers to intelligibility related to associations: Does the patient have "loose associations" in the sense of being circumstantial, tangential, or incoherent? Older people may be circumstantial. They return to the subject but only after providing excessive detail. Tangentiality is a flow of thought directed away from the subject being inquired about, with no return to the point of departure. Patients with schizophrenia are often tangential. Pressure of speech and flight of ideas are seen in mania and in drug intoxication. The patient with pressured speech seems to be compelled to talk. Manic speech flits from idea to idea, sometimes linked by only the most tenuous connections. Unlike tangentiality, however, manic speech frequently has connections that can be surmised. Patients in manic episodes often rhyme or pun and make "clang" associations, using one word after another because they sound similar. They tend to be overinclusive, including irrelevant and extraneous details. Patients with somatization disorder or borderline personality disorder can be almost maddenly circumstantial (providing excessive detail of little clinical importance) while at the same time being quite vague (lacking specific information being sought); when severe, this "nonpsychotic thought disorder" pattern (4) can be mistaken for the tangentiality of formal thought disorder observed in patients with psychosis.

Derailment, often seen in schizophrenia, is a form of speech in which it is impossible to follow the logic of the associations. Patients with schizophrenia may invent new words (neologisms) that presumably have a private meaning. Sometimes patients with schizophrenia display poverty of thought, conveying little information with their words. *Echolalia* refers to occasions when the patient repeats words back to the interviewer. Other abnormal speech patterns associated with schizophrenia (as well as dementia) are perseveration, in which the patient seems incapable of changing topics, and blocking, in which the flow of thought is suddenly stopped, often followed by a new and unrelated thought.

Patients who persistently display any of these symptoms (excluding poverty of thought) are said to have a *formal thought disorder*, meaning that the structure or form of thinking is disordered.

Content of thought refers to what the patient thinks and talks about. This category comprises hallucinations, delusions, obsessions, compulsions, phobias, suicidal/homicidal thoughts, and preoccupations deemed relevant to the psychiatric problem.

Delusions are fixed false beliefs neither amenable to logic or social pressure nor congruent with the patient's culture. They should be distinguished from *overvalued* ideas; fixed notions that most people consider false but that are not entirely unreasonable or that cannot be disproved, such as certain superstitions. Delusions occur in delirium/dementia, schizophrenia, affective disorders, and various intoxications.

Jaspers (2) believed the *subject* of the delusion had diagnostic significance. If the delusional ideas were "understandable," they more likely occurred in depressed patients. Understandable delusions included those in which persons were convinced they had a serious life-threatening illness such as cancer, were impoverished, or were being persecuted because they were bad persons. Jaspers pointed out that healthy, prosperous, and likable people often worry about their health, finances, and approval by others. Such delusions are thus understandable.

Delusions that are *not* understandable are seen in schizophrenia, according to Jaspers. Schizophrenic delusions tend to be bizarre; for example, one's acts are controlled by outside forces (delusions of control or influence) or one believes that one is Jesus or Napoleon. Schizophrenia-like delusions occur often in amphetamine psychosis and, less commonly, in other intoxicated states (e.g., from cocaine or cannabis). The delusions of schizophrenia fall outside the ordinary person's experience: the examiner finds it difficult to identify with the schizophrenic's private world; hence, the term "autistic," derived from "auto," is often applied to schizophrenic thinking.

Religious delusions are sometimes hard to interpret. Religious beliefs often seem delusional to those who do not accept the beliefs but normal to those who do. Among fundamentalist religious people, truly pathological delusions are usually identified without difficulty by others in the congregation.

Content also encompasses perceptual disturbances. In *illusions*, real stimuli are mistaken for something else (e.g., a belt for a snake).

Hallucinations are perceptions without an external stimulus. *Auditory hallucinations* may consist of voices or noises. They are associated primarily with schizophrenia but occur in other conditions such as alcoholic hallucinosis and affective disorders. Visual hallucinations are most characteristic of organic disorders, especially delirious states. They also occur with psychedelic drug use and in schizophrenia. (Certain hallucinations are more common in some conditions, but no type of hallucination is found exclusively in any illness.) *Hypnagogic hallucinations* arise in the period between sleep and wakefulness, especially when falling asleep. *Hypnopompic hallucinations* occur when awakening from sleep. These sleep cycle hallucinations are normal except when they are a symptom of narcolepsy.

Olfactory hallucinations are sometimes associated with complex partial seizures that involve the temporal lobes. *Haptic* (tactile) *hallucinations* occur in schizophrenia and also in cocaine intoxication and delirium tremens. The sensation of insects crawling in or under one's skin (formication) is particularly common in cocaine intoxication, but it also happens in delirium tremens.

In *extracampine hallucinations*, the patient sees objects outside the sensory field (e.g., behind his head). In *autoscopic hallucinations*, the patient visualizes himself projected into space. The patient occasionally has a *doppelgänger* (sees his double). Other perceptual distortions include *depersonalization* (the feeling that one has changed in some bizarre way) and *derealization* (the feeling that the environment has changed).

In one study of nonpsychiatric patients, 40% reported hallucinations, particularly seeing dead relatives. They had no other psychiatric symptoms and the hallucinations were not judged to be clinically important. Thus, a history of transient hallucinations or other perceptual disturbances, which occur occasionally during exhaustion or grief, does not necessarily signify the presence of psychosis. Such disturbances must be interpreted in the context of the overall clinical picture.

Affect and Mood

Affect refers to a patient's outwardly (externally) expressed emotion, which may or may not be appropriate to her reported mood and content of thought. For example, if a person smiles happily while telling of people trying to poison her, the affect would be described as inappropriate. If one describes unbearable pain but looks as if she were discussing the weather, the affect again would be inappropriate.

Affect is sometimes referred to as "flat," meaning that the usual fine modulation in facial expression is absent. Patients with schizophrenia sometimes have a flat affect, but so do patients taking neuroleptic medications, and depressed patients may show little change of expression while speaking.

"Flat affect" is probably the most overused and misused term in the psychiatric examination. It should only be used if the affect is extremely "flat" or "blunted." Inappropriate and flat affects are especially associated with schizophrenia.

Sometimes patients with hysteria have an inappropriate affect in that they describe excruciating pain and other extreme distress with the same indifference or good cheer with which they would describe a morning of shopping. (The French call this *la belle indifférence*.)

Mood refers to what the patient says about his internal emotional state. "I am sad," "I am happy," and "I am angry" are examples. Mood and affect are sometimes labile, meaning there is rapid fluctuation between manifestations of happiness, sadness, anger, and so on. *Labile* affect is often seen in patients with mania, somatization disorder, and delirium/dementia.

Memory and Intellectual Functioning

Subsumed under memory is orientation, meaning orientation for person, place, and time. To be disoriented for time, the patient should be more than 1 day off the correct day of the week and more than several days off the current date. Misidentifying people (e.g., thinking the nurse is one's aunt) is a clear case of disorientation, as is giving the wrong year or the wrong city and wrong hospital where one is currently. This part of the mental status is exceedingly important because, if a patient has a gross memory impairment (and is not malingering), he or she almost always has an organic disorder and all other psychiatric symptoms may be explainable in this context. (The exceptions are substance dependence and pseudodementia.)

There are many tests for memory and intellectual functioning. Memory can be subdivided into immediate, short-term, recent, and remote memory.

Immediate memory can be tested by asking the patient to repeat a series of digits. Serially subtracting 7 from 100 is a test of immediate memory (assuming the person's arithmetic was ever adequate for the task) as are tests of attention and concentration. Short-term memory loss can be tested by asking patients to remember three easy words you have spoken or showing them three objects and then, 5 to 15 minutes later, asking them to repeat what they heard or saw. A short-term memory deficit is the *sine qua non* of Korsakoff's syndrome (see also Chapter 13). Recent memory refers to recall of events occurring in recent days, weeks, or months; remote memory involves recall of events occurring many years before, such as the winner of a long-ago presidential election. In early dementia, recent memory is usually more severely impaired than remote memory.

As noted earlier, tests of intellectual functioning should be interpreted with the patient's background, education, cooperativeness, and mood state in mind. A history major should be able to name seven presidents, but a "normal" person with a 3rd-grade education may not be able to do so. Depressed patients may be too slowed down or distractible to concentrate. One approach would be to questions that are crafted to the particular situation that the examiner opines the patient should be able to answer. Another approach might be to ask the patient about his or her interests and then test the patient's fund of information in those areas.

Insight and Judgment

A person who has insight will know whether he is (or was) psychiatrically ill. If he says, for example, that the voices are "real," he lacks insight. If he says it was simply his imagination playing tricks on him, he has insight. If he says there is nothing wrong with him but that his evil uncle has arranged for his hospitalization because of a Communist conspiracy, he may or may not have insight. (Even paranoids, as the saying goes, sometimes have real enemies.) Psychosis and delirium/dementia are associated with lack of insight.

The term "judgment" is used here in the same sense as "competence" is used in a court of law: a competent person is able to understand the nature of the charges and to cooperate with counsel. It implies that a person is realistic about his limitations and life circumstances. A good question to ask is, "What are your plans when you leave the hospital?" If the patient says that he plans to start a chain of restaurants and has no money, this displays impaired judgment. Severe impairment of judgment is seen most often in dementia and psychotic disorders.

Excluding Psychiatric Disorders

Sometimes for all physicians and often for nonpsychiatric physicians, examination of the "mind" must be accomplished quickly, lest the liver, lungs, heart, and deep tendon reflexes be slighted. For the major disorders described in this book (and the less valid ones), a single question may suffice to strongly suggest ruling out the possibility the patient has the disorder. Some disorders will be missed, but one or two questions will identify the great majority of patients who do *not* have a particular psychiatric illness:

> *Depression*: Although it seems obvious, just ask the patient if he or she has periods of feeling down or depressed for days on end. Rare is the seriously depressed individual who will deny these feelings.
>
> *Mania*: Ask if the patient has ever had elevated mood or felt too good for days at a time. People with a history of mania love to reflect on past times when they felt "really good."
>
> *Schizophrenia*: Ask if the patient has ever heard or seen things that other people did not hear or see. Ask if he has ever been afraid of being poisoned or controlled by external forces. Hallucinations sometimes occur in normal people, but the presence of both hallucinations and delusions in a person with more or less normal mood suggests schizophrenia.
>
> *Panic disorder*: Has the patient ever thought she was having a heart attack that did not occur? Does she ever become intensely apprehensive for no apparent reason? Patients with panic disorder report both. At church, does she find a seat on the aisle close to the back? Patients with panic disorder almost always do. They feel the need to make a quick exit if a panic attack seems impending.
>
> *Posttraumatic stress disorder*: Was the patient involved in, or eyewitness to, a violent or physically traumatic event? After such an experience, did the patient develop new problems with jumpiness or sleeplessness, or intrusive memories of the experience? Are reminders of the event so upsetting that the patient will go to great lengths to avoid them?
>
> *Somatization disorder*: Mostly women. Inquire in a neutral manner roughly how many doctors the patient has consulted for various symptoms and what surgical procedures she has had. If the patient has consulted few physicians and has all of her abdominal and pelvic structures intact, it is unlikely that the patient has somatization disorder.

Obsessive-compulsive disorder: Does the patient, sitting in a waiting room, count things, such as the number of tiles on the floor? Does the patient repeatedly check a door to see if it is locked or an oven to see if it is turned off? Counting and checking are so common in this disorder that, if absent, the diagnosis should be questioned.

Phobic disorders: Does the patient avoid certain situations or things because they frighten him or her? Is the fear unreasonable?

Alcohol dependence: Has the patient ever stopped drinking for a period of time? If so, and the reason is not medical or a desire to lose weight, the patient probably stopped because he was worried about his drinking. At this point, the clinician can ask why he was worried, and this may break down the denial that is characteristic of alcoholism. Almost every patient with alcohol dependence has stopped, or tried to stop, at some time in his life. This is a better approach than asking, "Do you drink too much?"

Drug dependence: "Have you ever worried about a drug habit?" is probably as good an opener as any.

Antisocial personality (sociopathy): Ask if the patient was frequently truant in grade and high school. Rare is the sociopath who did not cut classes and get in trouble with school authorities as a teenager.

Borderline personality disorder: Ask if the patient suffers from reactive mood swings characterized by brief intense episodes of dysphoria, or irritability or anxiety lasting a few minutes, hours, or days. If not, only a rare chance of the disorder.

Dementia: Ask if the patient forgets where she parks her car. If this happens often, there should be some concern about her memory. Or simply ask, "How is your memory?" Many people with memory problems are relieved to have the chance to talk about them.

Anorexia nervosa: If the person is intelligent, ask her (and it is usually a her) if she has ever been told she had anorexia nervosa. Patients with this disorder usually know their diagnosis; the disorder is well described in popular media. Does the patient stuff herself (or himself) with food and then induce vomiting? This practice, called "bulimia," often goes with anorexia in both sexes.

Another question: "Are you the right weight?" If the patient is five foot seven inches, weighs 92 pounds, is not a model, and says, "I'm too fat," the diagnosis is strongly suggested.

Sexual problems: "Do you have any sexual issues?" is usually sufficient. This is a neutral approach to sexual problems.

These questions when answered in the negative will eliminate most people who have the above disorders. There will be few false-negatives. There will be many false-positives. (Some people who do not have depression or anxiety disorders sleep poorly and sit at the back of churches.) But for the physician trying to rule out disorders, false-positives are much less important. They simply mean probing is required. Probing takes time, and referral to a psychiatrist may be in order.

Suggestions for Presenting Cases

There is obviously a good deal of latitude in presenting case histories for teaching purposes. Different institutions and different teachers within the institutions will have their own advice on the subject. However, discussions with these teachers reveal some agreement about certain points. Following are some general rules for presenting patients:

1. Do not read the history.
2. Do not exceed 10 to 15 minutes (allowing for interruptions).
3. Start with *identifying data*: name, age, race, marital status, vocation.
4. Provide a clue to the problem you will highlight, for example, "This patient presents a diagnostic problem," "He has not responded to standard treatments," "She comes from an unusual family." Such clues offer a framework for your audience into which the rest of the presentation will fit.
5. Avoid dates. Open with "Patient was admitted to [hospital] _____ (days, weeks, months) ago. Do not refer to events occurring on December 3, 1937, but say, "At the age of 15, the patient _____." Instead of saying, "Between November and January of 1955 and 1956," say, "For a three-month period when the patient was twenty years old, he _____." It may be easier for patients to remember events by dates, but the listener has to translate dates into ages and, for the unmathematically inclined, this may be difficult while concentrating on the presentation.
6. Begin with the *psychiatric history*. A good way to begin is, "The patient had no psychiatric problems until age _____ (or _____ days, weeks, or months ago) when he (slowly or rapidly) developed the following symptoms: _____," then list the symptoms in order of severity. Tell how long the symptoms persisted (for weeks, months, years, or to the present) and what happened as a result (hospitalization, other treatment, full or partial recovery).

Often, of course, establishing time of onset is difficult or impossible, particularly when dealing with a poor historian or a complicated case. The onset of illness in a mentally retarded person would be "from birth," which does not help much. But an attempt to establish onset can be of considerable help because different illnesses characteristically begin at different ages.

7. It is important to know whether the illness has been chronic, perhaps with fluctuations, or episodic with full remissions between episodes. If the patient has had more than one episode, describe subsequent episodes, briefly giving the same information that was given for the first episode. Symptoms and life events obviously are interrelated, but emphasize the symptoms rather than the life events unless the life events appear to be causally related to the symptoms.

8. A brief *family history* should include the following: whether a close blood relative of the patient had a serious psychiatric illness requiring treatment (and what the treatment was, if known), pertinent medical illnesses, and suicide, alcohol or drug problems.

9. *Social history* should include (very briefly) circumstances of upbringing, particularly whether the parents were divorced or separated or whether the patient was brought up by both parents; parental vocation; siblings; years of education and how well the patient did in school from the standpoint of grades and adjustment; military and employment history; marital history; and number and ages of children.

10. Review the *medical history* only as it is pertinent to the psychiatric problems. The same applies to the review of systems, physical findings, and laboratory results.

11. Give the *mental status* as it was obtained either on admission or at the first opportunity to fully examine the patient. The mental status findings should be presented in the order provided in the previous section.

12. End the presentation with *course in hospital.* Tell how the patient has been doing, whether he has improved, and what treatment he is receiving. In other words, bring the patient up to the present moment.

13. With rare exceptions, all this can be presented in 10 to 15 minutes. The trick is to keep in mind at all times the goal of the presentation. If it is diagnostic, the differential diagnosis and the points for and against each of the reasonably likely diagnoses should be given. If you start out

by saying the patient was psychiatrically well until the age of 60, dwelling on such diagnoses as mental retardation, schizophrenia, somatization disorder, or panic disorder is unlikely to be useful. Assuming the history is correct (though, granted, this is often a dubious assumption), people who are well until the age of 60 and then develop major psychiatric problems generally have either an affective disorder or delirium/dementia.

14. The reasons for presenting the history and mental status according to the above sequence are to avoid leaving out important information and to make it easier for the listeners to follow the narration. There are many variations on this format, and none is perfect. (People's lives are much more complicated than formats.) Unlike written psychiatric histories, however, oral presentations should not attempt to be comprehensive. They should touch on the following categories, but not all with equal emphasis.

HISTORY

Identifying data
Focus of the presentation
Psychiatric history
Family history
Social history
Medical history
Review of systems
Physical findings
Laboratory results

MENTAL STATUS

Appearance and behavior
Form and content of thought
Affect and mood
Memory and intellectual functioning
Insight and judgment

REFERENCES

1. American Psychiatric Association. *Diagnostic and Statistical Manual of Mental Disorders*, 4th edition, text revision. Washington, DC: Author, 2000.

2. Jaspers, K. *General Psychopathology.* Chicago: University of Chicago Press, 1963.

3. Kraepelin, E. *Dementia Praecox and Paraphrenia* (Barclay, R. M., Robertson, G. M., trans.). Edinburgh: E. & S. Livingstone, 1919.

4. North, C. S., Kienstra, D. M., Osborne, V. A., Dokucu, M. E., Vassilenko, M., Hong, B., Wetzel, R. D., and Spitznagel, E. L. Interrater reliability and coding guide for nonpsychotic formal thought disorder. Percept. Mot. Skills, 103:395–411, 2006.

5. Sydenham, T. *Selected Works of Thomas Sydenham, M.D.* London: John Bales & Sons, Danielson, 1922.

Index